# First Trimester Ultrasound Diagnosis of Fetal Abnormalities

# First Trimester Ultrasound Diagnosis of Fetal Abnormalities

**Alfred Abuhamad, MD**

Professor of Obstetrics & Gynecology
Professor of Radiology
Chairman, Department of Obstetrics & Gynecology
Vice Dean for Clinical Affairs
Eastern Virginia Medical School
Norfolk, Virginia

**Rabih Chaoui, MD**

Professor of Obstetrics & Gynecology
Prenatal Diagnosis and Human Genetics Center
Berlin, Germany

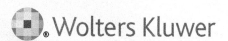

Philadelphia • Baltimore • New York • London
Buenos Aires • Hong Kong • Sydney • Tokyo

*Acquisitions Editor:* Chris Teja
*Product Development Editor:* Ashley Fischer
*Editorial Assistant:* Brian Convery
*Marketing Manager:* Rachel Mante Leung
*Senior Production Project Manager:* Alicia Jackson
*Design Coordinator:* Joan Wendt
*Artist/Illustrator:* Patricia Gast
*Manufacturing Coordinator:* Beth Welsh
*Prepress Vendor:* S4Carlisle Publishing Services

First edition

12   11   10

Printed in the United States of America

**Library of Congress Cataloging-in-Publication Data**

Names: Abuhamad, Alfred, author. | Chaoui, Rabih, author.
Title: First trimester ultrasound diagnosis of fetal abnormalities / Alfred
   Abuhamad, Rabih Chaoui.
Description: 1st edition. | Philadelphia: Wolters Kluwer Heath, [2018] |
   Includes bibliographical references and index.
Identifiers: LCCN 2017023493 | ISBN 9781451193725
Subjects: | MESH: Fetus—abnormalities | Fetal Diseases—diagnostic imaging |
   Ultrasonography, Prenatal | Pregnancy Trimester, First
Classification: LCC RG626 | NLM WQ 209 | DDC 618.3/2—dc23 LC record
   available at https://lccn.loc.gov/2017023493

LWW.com

## Dedication

May the knowledge gained from this book expand the use of high-quality
ultrasound examinations in the first trimester of pregnancy in order
to improve prenatal diagnosis, provide for compassionate
counseling, and optimize pregnancy outcomes.


We dedicate this book to our parents for their unwavering support
and commitment to excellence throughout the years, and to


*Sharon, Sami, and Nicole*
*Kathleen, Amin, and Ella,*


*With love.*

# Preface

It is with great pleasure that we introduce this first edition of *First Trimester Ultrasound Diagnosis of Fetal Abnormalities*, a product of substantial work on the rapidly evolving field of ultrasound in early gestation. This book represents the most up-to-date and comprehensive reference on this subject and is illustrated with the best ultrasound images that the current technology allows. In keeping with our prior projects, we opted to write this book in its entirety without outside collaboration in order to provide an easy-to-read style and to present a systematic and methodical approach to this subject.

Our main goal as we embarked on this project was to produce a comprehensive reference on ultrasound in the first trimester of pregnancy, based upon our collective clinical expertise in this field. For this purpose we divided the book into two main sections: the first section addressed the general aspects of the first trimester ultrasound and the second section, divided by organ systems, presented first trimester ultrasound findings in normal and abnormal conditions. In the general aspect section, we included chapters on existing guidelines to fetal imaging in the first trimester, the physical principles, bioeffects and technical aspects of the first trimester ultrasound, first trimester fetal biometry and pregnancy dating, first trimester screening for chromosomal aneuploidies, and the role of the first trimester ultrasound in multiple pregnancies. Of particular importance is the chapter on the detailed first trimester ultrasound (Chapter 5) in the general aspect section, which presents the authors' perspectives on a new detailed, comprehensive, and systematic approach to ultrasound imaging in early gestation, modeled following the detailed second trimester ultrasound examination. In the second part of the book, we included chapters dedicated to various organ systems such as the fetal central nervous system, face and neck, chest, heart, gastrointestinal, urogenital, and skeletal. The last chapter of the book focuses on the placenta and umbilical cord.

Over the past fifteen years, the advent of high-resolution transvaginal and transabdominal ultrasound and the widespread adoption of first trimester risk assessment with nuchal translucency evolved the field of ultrasound imaging in early gestation. Accumulating knowledge now suggests that the role of the first trimester ultrasound is expanding as it currently plays a critical role in pregnancy risk assessment and in the early detection of major fetal malformations.

Much credit to the evolving role of the first trimester ultrasound over the past decades is owed to Professor Kypros Nicolaides who revolutionized and introduced the role of the first trimester ultrasound with expansion of aneuploidy screening, standardization of the approach to the ultrasound examination, and providing substantial evidence on the role of the first trimester ultrasound in detection of major fetal malformations and in pregnancy risk assessment. The progress in this field over the past years has primarily resulted from the foundation laid by Professor Nicolaides.

This book would not have been a reality without the support of several people. First and foremost, our families who unselfishly allowed us to spend long evenings and weekends away from them in completing this task, the artistic talents of Ms. Patricia Gast who performed all the superb drawings in this book in an efficient and accurate manner, and the professional editorial and production teams at Wolters Kluwer. We also would like to acknowledge and thank Dr. Elena Sinkovskaya for her contribution to Chapter 15 on the placenta and umbilical cord.

We hope that this book provides the knowledge and necessary tools to expand the high-quality use of first trimester ultrasound in pregnancy.

*Alfred Abuhamad, MD*
*Rabih Chaoui, MD*

# Table of Contents

# First Trimester Ultrasound: General Aspects

# CHAPTER 1

# Guidelines to Fetal Imaging in the First Trimester

## INTRODUCTION

In the late 1980s and early 1990s, ultrasound evaluation of the fetus at less than 16 weeks of gestation was made possible by the advent of high-resolution transvaginal transducers.[1–7] With the introduction of transvaginal ultrasound, several reports evaluated the feasibility of this approach in the first trimester and demonstrated the ability to assess normal and abnormal anatomy of the fetal brain, heart, kidneys, and other organs.[1–7] The observation of the relationship between the presence of increased fluid in the fetal neck region in the first trimester and chromosomal abnormalities resulted in the establishment of nuchal translucency (NT) as an ultrasound screening tool for aneuploidy.[8–10] Largely through the efforts of Dr. Nicolaides and his coworkers, the NT measurement was standardized and a first trimester screening strategy program was established.[10–13] Consistency and reliability of NT was ensured through standardization of measurement and with the establishment of quality assurance programs.[14,15] Over the past two decades, the first trimester NT ultrasound examination has evolved beyond aneuploidy screening and now includes an evaluation of fetal anatomy in early gestation. Recently published guidelines reflect this development.[16,17] Familiarization with existing standardization of measurements and with national/international guidelines is an important step in the performance of the first trimester ultrasound examination. Given that knowledge in this field is evolving at a rapid pace, we recommend that ultrasound practitioners stay abreast of the literature on this subject. In this chapter, we present information on standardization of ultrasound measurements in the first trimester and report on existing guidelines. It is important to note that with new evidence, guidelines change over time and the readers are encouraged to refer to the most current version as reference.

## DEFINITION OF TERMS

It is important to understand the various terms that are used in standardization of ultrasound practice. Guidelines, protocols, standards, and policies refer to the ultrasound examination itself (the NT screening or the first trimester anatomy survey). Certifications, credentialing, and qualifications refer to the personnel performing the ultrasound examinations including physicians, sonographers, and allied health personnel. Accreditation, on the other hand, refers to the ultrasound laboratory/unit where the examination is performed and thus requires evaluation of the qualifications of the personnel performing the ultrasound examination, the equipment that is being used for the ultrasound examination, compliance with existing examination guidelines, and quality assurance.

The last 20 years have shown that standardizing the approach to NT, nasal bone, tricuspid regurgitation, and ductus venosus in the first trimester has increased the reliability and reproducibility of these measurements.[13] Recently published guidelines on first trimester ultrasound incorporate the NT and emphasize the role that the first trimester ultrasound plays in the assessment of fetal anatomy.[16,17] In general, guidelines are consensus based and reflect on the scientific evidence at the time of guideline development. Guidelines reduce inappropriate variations in practice and provide a more rational basis for study referral. Guidelines also, when appropriately developed, provide a focus for quality control and a need for continuing medical education for the personnel performing the ultrasound examination. Guidelines may also identify shortcomings of scientific studies and suggest appropriate research topics on the subject.

## STANDARDIZATION OF MEASUREMENTS

### Nuchal Translucency

NT is the sonographic appearance of a collection of fluid under the skin behind the fetal neck and back in the first trimester of pregnancy.[13,14] Appropriate training of sonographers and physicians, and compliance with established standard ultrasound techniques, is essential to ensure uniformity of NT measurements among various operators.[13] NT image criteria have been developed for adequate measurements (Fig. 1.1).[14,18] Semi-automated methods of measuring NT thickness have also been developed by several ultrasound manufacturers in order to reduce operator-dependent bias in NT measurements (Fig. 1.2).[19] Table 1.1 summarizes the essential criteria for an adequate NT measurement. The role of NT in detecting fetal aneuploidies is discussed in Chapter 6.

## Nasal Bones

The nasal bones are hypoplastic or not ossified in the majority of fetuses with trisomy 21 and other aneuploidies in early gestation (Fig. 1.3).[13] Typically, one of the two nasal bones is imaged in a midsagittal plane of the fetus in the first trimester. It is important to note that the ultrasound assessment of the nasal bone is technically difficult and requires substantial expertise for optimal performance.[20] The correct assessment of the nasal bone was shown to improve the performance of combined first trimester screening for Down syndrome.[13] In the normal fetus between the 11th and early 12th week of gestation, the nasal bone may appear poorly ossified or absent.[14] In such cases, it is recommended to repeat the measurement one week later.[14] Table 1.2 summarizes the essential criteria for an adequate nasal bone assessment in the first trimester.

## Ductus Venosus

The ductus venosus is an important vessel in the fetus as it directs highly oxygenated blood from the umbilical vein, through the foramen ovale and into the systemic arterial circulation. Doppler waveforms of the ductus venosus primarily reflect right atrial preload. Abnormalities in the Doppler waveforms of the ductus venosus in the first trimester have been reported in association with fetal aneuploidies, cardiac defects, and other adverse pregnancy outcomes.[13] Ductus venosus waveforms can be assessed qualitatively by observing the A-wave component of the Doppler spectrum, which reflects the atrial kick portion of diastole. Normal ductus venosus Doppler waveforms show a positive A-wave (Fig. 1.4), whereas the presence of an absent or reversed A-wave defines abnormal ductus venosus waveforms. An alternative approach relies on the quantification of the ductus venosus waveforms by using indices such as the pulsatility index for veins as a continuous variable.[14] We do not recommend routine assessment of ductus venosus flow in all pregnancies, but rather in pregnancies at increased risk for congenital heart disease or in pregnancies with an intermediate risk for aneuploidy.[14]

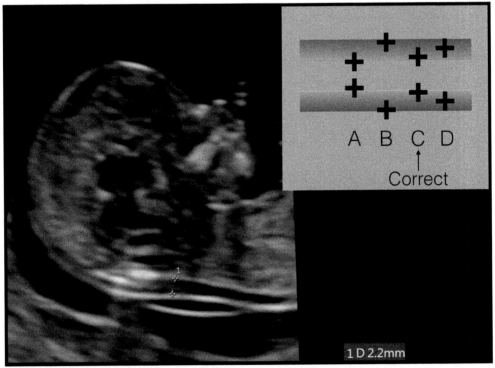

**Figure 1.1:** Midsagittal view of a fetus at 13 weeks of gestation showing the nuchal translucency (NT) thickness measurement according to the recommended standards as listed in Tables 1.1 and 1.7. The schematic diagram in the figure shows the correct (C) and incorrect (A, B, D) placement of the calipers for NT measurements. In this example the NT measurement is 2.2 mm.

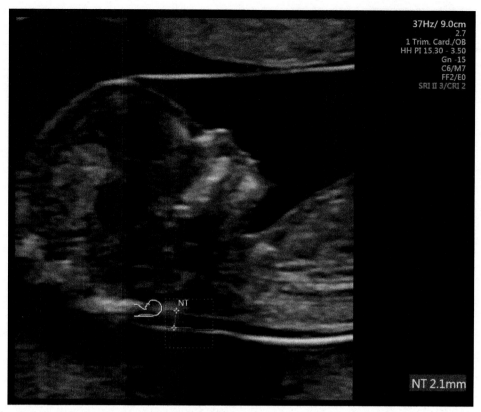

**Figure 1.2:** Midsagittal view of a fetus at 12 weeks of gestation showing the semiautomatic measurement of the nuchal translucency (NT) thickness. In the semiautomatic approach, the examiner places a box around the region of interest (*dash box*) and the software recognizes the largest NT size and places the calipers accordingly. This approach decreases the subjectivity of the measurement and increases its accuracy. In this example the NT measurement is 2.1 mm.

**Table 1.1 •** Criteria for the Standardized Measurement of Nuchal Translucency (NT) According to the Fetal Medicine Foundation-United Kingdom[14]

Gestational age should be between 11 and 13 +6 weeks.

The fetal crown-rump length should be between 45 and 84 mm.

The magnification of the image should be such that the fetal head and thorax occupy the whole screen.

A midsagittal view of the face should be obtained. This is defined by the presence of the echogenic tip of the nose and rectangular shape of the palate anteriorly, the translucent diencephalon in the center, and the nuchal membrane posteriorly.

The fetus should be in a neutral position, with the head in line with the spine.

Care must be taken to distinguish between fetal skin and amnion.

The widest part of translucency must always be measured.

Measurements should be taken with the inner border of the horizontal line of the calipers placed on the line that defines NT thickness

It is important to turn the gain down to avoid the mistake of placing the caliper on the fuzzy edge of the line.

More than one measurement must be taken and the maximum one that meets all the above criteria should be recorded in the database.

The semi-automated technique may also be used.

Nuchal cord: Use the mean of NT from above and below the cord

Nicolaides KH. The fetal medicine foundation. Available from: https://fetalmedicine.org. Accessed March 1, 2017.

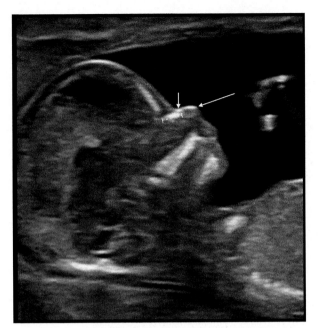

**Figure 1.3:** Midsagittal view of a fetus at 13 weeks of gestation showing the display of the nasal bone according to the recommended standards as shown in Table 1.2. *Yellow* calipers measure the nasal bone. Note the presence of two other echogenic lines, superior to the nasal bone, representing the nasal skin (*short arrow*) and the tip of the nose (*long arrow*).

---

**Table 1.2 • Criteria for the Standardized Measurement of the Nasal Bone (NB) According to the Fetal Medicine Foundation-United Kingdom[14]**

Gestational age should be between 11 and 13 +6 weeks.

The magnification of the image should be such that the fetal head and thorax occupy the whole screen.

A midsagittal view of the face should be obtained. This is defined by the presence of the echogenic tip of the nose and rectangular shape of the palate anteriorly, the translucent diencephalon in the center, and the nuchal membrane posteriorly. Minor deviations from the exact midline plane would cause non-visualization of the tip of the nose and visibility of the zygomatic process of the maxilla.

The ultrasound transducer should be held parallel to the direction of the nose and should be gently tilted from side to side to ensure that the NB is seen separate from the nasal skin.

The echogenicity of the NB should be greater than the skin overlying it. In this respect, the correct view of the NB should demonstrate three distinct lines: the first two lines are horizontal and parallel to each other; the top line represents the skin and the bottom one the NB. A third line represents the tip of the nose.

When the NB line appears as a thin line, less echogenic than the overlying skin, it suggests that the NB is not yet ossified, and it is therefore classified as being absent.

---

Nicolaides KH. The fetal medicine foundation. Available from: https://fetalmedicine.org. Accessed March 1, 2017.

Table 1.3 summarizes essential criteria for the adequate assessment of ductus venosus Doppler waveforms.

## Tricuspid Regurgitation

Color and pulsed Doppler of the tricuspid valve can be obtained in the apical four-chamber view of the fetal heart by placing the color Doppler box and the pulsed Doppler sample volume over the valve at the level of the annulus (Fig. 1.5). Tricuspid regurgitation in the first trimester is a common finding in fetuses with aneuploidies (trisomies 21, 18, and 13) and in those with major congenital heart malformations.[14] Trivial tricuspid regurgitation, defined by the presence of a small regurgitant jet at the valve annulus, is a common finding in the first trimester and has been reported in the majority of normal fetuses.[21] Table 1.4 lists essential criteria for defining tricuspid regurgitation in screening for fetal aneuploidy and congenital heart disease. Tricuspid regurgitation, as defined in Table 1.4, is found in about 1% of euploid fetuses, in 55% of fetuses with trisomy 21, and in one-third of fetuses with trisomy 18 and trisomy 13.[14] Similar to the ductus venosus, we do not recommend routine assessment of the tricuspid valve for tricuspid regurgitation in all pregnancies, but rather in pregnancies at increased risk for congenital heart disease or in pregnancies with an intermediate risk for aneuploidy.[14]

## PRACTICE GUIDELINES FOR THE PERFORMANCE OF THE FIRST TRIMESTER OBSTETRIC ULTRASOUND EXAMINATION

Practice guidelines in ultrasound imaging are created to better define an ultrasound examination and to provide for more standardization in its indications, approach, and content. Typically practice guidelines are evidence based and consensus driven. There are two types of ultrasound examinations in obstetrics—screening or routine examinations that are offered to all pregnant women irrespective of risk and targeted examinations that are indication driven and offered to pregnant women with increased risk. The second trimester morphology ultrasound examination has become a screening examination in most countries and is offered routinely to all pregnant women. The fetal echocardiogram, on the other hand, is a targeted ultrasound examination that is offered to pregnant women at increased risk for congenital heart disease. The first trimester ultrasound examination is now considered a screening examination in many countries but is still indication driven in others.[22] As more data accumulate on the value of the first trimester ultrasound in the assessment of fetal malformations, and more expertise develops in the performance of the examination, the authors believe that the first trimester ultrasound examination will be routinely offered to all pregnant women where local resources allow. The role of

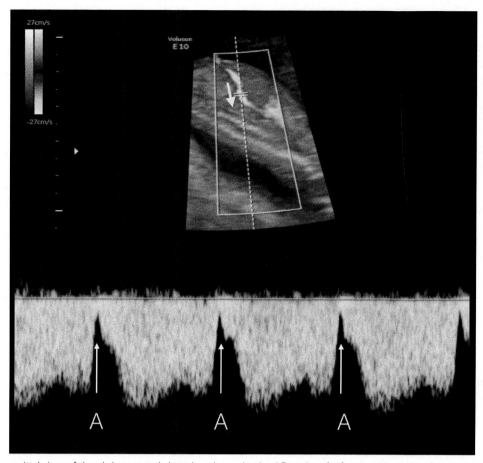

**Figure 1.4:** Parasagittal view of the abdomen and chest in color and pulsed Doppler of a fetus at 13 weeks of gestation with the pulsed Doppler sample volume placed at the ductus venosus. Note that the insonation angle is almost parallel to the direction of blood flow in the ductus venosus (*arrow*). Criteria for optimal display of ductus venosus Doppler waveforms are shown in Table 1.3. *A* represents the atrial contraction phase of the cardiac cycle in the Doppler waveform.

**Table 1.3 • Criteria for the Standardized Measurement of the Ductus Venosus (DV) flow According to the Fetal Medicine Foundation-United Kingdom[14]**

Gestational age should be between 11 and 13 +6 weeks.

The examination should be undertaken during fetal quiescence

The magnification of the image should be such that the fetal head and thorax occupy the whole screen.

A right ventral midsagittal view of the fetal trunk should be obtained and color flow mapping should be undertaken to demonstrate the umbilical vein, DV, and fetal heart.

The pulsed Doppler sample volume should be small (0.5–1.0 mm) to avoid contamination from the adjacent veins, and it should be placed in the yellowish aliasing area.

The insonation angle should be less than 30 degrees.

The filter should be set at a low frequency (50–70 Hz) so that the A-wave is not obscured.

The sweep speed should be high (2–3 cm/s) so that the waveforms are spread allowing better assessment of the A-wave.

The DV PIV is measured by the machine, after manual tracing of the outline of the waveform.

Nicolaides KH. The fetal medicine foundation. Available from: https://fetalmedicine.org. Accessed March 1, 2017.
PIV, pulsatility index for veins.

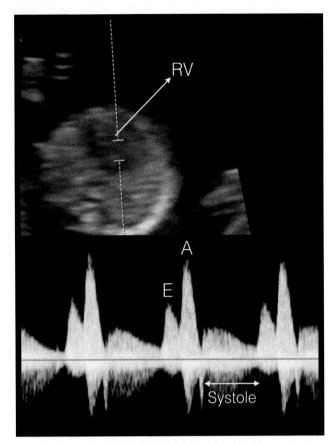

Figure 1.5: Axial plane of the fetal chest in a fetus at 13 weeks of gestation showing placement of the pulsed Doppler sample volume for tricuspid Doppler flow assessment. Note that the sample volume is placed over the valve to cover inflow and regurgitation when present. In this example, there is no tricuspid regurgitation in systole (*double arrow*) and the Doppler spectrum is normal with *E* corresponding to early diastole and *A* corresponding to the atrial kick portion of diastole. Criteria for pulsed Doppler of the tricuspid valve are shown in Table 1.4. RV, right ventricle.

the first trimester ultrasound is evolving from pregnancy dating and aneuploidy screening to the first look at fetal anatomy to detect major malformations. Guidelines for the performance of the first trimester ultrasound were published recently. In the following sections, we present highlights of existing first trimester ultrasound guidelines from the International Society of Ultrasound in Obstetrics and Gynecology (ISUOG), the American Institute of Ultrasound in Medicine (AIUM), and the German Society of Ultrasound in Medicine (DEGUM).[16,17,23]

## First Trimester Ultrasound— Guidelines from the International Society of Ultrasound in Obstetrics & Gynecology

The ISUOG published in 2013 the practice guidelines for the performance of the first trimester ultrasound scan.[16] These guidelines are comprehensive and discuss the early dating scan before 11 weeks of gestation, the aneuploidy screening with NT measurement, and the anatomic survey.[16]

### Table 1.4 • Criteria for the Standardized Measurement of the Tricuspid Flow According to the Fetal Medicine Foundation-United Kingdom[14]

Gestational age should be between 11 and 13 +6 weeks.

The magnification of the image should be such that the fetal thorax occupies most of the image.

An apical four-chamber view of the fetal heart should be obtained.

A pulsed-wave Doppler sample volume of 2.0 to 3.0 mm should be positioned across the tricuspid valve so that the angle to the direction of flow is less than 30 degrees from the direction of the interventricular septum.

Tricuspid regurgitation is diagnosed if it is found during at least half of the systole and with a velocity of over 60 cm/s, because aortic or pulmonary arterial blood flow at this gestation can produce a maximum velocity of 50 cm/s.

The sweep speed should be high (2–3 cm/s) so that the waveforms are widely spread for better assessment.

The tricuspid valve could be insufficient in one or more of its three cusps, and therefore the sample volume should be placed across the valve at least three times, in an attempt to interrogate the complete valve.

Nicolaides KH. The fetal medicine foundation. Available from: https://fetalmedicine.org. Accessed March 1, 2017.

## Purpose of the First Trimester Ultrasound Scan

ISUOG guidelines describe the purpose of the first trimester ultrasound examination as follows:

> In early pregnancy, it is important to confirm viability, establish gestational age accurately, determine the number of fetuses and, in the presence of a multiple pregnancy, assess chorionicity and amnionicity. Towards the end of the first trimester, the scan also offers an opportunity to detect gross fetal abnormalities and, in health systems that offer first-trimester aneuploidy screening, measure the nuchal translucency thickness (NT).

The guidelines also discuss the ultrasound equipment to be used (summarized in **Table 1.5**).

### Biometry

The minimal required biometric measurements according to ISUOG include the crown-rump length, the biparietal diameter, or head circumference. Other measurements can also be performed including the abdominal circumference (AC), the femur length (FL), or others. Nomograms in the first trimester are currently available for most of the biometric measurements that can be performed in the second trimester.

**Table 1.5 • Requirements for the Ultrasound Equipment in First Trimester Scanning According to the International Society of Ultrasound in Obstetrics and Gynecology (ISUOG)[16]**

Real-time, gray-scale, two-dimensional (2D) ultrasound

Transabdominal and transvaginal ultrasound transducers

Adjustable acoustic power output controls with output display standards

Freeze frame and zoom capabilities

Electronic calipers

Capacity to print/store images

Regular maintenance and servicing

Salomon LJ, Alfirevic Z, Bilardo CM, et al. ISUOG practice guidelines: performance of first-trimester fetal ultrasound scan. *Ultrasound Obstet Gynecol.* 2013;41:102–113.

ISUOG guidelines state that there is no reason to measure the AC or FL as part of the routine first trimester scan.[16] The role of biometry and dating in the first trimester is discussed in more detail in Chapter 4.

## Nuchal Translucency

ISUOG guidelines state the following regarding NT measurement in the first trimester:

A reliable and reproducible measurement of NT requires appropriate training. A rigorous audit of operator performance and constructive feedback from assessors has been established in many countries and should be considered essential for all practitioners who participate in NT-based screening programs. However, even in the absence of NT-based screening programs, qualitative evaluation of the nuchal region of any fetus is recommended and, if it appears thickened, expert referral should be considered.[16]

## Assessment of Fetal Anatomy

ISUOG guidelines emphasize the importance of the early anatomic survey and present the pros and cons of the first trimester ultrasound for fetal anatomy assessment. ISUOG guidelines also state that advantages of the early anatomy scan include early detection and exclusion of many major anomalies, early reassurance to at-risk mothers, earlier genetic diagnosis, and easier pregnancy termination if appropriate.[16] The limitations of early anatomic assessment are also discussed in the ISUOG guidelines and include the need for trained and experienced personnel, uncertain cost/benefit ratio, and the need for a second trimester ultrasound, as some anomalies develop later on in pregnancy and cannot be excluded early in gestation. Table 1.6 lists the fetal anatomic areas and organs that can be assessed in the first trimester.

**Table 1.6 • Suggested Anatomic Assessment at Time of 11 to 13 + 6-week Scan According to the International Society of Ultrasound in Obstetrics and Gynecology (ISUOG)[16]**

| Anatomic Region | What to Look for |
|---|---|
| Head | Present, cranial bones, midline falx, choroid plexus fill ventricles |
| Neck | Normal appearance, nuchal translucency thickness (if accepted after informed consent and trained/certified operator available)[a] |
| Face | Eyes with lens[a], nasal bone[a], normal profile/mandible[a], intact lips[a] |
| Spine | Vertebrae (longitudinal and axial)[a], intact overlying skin[a] |
| Chest | Symmetrical lung fields, no effusions or masses |
| Heart | Cardiac regular activity, four symmetrical chambers[a] |
| Abdomen | Stomach present in left upper quadrant, bladder[a], kidneys[a] |
| Abdominal wall | Normal cord insertion, no umbilical defects |
| Extremities | Four limbs each with three segments, hands and feet with normal orientation[a] |
| Placenta cord | Size and texture |
| Cord | Three-vessel cord[a] |

[a]Optional structures

Salomon LJ, Alfirevic Z, Bilardo CM, et al. ISUOG practice guidelines: performance of first-trimester fetal ultrasound scan. *Ultrasound Obstet Gynecol.* 2013;41:102–113.

## First Trimester Ultrasound — Guidelines from the American Institute of Ultrasound in Medicine

As of the date of this writing, the AIUM does not have specific guidelines dedicated for ultrasound in the first trimester. Ultrasound in the first trimester is discussed however in the document on the Practice Parameter for the Performance of Obstetric Ultrasound Examinations which is currently (2017) being revised.[23] In this document the AIUM states the following:

A standard obstetric sonogram in the first trimester includes evaluation of the presence, size, location, and number of gestational sac(s). The gestational sac is examined for the presence of a yolk sac and embryo/fetus. When an embryo/fetus is detected, it should be measured and cardiac activity recorded by a 2-dimensional video clip or M-mode imaging. Use of spectral Doppler imaging is discouraged. The uterus, cervix, adnexa, and cul-de-sac region should be examined.[23]

**Table 1.7 •** Parameters for Nuchal Translucency (NT) Measurements According to Nuchal Translucency Quality Review and the American Institute of Ultrasound in Medicine[15]

The margins of the NT edges must be clear enough for proper placement of the calipers

The fetus must be in the midsagittal plane

The image must be magnified so that it is filled by the fetal head, neck, and upper thorax

The fetal neck must be in a neutral position, not flexed, and not hyperextended

The amnion must be seen as separate from the NT line

The "+" calipers on the ultrasound must be used to perform the NT measurement

Electronic calipers must be placed on the inner borders of the nuchal line space with none of the horizontal crossbar itself protruding into the space

The calipers must be placed perpendicular to the long axis of the fetus

The measurement must be obtained at the widest space of the NT

Cuckle H, Platt LD, Thornburg LL, et al. Nuchal Translucency Quality Review (NTQR) program: first one and half million results. *Ultrasound Obstet Gynecol.* 2015;45:199–204.

The document also reports on NT screening as performed for individual risk assessment for aneuploidy. The NT prerequisites as listed by the AIUM are shown in Table 1.7. The AIUM document does not currently provide any details on the assessment of fetal anatomy in the first trimester. Based upon the existing practice parameter for obstetric ultrasound examination, the AIUM recommends that the first trimester ultrasound currently remains indication driven and not routinely offered to all low-risk pregnancies.[23]

## First Trimester Ultrasound— Guidelines from the German Society of Ultrasound in Medicine

The DEGUM published in 2016 an update of the guidelines of the first trimester ultrasound scan, dedicated to ultrasound specialists.[17] Prerequisites for the NT measurements are not only technical as recommended by the Fetal Medicine Foundation, but include the process of informed consent and patient counseling according to existing genetic laws.[17] The document emphasizes the role of an early anatomic survey performed by a specialist as an integral part of the first trimester ultrasound, especially in the era of the noninvasive prenatal testing (see Chapter 6). The minimum anatomic requirements in the first trimester for the assessment of the fetus are summarized in Table 1.8 and are slightly different from those listed in the ISUOG guidelines.

## CONCLUSIONS

The first trimester ultrasound has evolved over the years to become an integral part of obstetric scanning in many modalities around the world. Beyond the confirmation of an intrauterine location of a gestational sac, viability of an embryo or a fetus, accurate pregnancy dating, determination

**Table 1.8 •** Ultrasound Standard Views of the Fetal Anatomy and Optional Parameters According to the German Society of Ultrasound in Medicine Guidelines (DEGUM)[17]

|  | Standard Views | Optional Parameters |
| --- | --- | --- |
| Skull/brain | Bone of the skull, falx cerebri, choroid plexus | Intracranial translucency, brainstem |
| Face | Profile | Eyes, maxillary and mandible, lips |
| Neck | Nuchal translucency (NT)[a] | Nasal bone (NB)[a] |
| Spine |  | Outline |
| Heart/thorax | Position, contour, four-chamber view, lungs | Outflow tracts (color), three-vessel trachea view, tricuspid flow (TR)[a] |
| Abdomen | Stomach, abdominal wall | Diaphragm, DV flow[a], umbilical arteries, and urinary bladder |
| Extremities | Arms, legs | Hands and feet (femur, tibia, fibula, humerus, radius, ulna) |
| Urogenital tract | Urinary bladder | Kidneys |
| Placenta | Chorionicity, amnionicity (multiple gestation), structure | Position, insertion of umbilical cord, uterine arteries[a] |

[a]After counseling and consenting according to German law on genetics and certification through the Fetal Medicine Foundation (FMF).

Kaisenberg von C, Chaoui R, Häusler M, et al. Quality Requirements for the early Fetal Ultrasound Assessment at 11-13+6 Weeks of Gestation (DEGUM Levels II and III). *Ultraschall Med.* 2016;37:297–302.

of placental chorionicity in multiple pregnancies, the first trimester ultrasound has evolved to become a comprehensive early anatomic survey when performed by experienced personnel. This book presents the collective experience in the first trimester ultrasound examination in two prenatal diagnosis centers. Our experience is also supported by studies and case reports from the literature. Following chapters in this book present various topics related to the first trimester ultrasound examination to include bioeffects of ultrasound, fetal biometry, aneuploidy screening, image optimization, multiple pregnancies, and detailed assessment of the normal and abnormal anatomy of various fetal organ systems.

## REFERENCES

1. Achiron R, Achiron A. Transvaginal ultrasonic assessment of the early fetal brain. *Ultrasound Obstet Gynecol.* 1991;1:336–344.
2. Achiron R, Tadmor O. Screening for fetal anomalies during the first trimester of pregnancy: transvaginal versus transabdominal sonography. *Ultrasound Obstet Gynecol.* 1991;1:186–191.
3. Blaas HG, Eik-Nes SH, Kiserud T, et al. Early development of the forebrain and midbrain: a longitudinal ultrasound study from 7 to 12 weeks of gestation. *Ultrasound Obstet Gynecol.* 1994;4:183–192.
4. Bronshtein M, Blumenfeld Z. Transvaginal sonography-detection of findings suggestive of fetal chromosomal anomalies in the first and early second trimesters. *Prenat Diagn.* 1992;12:587–593.
5. Bronshtein M, Siegler E, Eshcoli Z, et al. Transvaginal ultrasound measurements of the fetal heart at 11 to 17 weeks of gestation. *Am J Perinatol.* 1992;9: 38–42.
6. Gembruch U, Knopfle G, Chatterjee M, et al. First-trimester diagnosis of fetal congenital heart disease by transvaginal two-dimensional and Doppler echocardiography. *Obstet Gynecol.* 1990;75:496–498.
7. Rottem S, Bronshtein M. Transvaginal sonographic diagnosis of congenital anomalies between 9 weeks and 16 weeks, menstrual age. *J Clin Ultrasound.* 1990;18:307–314.
8. Szabó J, Gellén J. Nuchal fluid accumulation in trisomy-21 detected by vaginosonography in first trimester. *Lancet.* 1990;336:1133.
9. Schulte-Vallentin M, Schindler H. Non-echogenic nuchal oedema as a marker in trisomy 21 screening. *Lancet.* 1992;339:1053.
10. Nicolaides KH, Azar G, Byrne D, et al. Fetal nuchal translucency: ultrasound screening for chromosomal defects in first trimester of pregnancy. *BMJ (Clin Res Ed).* 1992;304:867–869.
11. Snijders RJ, Johnson S, Sebire NJ, et al. First-trimester ultrasound screening for chromosomal defects. *Ultrasound Obstet Gynecol.* 1996;7: 216–226.
12. Nicolaides KH, Brizot ML, Snijders RJ. Fetal nuchal translucency: ultrasound screening for fetal trisomy in the first trimester of pregnancy. *Br J Obstet Gynaecol.* 1994;101:782–786.
13. Nicolaides KH. Screening for fetal aneuploidies at 11 to 13 weeks. *Prenat Diagn.* 2011;31:7–15.
14. Nicolaides KH. The fetal medicine foundation. Available from: https://fetalmedicine.org. Accessed March 1, 2017.
15. Cuckle H, Platt LD, Thornburg LL, et al. Nuchal Translucency Quality Review (NTQR) program: first one and half million results. *Ultrasound Obstet Gynecol.* 2015;45:199–204.
16. Salomon LJ, Alfirevic Z, Bilardo CM, et al. ISUOG practice guidelines: performance of first-trimester fetal ultrasound scan. *Ultrasound Obstet Gynecol.* 2013;41:102–113.
17. Kaisenberg von C, Chaoui R, Häusler M, et al. Quality Requirements for the early Fetal Ultrasound Assessment at 11-13+6 Weeks of Gestation (DEGUM Levels II and III). *Ultraschall Med.* 2016;37:297–302.
18. Abuhamad A. Technical aspects of nuchal translucency measurement. *Semin Perinatol.* 2005;29:376–379.
19. Moratalla J, Pintoffl K, Minekawa R, et al. Semi-automated system for measurement of nuchal translucency thickness. *Ultrasound Obstet Gynecol.* 2010;36:412–416.
20. Cicero S, Longo D, Rembouskos G, et al. Absent nasal bone at 11-14 weeks of gestation and chromosomal defects. *Ultrasound Obstet Gynecol.* 2003;22:31–35.
21. Yagel S. Mild tricuspid regurgitation: a benign fetal finding at various stages of gestation. *Ultrasound Obstet Gynecol.* 2006;27:102–103.
22. Reddy UM, Abuhamad AZ, Levine D, et al. Fetal imaging: Executive summary of a Joint Eunice Kennedy Shriver National Institute of Child Health and Human Development, Society for Maternal-Fetal Medicine, American Institute of Ultrasound in Medicine, American College of Obstetricians and Gynecologists, American College of Radiology, Society for Pediatric Radiology, and Society of Radiologists in Ultrasound Fetal Imaging Workshop. *J Ultrasound Med.* 2014;33(5):745–757.
23. American Institute of Ultrasound in Medicine. AIUM practice guideline for the performance of obstetric ultrasound examinations. *J Ultrasound Med.* 2013;32:1083–1101.

# CHAPTER 2

# Physical Principles and Bioeffects of First Trimester Ultrasound

## INTRODUCTION

Recent advances in ultrasound technology along with a growing body of literature expanded the role of obstetric ultrasound in the first trimester. Currently, first trimester ultrasound is considered an important element of pregnancy care and is clinically used to accurately date a pregnancy, assess for risk of aneuploidy, and screen for major fetal malformations. Understanding the basic physical principles of ultrasound is essential for knowledge of instrument control and also for the safety and bioeffects of this technology. In this chapter, we present the basic concepts of the physical principles of ultrasound, define important terminology, and review its safety and bioeffects, especially with regard to its use in the first trimester of pregnancy. Following chapters will present the role of first trimester ultrasound in pregnancy dating and in screening for fetal malformations.

## PHYSICAL CHARACTERISTICS OF SOUND

Sound is a mechanical wave that travels in a medium in a longitudinal and straight-line fashion by transmitting its energy from one molecule to another. Sound therefore cannot travel in vacuum as it requires a medium for energy transfer. When sound travels through a medium, the molecules of that medium are alternately compressed (squeezed) and rarefied (stretched). It is important to note that the molecules oscillate but do not move as the sound wave passes through them. Seven acoustic parameters describe the characteristics of a sound wave and are listed in Table 2.1. In this chapter, we will briefly discuss the frequency, power, and intensity of sound given their importance to safety of ultrasound. For more details and a broader discussion on ultrasound physics, the readers are directed to references on this subject.[1–3]

The frequency of a sound wave is the number of cycles that occurs in 1 second. The unit Hertz is 1 cycle per second. *Frequency* is an important characteristic of sound in ultrasound imaging as it affects penetration of sound and image quality.

In general, higher ultrasound frequencies provide better image quality at the expense of tissue penetration. *Power* and *intensity* of the ultrasound beam relate to the strength of a sound wave. *Power* is the rate of energy transferred through the sound wave and is expressed in Watts. *Power* can be altered up or down by a control on the ultrasound machine. Intensity is the concentration of energy in a sound wave and thus is dependent on the power and the cross-sectional area of the sound beam. The *intensity* of a sound beam is thus calculated by dividing the power of a sound beam (Watts) by its cross-sectional area (cm$^2$), expressed in units of W per cm$^2$.

The sound source, which is the ultrasound machine and/or the transducer, determines the frequency, power, and intensity of the sound. The propagation speed of sound in soft tissue is constant at 1,540 m per second. The propagation speed of sound is fastest in bone and is slowest in air. This is why the use of medical ultrasound is limited in anatomic regions involving air, such as the lungs or large bowels.

Sound is classified based upon the ability of the human ear to hear it. Sounds sensed by young healthy adult human ears are in the range of 20 to 20,000 cycles per second or Hertz, abbreviated as Hz, and this range is termed the audible sound (range of 20 to 20,000 Hz). If the frequency of a sound is less than 20 Hz, it cannot be heard by humans and is defined as infrasonic or infrasound. If the frequency of sound is higher than 20,000 Hz or 20 kHz, it cannot be heard by humans and

**Table 2.1 • Characteristics of a Sound Wave**

Frequency
Period
Amplitude
Power
Intensity
Wavelength
Propagation speed

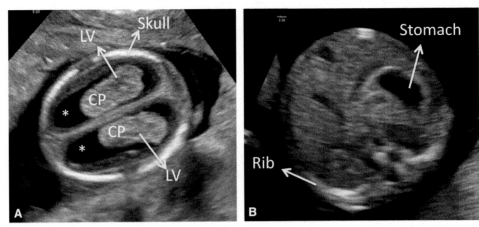

**Figure 2.1:** Ultrasound image of a fetal head **(A)** and abdomen **(B)** at 13 weeks of gestation. Note the hyperechoic bones of the skull and anechoic fluid (*asterisk*) within the lateral ventricles (LV). Note that the echogenicity of the choroid plexuses (CP) is less than bone. In **B**, the hyperechoic rib and anechoic fluid within the fetal stomach are seen.

is called ultrasonic or ultrasound. Typical frequencies used in medical ultrasound are 2 to 10 MHz (mega [million] Hertz). Ultrasound frequencies that are commonly used in obstetrics and gynecology are between 3 and 10 MHz.

## ULTRASOUND WAVES

Ultrasound waves are generated from tiny piezoelectric crystals packed within ultrasound transducers. When an alternate current is applied to these crystals, they contract and expand at the same frequency at which the current changes polarity and generate an ultrasound beam. The ultrasound beam traverses into the body at the same frequency generated. Conversely, when the ultrasound beam returns to the transducer, these crystals change in shape and this minor change in shape generates a tiny electric current that is amplified by the ultrasound machine to generate an ultrasound image on the monitor. The piezoelectric crystals within the transducer therefore transform electric energy into mechanical energy (ultrasound) and vice versa. A rubber covering on the ultrasound transducer protects the crystal and helps to decrease the resistance to sound transmission (impedance) from the crystals to the body and vice versa. In order to minimize the impact of air, a watery gel is applied on the skin of the patient to facilitate transfer of sound to and from the transducer.

## THE ULTRASOUND IMAGE

Modern ultrasound equipment create a graded gray scale ultrasound image by sending multiple sound pulses from the transducer at slightly different directions and analyzing return-ing echoes received by the crystals. The details of this process are beyond the scope of this chapter, but it is important to note that tissues that are strong reflectors of the ultrasound beam, such as bone or air, will result in a strong electric current generated by the piezoelectric crystals, which will appear as a

hyperechoic image (bright) on the monitor (**Fig. 2.1**). On the other hand, weak reflectors of ultrasound beam, such as fluid or soft tissue, will result in a weak current, which will appear as a hypoechoic or anechoic image (dark) on the monitor (**Fig. 2.1**). The ultrasound image is thus created from a sophisticated analysis of returning echoes in a gray scale format. Given that the ultrasound beam travels in a longitudinal format, in order to get the best possible image, keep the angle of incidence of the ultrasound beam perpendicular to the object of interest, as the angle of incidence is equal to the angle of reflection.

## ULTRASOUND MODES

### B-Mode Ultrasound

B-mode ultrasound, which stands for "Brightness mode," is also known as two-dimensional (2D) imaging and is commonly

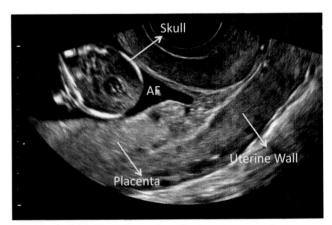

**Figure 2.2:** Variations in gray scale in a 2D transvaginal ultrasound image in the first trimester. Note the hyperechoic bones of the fetal skull, hypoechoic tissue of the uterus, and anechoic amniotic fluid (AF). The placenta is seen on the posterior uterine wall and is slightly more echogenic than the uterine wall. The intensity of the returning beam determines echogenicity.

used to describe any form of gray scale display of an ultrasound image. The image is created based upon the intensity of the returning ultrasound beam, which is reflected in a variation of shades of gray that form the ultrasound image (Fig. 2.2). It is important to note that B-mode is obtained in real time, an important and fundamental characteristic of ultrasound imaging. B-mode, or gray scale imaging, is the fundamental imaging modality for ultrasound in the first trimester and as discussed later in this chapter, it carries the least amount of energy.

## M-Mode Ultrasound

M-mode ultrasound, which stands for "Motion mode," is a display that is frequently used in early gestation to assess the motion of the fetal cardiac chambers and valves in order to document cardiac activity. The M-mode originates from a single beam penetrating the body with a high pulse repetition frequency. The display on the monitor shows the time of the M-mode display on the x-axis and the depth on the y-axis (Fig. 2.3).

## Spectral (Pulsed) Doppler

Spectral (pulsed) Doppler modes are ultrasound displays that are dependent on the Doppler principle (effect). The Doppler principle describes the apparent variation in frequency of a sound wave as the source of the wave approaches or moves away, relative to an observer. This apparent change in frequency, or what is termed the frequency shift, is proportional to the speed of movement of the sound emitting or reflecting object(s), such as red blood cells within a vessel. This frequency shift is displayed in a graphic form as a time-dependent plot. In this display, the vertical axis represents the frequency shift and the horizontal axis represents the temporal change of this frequency shift as it relays to the events of the cardiac cycle (Fig. 2.4). This frequency shift is highest during systole, when the blood flow is fastest and lowest during end diastole, when the blood flow is slowest in the peripheral circulation (Fig. 2.4). Given that the velocity of flow in a particular vascular bed is inversely proportional to the downstream impedance to flow, the frequency shift therefore derives information on the downstream impedance to flow of the vascular bed under study. The frequency shift is also dependent on the cosine of the angle that the ultrasound beam makes with the targeted blood vessel (see formula in Fig. 2.4). Given that the insonation angle (angle of incidence) is difficult to measure in clinical practice, indices that rely on ratios of frequency shifts were developed to quantitate Doppler waveforms.

In spectral Doppler mode, quantitative assessment of vascular flow can be obtained at any point within a blood vessel by placing a sample volume or the gate within the vessel (Fig. 2.4). The operator controls the velocity scale, wall

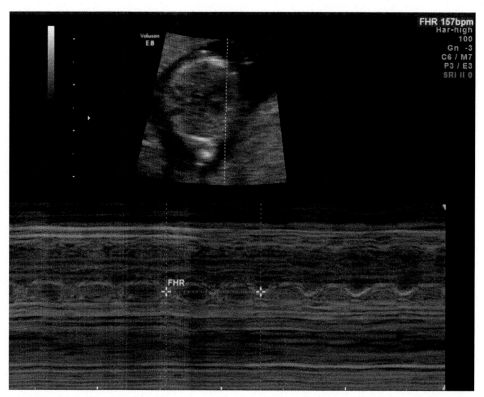

**Figure 2.3:** M-mode ultrasound of the fetal heart in a fetus at 12 weeks of gestation. Note that the M-mode line intersects the heart and the cardiac activity is displayed on the M-mode spectrum. This represents the preferred method (along with saving a movie clip in B-mode) for documentation of cardiac activity in the first trimester, as it is associated with less energy than spectral Doppler. Note that the fetal heart rate is measured at 157 beats per minute.

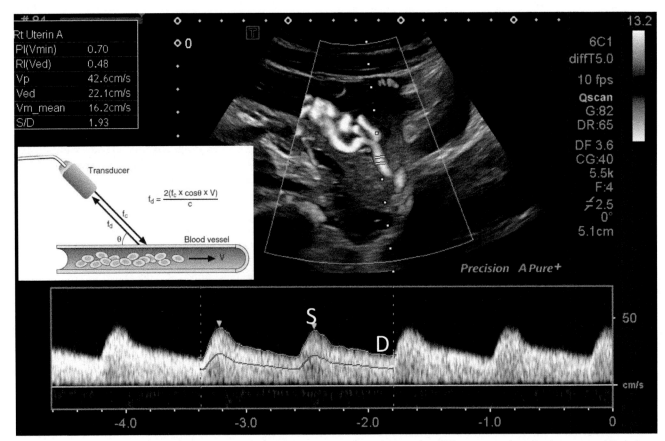

**Figure 2.4:** Spectral Doppler velocimetry of the maternal uterine artery in early gestation. "S" corresponds to the frequency shift during peak systole and "D" corresponds to the frequency shift during end diastole. The Doppler effect formula is also shown in *white background* with $f_c$ corresponding to the ultrasound frequency, $f_d$ corresponding to the frequency shift, V is the velocity of flow, $\cos\theta$ represents cosine of the angle of incidence, and c is a constant related to the milieu that the ultrasound beam is traversing. Spectral Doppler of the uterine arteries are not associated with added risk to the embryo/fetus as the sample gate is placed on the uterine vessels outside of the gestational sac.

filter, and the angle of incidence. Flow toward the transducer is displayed above the baseline and flow away from the transducer is displayed below the baseline. In spectral Doppler mode, only one crystal is typically necessary and it alternates between sending and receiving ultrasound pulses.

## Color Doppler

Color Doppler mode or Color flow mode is a mode that is superimposed on the real-time B-mode image. This mode is used to detect the presence of vascular flow within the tissue being insonated (Fig. 2.5). By convention, if the flow is toward the transducer it is colored red and if the flow is away from the transducer it is colored blue. Low velocity scales and filters are reserved for low impedance vascular beds such as placental flow (Fig. 2.5) and high velocity scales and filters are reserved for high impedance circulation such as intracardiac flow (Fig. 2.6). In order to optimize the display of color Doppler, the angle of insonation should be as parallel to the direction of blood flow as possible. If the angle of insonation approaches 90 degrees, no color flow will be displayed given that the "Doppler effect" is dependent on the cosine of the

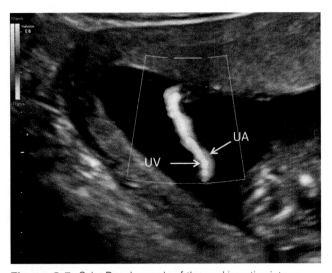

**Figure 2.5:** Color Doppler mode of the cord insertion into an anterior placenta in a pregnancy at 12 weeks of gestation. Note that blood in the umbilical vein (UV) is colored *blue* (away from the placenta) and blood in the umbilical arteries (UA) is colored *red* (toward the placenta).

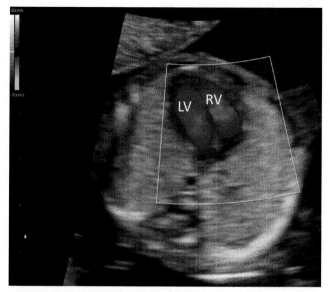

Figure 2.6: Color Doppler mode of the four-chamber view of the fetal heart at 14 weeks of gestation. Blood flow in the fetal heart has high velocity and thus is detected on a high velocity scale (here at 33 cm per second). LV, left ventricle; RV, right ventricle.

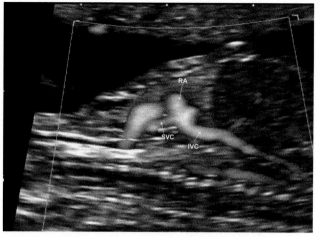

Figure 2.8: High definition color Doppler ultrasound of a parasagittal view of the fetal chest and abdomen at 13 weeks of gestation demonstrating the inferior vena cava (IVC) and superior vena cava (SVC) entering the right atrium (RA). High definition color Doppler or power color Doppler allows for a clear display of fetal vasculature in the first trimester. See text for details.

angle of insonation, and cosine of 90 degrees is equal to zero (Fig. 2.7). Characteristics and optimization of color Doppler in the first trimester are discussed in detail in Chapter 3.

## Power or High Definition Doppler Mode

Power or high definition Doppler mode is a sensitive mode of Doppler that is available on some high-end ultrasound equipment

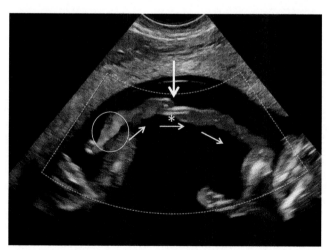

Figure 2.7: Blood flow in an umbilical cord at 13 weeks of gestation showing the Doppler effect. *Yellow arrows* show the direction of blood flow in the umbilical arteries. Note the absence of blood flow on color Doppler (*asterisk*) where the ultrasound beam (*white arrow*) images the cord with an angle of insonation equal to 90 degrees (cosine of 90 degrees = 0). The *circle* shows area of blood flow with an angle of insonation almost parallel to the ultrasound beam and thus displays the brightest color corresponding to the highest velocities.

and is helpful in cardiac imaging in the first trimester (Fig. 2.8). The strength (amplitude) of the reflected signal is primarily processed. Power Doppler mode is less affected by the angle of insonation than the traditional color or spectral Doppler.

## BIOEFFECTS AND SAFETY OF ULTRASOUND

Ultrasound is a form of energy and its output varies based upon the mode applied. As the ultrasound wave traverses through tissue, the absorption of energy results in heat dissipation, referred to as the thermal effect of ultrasound. The passage of the ultrasound waveform through tissue also produces a direct mechanical effect from the succession of positive and negative pressures. The thermal and mechanical effects of ultrasound are reflected in two important indices for measurement of bioeffects of ultrasound: the thermal index (TI) and the mechanical index (MI). The MI gives an estimation of the cavitation effect of ultrasound, which results from the interaction of sound waves with microscopic, stabilized gas bubbles in the tissues. The TI is a predictor of maximum temperature increase under clinically relevant conditions and is defined as the ratio of the power used over the power required to produce a temperature rise of 1°C. The TI is reported in three forms—thermal index soft (TIS) tissue assumes that sound is traveling in soft tissue and is primarily useful in the first trimester; thermal index bone (TIB) assumes that sound is at or near bone, useful in late second and third trimester; thermal index cranial (TIC) assumes that the cranial bone is in the sound beam's near field, used for examination in adult patients. Other energy effects of ultrasound include physical (shock wave) and chemical (release of free radicals) effects on tissue.

In obstetrical scanning, the thermal effect (TI) of ultrasound is of more concern than the mechanical effect (MI). Hyperthermia has been shown to have a teratogenic effect on the developing embryo in various species.[4,5] As the thermal effect results in an increase in temperature in the insonated tissue, caution should be undertaken to limit embryo and fetal exposure to the minimal time that is needed for diagnostic purposes and the benefit to the patient must always outweigh the risk. A general threshold of 1.5°C above normal physiologic levels is suggested as a safe threshold for diagnostic imaging.[6]

In 1992, the output display standard (ODS) was mandated for all diagnostic ultrasound devices. In this ODS, the manufacturers are required to display in real time the TI and the MI on the ultrasound screen with the intent of making the user aware of the bioeffects of ultrasound examination (Fig. 2.9). The user has to be aware of the power output and make sure that reasonable levels are maintained. Despite the lack of epidemiologic studies of confirmed harmful bioeffects from exposure to diagnostic ultrasound, the potential benefit and risk of the ultrasound examination should be assessed and the principle of ALARA (as low as reasonably achievable) should be always followed, particularly when adjusting controls of the ultrasound equipment in order to minimize the risk. This implies that the ultrasound power should be kept as low as possible and the time of ultrasound exposure as short as possible within the scope of the clinical ultrasound examination. Always keep track of the TI and MI values on the ultrasound screen, and keep the TI below 1 and MI below 1 for obstetrical ultrasound imaging.

Bioeffects and safety of ultrasound is an important topic, especially as it relates to the developing embryo and fetus in early gestation. Guiding principles on this topic suggest that the benefit of ultrasound should always be weighed against its risk when ultrasound is performed in early gestation. Acoustic outputs of B-mode and M-mode are generally not high enough to produce deleterious effects. Their use therefore appears to be safe, for all stages of pregnancy.[7] Pulsed Doppler however focuses the ultrasound beam's energy on a small anatomic target and thus it should not be used routinely in the first trimester.[8] Its use in the first trimester should be limited to clinical situations with clear pregnancy benefit. When performing Doppler ultrasound, the displayed TI should be ≤1.0 and exposure time should be kept as short as possible (usually no longer than 5 to 10 minutes) and should not exceed 60 minutes.[8] The use of 3D and 4D ultrasound is associated in general with low TI, comparable to that of B-mode, and is considered as safe as B-mode for obstetrical scanning.[9]

When attempting to obtain fetal heart rate with a diagnostic ultrasound system, the American Institute of Ultrasound in Medicine (AIUM) recommends using M-mode at first, because the time-averaged acoustic intensity delivered to the fetus is lower with M-mode than with spectral Doppler.[10] If this is unsuccessful, spectral Doppler ultrasound may be used with the following guidelines: use spectral Doppler only briefly (e.g., 4 to 5 heart beats) and keep the TI (TIS for soft tissues in the first trimester) as low as possible, preferably below 1 in accordance with the ALARA principle. It is important to note however that documentation of cardiac activity in early gestation can also be achieved by saving a movie clip in B-mode.

No independently confirmed adverse effects caused by exposure from present diagnostic ultrasound instruments have been reported in human patients in the absence of contrast agents.[11] Biological effects (such as localized pulmonary bleeding) have been reported in mammalian systems at diagnostically relevant exposures,[12] but the clinical significance of such effects is not yet known.

National and international ultrasound societies have developed official statements that relate to the use of medical ultrasound in obstetrics.[7,8,10–16] It is important to note that official societal statements tend to be updated from time to time and the reader should consult with the society's website for the most recent versions. Ultrasound examinations should be used by qualified health professionals to provide medical benefit to the patient. Ultrasound exposures during examinations should always be as low as reasonably achievable (ALARA).[16] Knowledge of the bioeffects of ultrasound, the ALARA principle, and the output display standard is required learning for healthcare workers involved in ultrasound imaging.

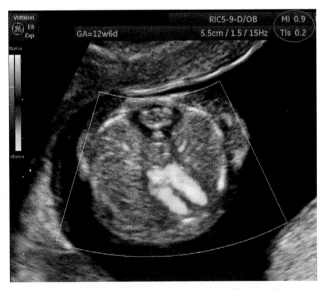

**Figure 2.9:** An ultrasound examination of the four-chamber view at 13 weeks of gestation in color Doppler. Note the display of MI and TIs in the *red circle*. Mechanical index (MI) and thermal index soft (TIS) tissue. TIS is useful in the first trimester given the absence of ossified bony structures. See text for details.

## REFERENCES

1. Miele F. *Ultrasound Physics and Instrumentation.* 5th ed. Brampton, Canada: Miele Enterprises; 2013.
2. Edelman SK. *Understanding Ultrasound Physics.* 4th ed. Tenafly, NJ: E.S.P. Ultrasound; 2012.
3. Kremkau FW. *Diagnostic Ultrasound: Principles & Instruments.* 8th ed. Philadelphia: Saunders; 2010.
4. Edwards MJ, Saunders RD, Shiota K. Effects of heat on embryos and fetuses. *Int J Hyperthermis.* 2003;19(3):295–324.

5. Clarren SK, Smith DW, Harvey MA, et al. Hyperthermia—a prospective evaluation of a possible teratogenic agent in man. *J Pediatr.* 1979;95(1):81–83.

6. Barnett SB. WFUMB symposium on safety of ultrasound in medicine. Conclusions and recommendations on thermal and non-thermal mechanisms for biological effects of ultrasound. *Ultrasound Med Biol.* 1998;24(suppl 1):8.

7. International Society of Ultrasound in Obstetrics and Gynecology. Official statement on safety. *Ultrasound Obstet Gynecol.* 2003;21:100.

8. International Society of Ultrasound in Obstetrics and Gynecology. Official statement on the safe use of Doppler in the 11 to 13+6 week fetal ultrasound examination. *Ultrasound Obstet Gynecol.* 2011;37:628.

9. Sheiner E, Hackmon R, Shoham-Vardi I, et al. A comparison between acoustic output indices in 2D and 3D/4D ultrasound in obstetrics. *Ultrasound Obstet Gynecol.* 2007;29(3):326–328.

10. American Institute of Ultrasound in Medicine. Official statement on measurement of fetal heart rate, 2011. http://www.aium.org/official Statements/43. Accessed March 11, 2016.

11. American Institute of Ultrasound in Medicine. Official statement on Conclusions regarding epidemiology for obstetric ultrasound, 2010 http://www.aium.org/officialStatements/34. Accessed March 11, 2016.

12. American Institute of Ultrasound in Medicine. Official statement on mammalian biological effects of ultrasound in vivo, 2015. http://www.aium.org/officialStatements/9. Accessed March 11, 2016.

13. American Institute of Ultrasound in Medicine. Official statement on the Safe Use of Doppler Ultrasound During 11–14 week scans (or earlier in pregnancy), 2016, http://www.aium.org/officialStatements/42. Accessed March 11, 2016.

14. American Institute of Ultrasound in Medicine. Official statement on prudent use in pregnancy, 2012. http://www.aium.org/officialStatements/33. Accessed March 11, 2016.

15. International Society of Ultrasound in Obstetrics and Gynecology. Official statement on non-medical use of ultrasound. *Ultrasound Obstet Gynecol.* 2009;33(5):617.

16. American Institute of Ultrasound in Medicine. Official statement on as low as reasonably achievable principal, 2008. http://www.aium.org/officialStatements/16. Accessed March 11, 2016.

# CHAPTER 3

# Technical Aspects of the First Trimester Ultrasound Examination

## INTRODUCTION

Over the past two decades the detailed ultrasound examination of a fetus before the 16th week of gestation was made possible by two important events: the widespread adoption of first trimester risk assessment with nuchal translucency (NT) and the improvement in ultrasound imaging with enhanced resolution and image processing. High-resolution transabdominal and transvaginal transducers provide images of the fetus in the first trimester with such quality that allows for detailed anatomic evaluation. In addition, the use of sensitive color and high-definition power Doppler improved the visualization of the fetal cardiovascular system, including small peripheral vessels. The widespread use of three-dimensional (3D) ultrasound technology added a new approach to fetal imaging through the acquisition, display, and post-processing of 3D volumes. The embryo can now be imaged on ultrasound from about the sixth week of gestation and detailed anatomic evaluation of the fetus can be performed from about the 12 weeks of gestation onward. This chapter provides an overview of the technical aspects of ultrasound examination in the first trimester.

## TWO-DIMENSIONAL GRAY SCALE ULTRASOUND

The quality of the two-dimensional (2D) ultrasound image is dependent on several factors including the choice of transducers, system settings (image presets), access to the anatomic region of interest, and magnification of the target region of interest (see Table 3.1).

### Ultrasound Transducers

Ultrasound manufacturers offer a wide range of transducers to choose from. Only a few transducers are optimally suited for imaging the first trimester pregnancy however. Most obstetric transducers have a frequency range between 2 and 12 MHz.

Transabdominal and transvaginal transducers that are used in the first trimester of pregnancy are discussed in detail in the following sections.

### Transabdominal Transducers

Two groups of transabdominal transducers are used in obstetric scanning: transducers with low frequency range (2 to 5 MHz), which allow for good tissue penetration of sound and acceptable image resolution, and transducers with high frequency range (5 to 9 MHz), which allow for improved resolution but with limited tissue penetration of sound. The authors recommend the use of high frequency range transducers in the first

---

**Table 3.1 • Image Optimization for Two-Dimensional Ultrasound in Gray Scale in the First Trimester**

- Choose a high frequency transducer when possible
- Consider using linear and transvaginal high-resolution transducers
- Use the other hand to gently manipulate the uterus when performing a transvaginal ultrasound
- Combine harmonic imaging, compound imaging, and speckle reduction when possible
- Narrow the image sector
- Reduce the image depth
- Magnify the region of interest in order to fill one-third to half of the ultrasound image
- Use one focal zone positioned at the level of the region of interest
- Adapt the dynamic range to have a high or low contrast image
- Adjust image resolution
- Use cine loop to return back to images stored in the recorded loop for review

trimester when available and technically feasible, as this enables a detailed anatomic evaluation of the fetus in keeping with existing guidelines[1,2] (see Chapter 1). In the first trimester, the use of high frequency transducers provides adequate imaging, thus allowing for optimal nuchal and intracranial translucency evaluation along with clear visualization of fetal organs such as brain, heart, lungs, stomach, kidneys, and bladder. The general contour of the fetus with the surrounding amniotic fluid can be imaged (Fig. 3.1A), in addition to the skeletal system to include the skull, nasal bone, ribs, spine, and limbs (Fig. 3.1A–E). Limitations of transabdominal high frequency transducers are encountered when the fetus is deep in the pelvis. Recently, linear transducers, that are commonly used for soft tissue imaging in radiology, have been adapted to obstetric imaging.[3] These linear transducers are desirable because of their high resolution with good tissue penetration of sound. Unlike the curved array transducers, the linear transducers have ultrasound beams that are uniform throughout all tissue levels and do not diverge in deeper tissue. We have found

linear transducers to be well adapted for first trimester ultrasound imaging and can provide detailed anatomic evaluation of the fetus (Fig. 3.2) with comparable resolution to that of transvaginal transducers.[4]

### Transvaginal Transducers

When ultrasound imaging is suboptimal by the transabdominal approach due to an increased distance between the transducer and target anatomic region (Fig. 3.3A), or when a suspected abnormality is noted, the transvaginal approach is recommended (Fig. 3.3B and C). The main advantage of the transvaginal approach is the short distance of the ultrasound beam to the region of interest, thus allowing for the use of higher frequency transducers with better resolution (Fig. 3.4). Transvaginal transducers have in general a range between 5 and 12 MHz. In the experience of the authors, fetuses with crown-rump length (CRL) greater than 65 mm are often well imaged by transabdominal transducers, whereas fetuses

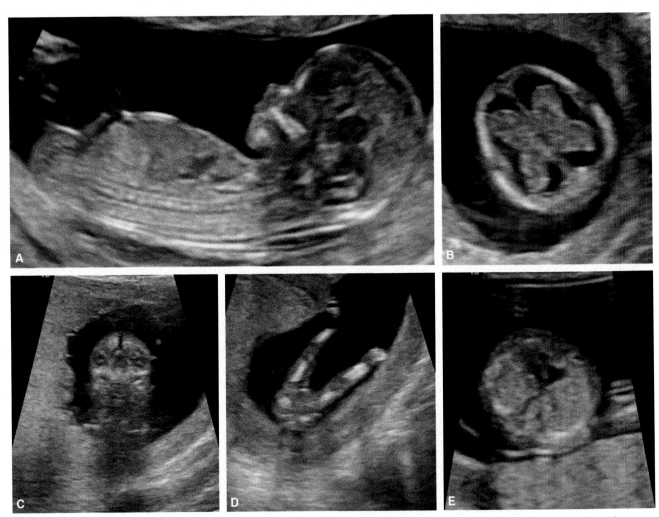

**Figure 3.1:** Various planes **(A–E)** obtained by a transabdominal curved array high-resolution transducer in fetuses at 12 to 13 weeks of gestation. Plane **A** represents a midsagittal view of the fetus obtained for measurement of crown-rump length, nuchal and intracranial translucency, and for visualization of the nasal bone. Plane **B** is an axial view of the head. Plane **C** is a frontal facial view. Plane **D** shows two lower limbs and plane **E** represents the four-chamber view.

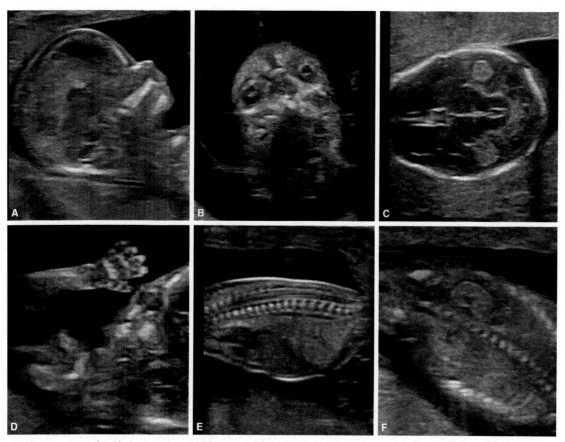

**Figure 3.2:** Various planes **(A–F)** obtained by a transabdominal high-resolution linear transducer in fetuses at 12 to 13 weeks of gestation. Compare with Figure 3.1. Plane **A** represents a midsagittal view of the fetal head. Plane **B** is a frontal facial view. Plane **C** shows the intracerebral structures. Plane **D** shows a hand with digits. Planes **E** and **F** show a sagittal and coronal view of the fetal spine respectively with fetal kidneys noted in plane **F**. Note the high resolution of these images as compared to images in Figure 3.1.

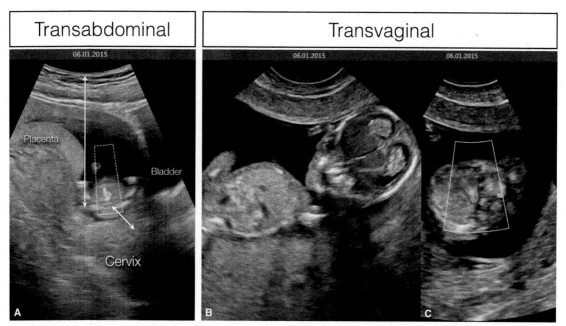

**Figure 3.3: A:** A fetus at 12 weeks of gestation scanned transabdominally with color Doppler at the three-vessel trachea view. Note that the image displays decreased resolution, primarily due to the long distance between the transducer and the region of interest; upper fetal chest in this case (*yellow arrow*). Note also that the fetus is deep in the pelvis and near the cervix (*white arrow*). **B:** A transvaginal view showing that the fetus is in a transverse lie, an ideal fetal position for a transvaginal ultrasound examination. **C:** A transvaginal ultrasound in color Doppler at the three-vessel trachea view showing improved resolution over the transabdominal approach in **A**. Planes **B** and **C** are obtained in the same fetus as plane **A**.

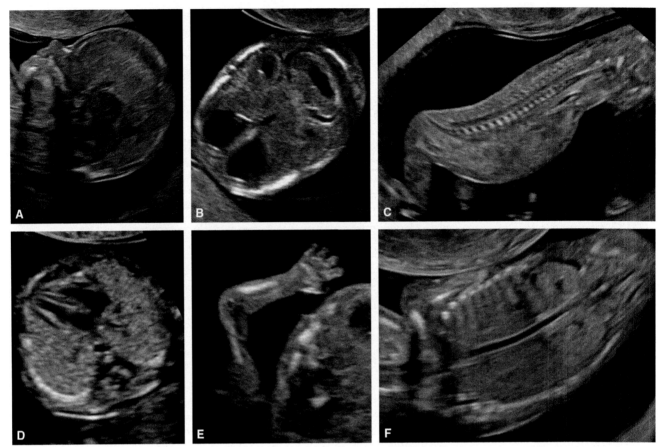

**Figure 3.4:** Various planes (**A–F**) obtained by a transvaginal high-resolution transducer in fetuses at 11 to 13 weeks of gestation. Compare with Figures 3.1 and 3.2. Plane **A** represents a midsagittal view of the fetal head. Plane **B** shows the intracerebral structures. Plane **C** shows a midsagittal view of the spine. Plane **D** is a four-chamber view of the fetal heart. Plane **E** shows a fetal hand with digits and plane **F** is a coronal view of the chest and abdomen showing the fetal kidneys. Note the high resolution of these images as compared to images in Figures 3.1 and 3.2.

between 10 and 12 weeks of gestation and embryos before 10 weeks of gestation are better imaged by the transvaginal approach. It has also been our experience that the NT and nasal bones are imaged easily with transabdominal transducers. **Figures 3.5 and 3.6** display the fetal abdomen and face respectively with the transabdominal curvilinear, transabdominal linear, and transvaginal transducers. Note that the three transducers provide adequate imaging of upper abdominal structures (Fig. 3.5), whereas the linear and transvaginal transducers provide superior imaging for complex anatomic regions such as the facial profile (Fig. 3.6).

## Image Presets

Image presets influence the quality of the displayed image on the monitor of the ultrasound system. The gray scale image presets should be adapted according to the selection of the transducer. For imaging in the first trimester, we generally recommend a high-resolution image with high line density, in combination with harmonic imaging. Despite recommendations to the contrary for NT measurements, we recommend compound imaging as well as speckle reduction, for imaging

of fetal anatomy in the first trimester. A wide image angle is recommended at the initial part of the ultrasound examination in order to measure the CRL and to assess for any gross abnormalities. The image angle however should be narrowed in order to examine selective anatomic regions of the fetus, such as the brain or heart. A narrow angle provides a higher image quality with good frame rate.

## Technical Skills

The technical skills of the operator performing the first trimester ultrasound examination play a critical role in the quality of images. In general, the operator performing the first trimester ultrasound should be well versed in the second trimester examination and should adapt its approach to early gestation. A systematic approach to the first trimester ultrasound, as shown in Chapter 5, standardizes the examination approach and provides consistency in image display. In contrast to ultrasound imaging in the second trimester, the small size of the fetus and the relatively flat maternal abdomen limits the insonation angles in early gestation. Increased mobility of the fetus in the first trimester however commonly overcomes this

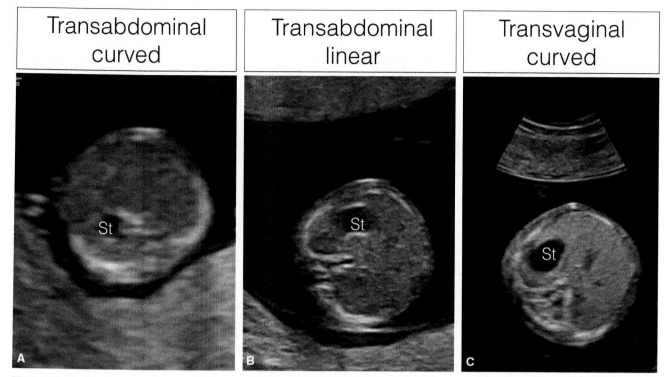

**Figure 3.5:** Axial views of the fetal abdomen at 12 weeks of gestation in three fetuses **(A–C)** using three different high-resolution transducers: **A**—transabdominal curved array, **B**—transabdominal linear, and **C**—transvaginal. Note the increased resolution in planes **B** and **C**. St, stomach.

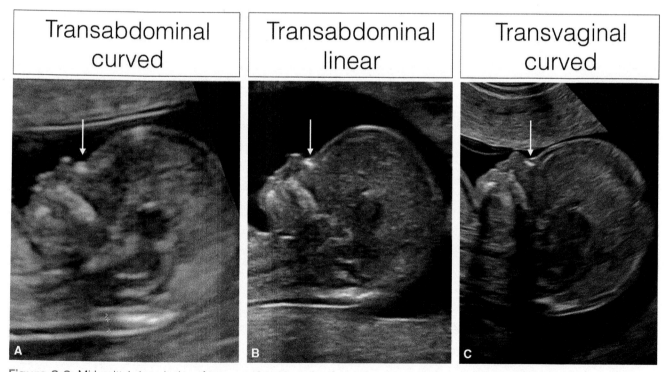

**Figure 3.6:** Midsagittal views in three fetuses at 12 to 13 weeks of gestation, imaged with three different high-resolution transducers: **A**—transabdominal curved array, **B**—transabdominal linear, and **C**—transvaginal. Note the increase in resolution and tissue characterization in **C** as compared to **A** and **B**. Also note that the nasal bone *(arrows)* has sharp borders in **B** and **C**, as compared to blurred borders in **A**. When fetal malformations are suspected, the transvaginal approach provides more detailed assessment of fetal anatomy in early gestation.

obstacle as it provides various approaches to imaging within a relatively short time frame. Asking the mother to cough or to walk around for few minutes can often lead the fetus to move and change position. Furthermore, applying gentle pressure with the transducer during the transabdominal ultrasound examination may shorten the distance to the fetus and improves imaging. With the transvaginal approach, the transducer should be inserted gently into the vaginal canal, thus making the examination well tolerated by most women.[5] Following the introduction of the transvaginal transducer, the operator should visualize the entire uterine cavity, including the fetus, without magnification. Following this overview, the region of interest can be magnified to optimize imaging and to get detailed anatomic assessment. Occasionally, a gentle manipulation of the uterus with the other hand placed on the maternal abdomen can lead to a change in the position of the fetus and brings the region of interest into the focus region.

## COLOR AND PULSED DOPPLER

Color and pulsed Doppler ultrasound has been useful in the evaluation of the first trimester pregnancy. The application of color Doppler has been shown to be helpful in the assessment of the fetal cardiovascular system (Fig. 3.7) and in guiding placement of pulsed Doppler for the study of fetal vasculature. It is important to note that color and pulsed Doppler application involves higher energy than conventional gray scale imaging and its prudent application in early gestation is

recommended. Respecting the ALARA (as low as reasonably achievable) principle (described in Chapter 2), and using color Doppler when indicated and in a standardized fashion, allow its safe application in the first trimester. Pulsed Doppler application across the tricuspid valve and ductus venosus (DV) has been used to assess aneuploidy risk and to screen for congenital heart disease. The authors however recommend the limited use of pulsed Doppler in the first trimester to specific indications, given its increased focused energy. In our experience, the prudent application of color Doppler selectively on few anatomic planes in the first trimester helps to complete the assessment of fetal anatomy. Color Doppler is especially important for the assessment of fetal cardiac anatomy in the first trimester (Fig. 3.8).

### Color Doppler Presets

The most common use of color Doppler in the first trimester is for the examination of the fetal heart and occasionally for the visualization of umbilical arteries, the umbilical vein, and the DV. Ideally the examiner has to be familiar with the optimization of the ultrasound equipment in order to properly examine the heart in early gestation.[6] Improper use of color Doppler of the fetal heart bears the risk of false-negative or false-positive diagnoses. The optimum color Doppler image is a compromise between image quality and frame rate. Optimizing the gray scale image is essential before the application of color Doppler. Choosing the smallest color box needed for your target anatomic region will ensure the highest frame rate possible for

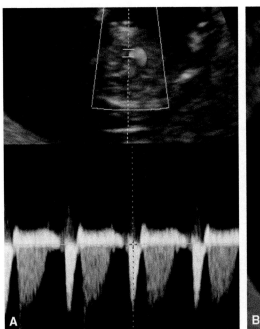 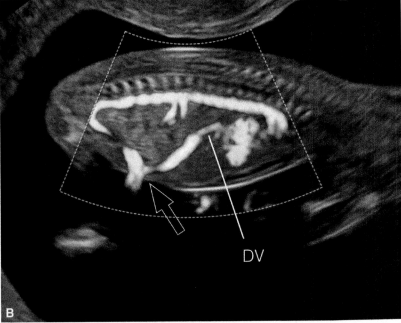

**Figure 3.7: A:** An axial plane of the fetal chest at 13 weeks with the application of pulsed-wave Doppler on the heart to demonstrate and document cardiac activity. The authors do not recommend this practice given the increased energy associated with pulsed-wave Doppler. It is recommended to use M-mode or to save a gray scale movie clip for this purpose (see Chapter 2). When color Doppler is indicated, an application of the color box over the fetus **(B)** can document cardiac activity and demonstrate an intact anterior abdominal wall (*arrow*) and a normal course of the ductus venosus (DV).

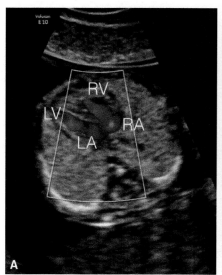
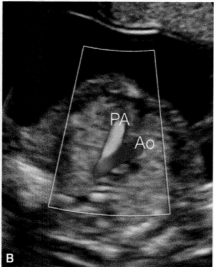
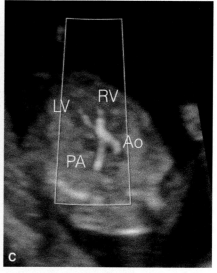

**Figure 3.8:** Images of the fetal heart at 11 to 13 weeks of gestation, examined with color Doppler ultrasound. **A:** Diastolic flow from both right (RA) and left (LA) atrium into the right (RV) and left (LV) ventricle, respectively. **B:** A normal three-vessel trachea view with aorta (Ao) and pulmonary artery (PA). **C:** An oblique view showing both left and right ventricular outflow tract in systole with the crossing of Ao and PA.

the ultrasound examination. Velocity scale or pulse repetition frequency is used to determine the range of mean velocities within the color box. For color Doppler interrogation of the cardiac chambers and the great vessels, a high velocity range (>30 cm per second) should be selected. For the examination of the umbilical arteries and veins, renal arteries, or other fetal peripheral vasculature, lower velocity ranges should be selected (5 to 20 cm per second). Table 3.2 summarizes the presets that we commonly use for color Doppler application in the first trimester. For a more comprehensive presentation on this subject, the readers are referred to our previous work on the optimization of the color Doppler ultrasound examination of the fetal heart.[4]

## Regions of Interest for Color Doppler Application

The same anatomic regions of interest examined in the second trimester can also be applied in the first trimester. It is important to note that not all second trimester anatomic regions have the same clinical importance or are easy to image on color Doppler

in the first trimester. We hereby present important anatomic regions for the first trimester color Doppler application.

### Heart and Great Vessels

The use of color Doppler is, in our opinion, essential for the reliable assessment of the heart and great vessels in the first trimester. The four-chamber and the three-vessel trachea views are relatively easy to obtain on color Doppler and provide for adequate screening for cardiac malformations in early gestation (Fig. 3.8).[4,7] In pregnancies at increased risk for congenital heart disease, obtaining additional planes such as the five-chamber view, the short-axis and aortic arch views provides for a comprehensive evaluation of the fetal heart in the first trimester. In selective cases, the demonstration of the pulmonary veins draining into the left atrium can be of importance as well as the demonstration of the course of the right subclavian artery. Detailed evaluation of first trimester normal and abnormal fetal cardiac anatomy is presented in Chapter 11.

### Abdominal Vessels

The axial plane in the lower abdomen allows for the demonstration of the two umbilical arteries surrounding the bladder, thus confirming a three-vessel umbilical cord (Figs. 3.9A and 3.10A). In the presence of a single umbilical artery, the site of the missing artery can be documented (Fig. 3.10B). An axial plane at the level of the mid-abdomen allows for the demonstration of the normal abdominal wall and its umbilical cord insertion, thus ruling out abdominal wall defects (Fig. 3.9B). In the midsagittal plane of the fetus (NT plane), color Doppler can be applied over the abdomen to visualize the course of the umbilical vein and DV toward the heart (Figs. 3.7B and 3.11). The narrow size and high blood flow velocities of the DV differentiate it from the umbilical vein. This midsagittal plane

| Table 3.2 • Image Optimization for Color Doppler Ultrasound in the First Trimester | | |
| --- | --- | --- |
| | **Fetal Heart** | **Peripheral Vasculature** |
| Velocity scale | High | Low |
| Color gain | Low | High |
| Color filter | High | Low |
| Color persistence | Middle | High |
| Color resolution | Middle | High |

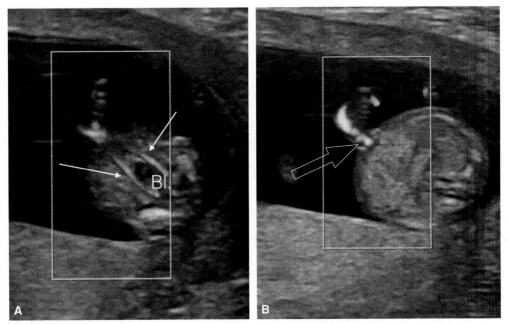

**Figure 3.9:** Transverse views in color Doppler of the fetal pelvis **(A)** and mid-abdomen **(B)** at 13 weeks of gestation using a linear high-resolution transducer. Note the two umbilical arteries (*arrows*) surrounding the bladder (Bl.) in **A** and the intact abdominal wall (*open arrow*) in **B**. Compare with Figure 3.10.

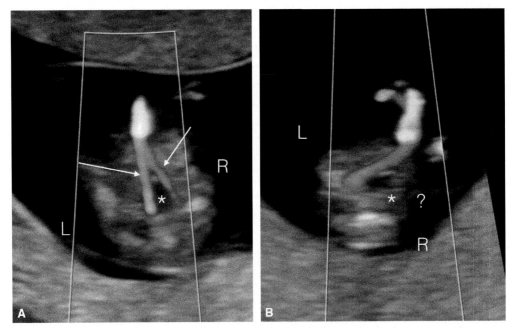

**Figure 3.10:** Transverse views in color Doppler of the fetal pelvis in two fetuses **(A and B)** at 12 weeks of gestation using a curvilinear transducer. Note in **A** the presence of two umbilical arteries (*arrows*) surrounding the bladder (*asterisk*). The absence of the right umbilical artery (?) to the right of the bladder (*asterisk*) is demonstrated in fetus **B**. L, left; R, right.

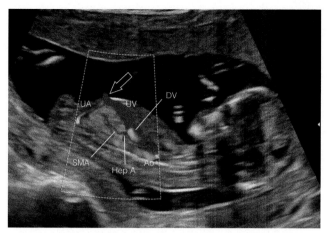

**Figure 3.11:** Sagittal plane of the fetal chest and abdomen in color Doppler in a fetus at 11 weeks of gestation demonstrating an intact anterior abdominal wall (*open arrow*) and the umbilical artery (UA) and umbilical vein (UV) at the insertion of the umbilical cord into the abdomen. This plane also demonstrates the normal course of the UV in the abdomen and shows the narrow ductus venosus (DV), connecting into the heart. This is the ideal plane for Doppler sampling of the DV in early gestation (see Fig. 3.17). From the descending aorta (Ao) posteriorly, the hepatic artery (Hep.A) and the superior mesenteric artery (SMA) are seen to emerge in perpendicular orientation to the aorta (see Fig. 3.7). The inferior vena cava is not seen in this plane as its anatomic course runs in the right abdomen.

can also be used to rule out agenesis of the DV or abnormal connections of the DV. In the same midsagittal view, two arteries appear to arise from the abdominal aorta, namely the hepatic artery superiorly and the superior mesenteric artery inferiorly (Figs. 3.7B and 3.11). In a slightly more angulated view, the inferior vena cava can be visualized ascending from the middle abdomen and draining into the right atrium[8,9] (Fig. 3.12). Interrupted inferior vena cava can be confirmed in this view when suspected in left atrial isomerism. Color Doppler applied to a coronal view of the posterior part of the abdomen demonstrates both renal arteries arising orthogonally from the abdominal aorta toward the renal pelves (Fig. 3.13). Detailed evaluation of first trimester normal and abnormal fetal gastrointestinal and urogenital anatomy is presented in Chapters 12 and 13, respectively.

## Placenta and Umbilical Cord

The assessment of the placental attachment and course of the umbilical artery is best demonstrated in the first trimester on color Doppler (Fig. 3.14). The presence of marginal or velamentous cord insertion can be easily suspected in the first trimester given that the full length of the placenta can be imaged in one view. When umbilical cord abnormalities are suspected in the first trimester, follow-up ultrasound

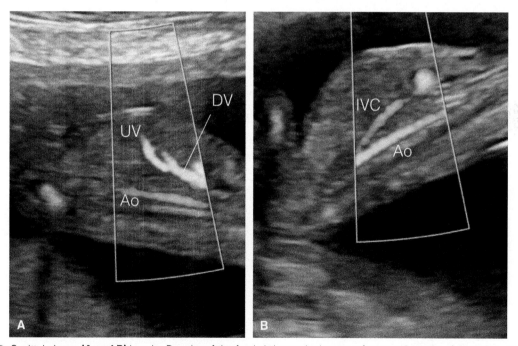

**Figure 3.12:** Sagittal planes **(A and B)** in color Doppler of the fetal abdomen in the same fetus at 13 weeks of gestation. Note in **A**, the ductus venosus (DV) in the mid-abdomen along with the descending aorta (Ao), seen posteriorly. The inferior vena cava (IVC) is not seen due to its anatomic course in the right abdomen. When the probe was reoriented in **B**, the IVC connecting to the heart along with the descending Ao is seen and the DV is not seen. Note the *blue color* in the aorta in **B** (flow away from transducer) due to transducer reorientation.

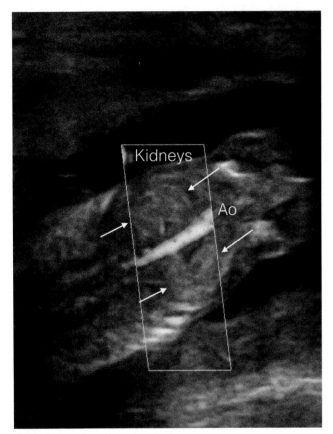

**Figure 3.13:** Coronal plane in color Doppler of the posterior abdomen and pelvis at 13 weeks of gestation showing the descending aorta (Ao) with the left and right renal arteries arising from the Ao and coursing into the kidneys (*arrows*).

examination in the second trimester is recommended to confirm such findings.

### Intracerebral Vessels

Several articles have reported on the course of the cerebral arteries and veins in the first trimester in normal and abnormal conditions.[10–13] Figure 3.15 shows the cerebral arteries and veins from an axial view at the base of the skull (Fig. 3.15A), demonstrating the circle of Willis and from the midsagittal view of the fetal head (Fig. 3.15B), demonstrating the anterior cerebral and pericallosal arteries. The application of color Doppler of the fetal head should be reserved for pregnancies at increased risk for central nervous system abnormalities.

## Regions of Interest for Pulsed Doppler

The application of pulsed (spectral) Doppler ultrasound in the first trimester is limited to the assessment of the maternal uterine arteries for evaluation of pregnancy risk and fetal vessels for aneuploidy risk assessment or for fetal malformations. It is important to note that pulsed Doppler application in the first trimester is associated with a potential risk to the fetus and should be performed when the benefit outweighs the risk (see Chapter 2).

### Uterine Arteries

Pulsed Doppler examination of the uterine arteries in the first trimester has been used to assess uteroplacental impedance and to integrate the results in the risk profiling for preeclampsia[14] (Fig. 3.16). This examination can be performed as part of general screening or targeted to women with a prior history of fetal growth restriction or preeclampsia. Given that the uterine arteries are lateral to the gestational sac, pulsed Doppler can be performed without concern of risk to the fetus.[15]

### The Umbilical Cord

Pulsed Doppler interrogation of the umbilical cord is rarely obtained before the 15th week of gestation. Pulsed Doppler should not be used for confirmation of cardiac activity, as the use of M-mode or a motion clip is preferred for that purpose.

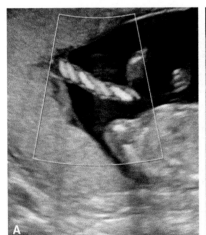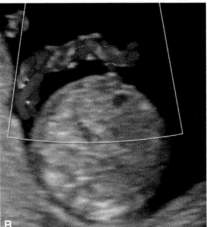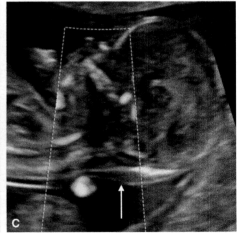

**Figure 3.14:** Color Doppler showing in **A** the placental cord insertion in a fetus at 13 weeks of gestation, in **B** a free loop of umbilical cord in a fetus at 13 weeks and in **C** nuchal cord in a fetus at 12 weeks of gestation resulting in a slight increase in nuchal translucency (*arrow*).

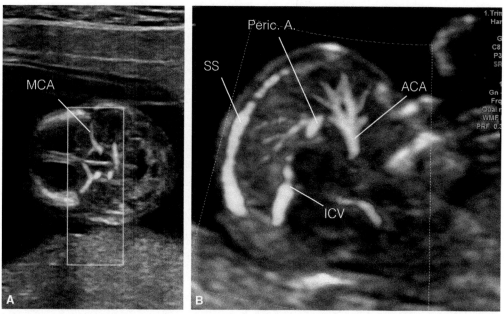

**Figure 3.15: A:** An axial plane of the fetal skull base at 13 weeks of gestation in color Doppler showing the circle of Willis with the middle cerebral artery (MCA). **B:** A midsagittal plane of the fetal head in color Doppler at 12 weeks of gestation showing the anterior cerebral artery (ACA), the proximal portion of the pericallosal artery (Peric.A.), and the internal cerebral vein (ICV) shown coursing posteriorly along the borders of the thalamus. Blood flow in the sagittal sinus (SS) is also demonstrated anteriorly.

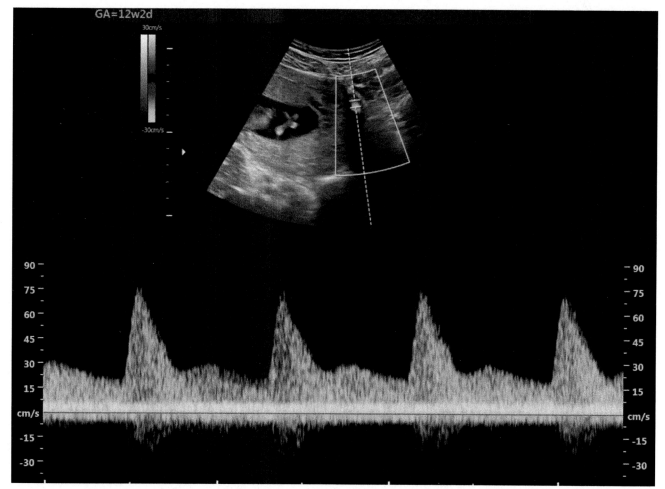

**Figure 3.16:** Color and spectral Doppler of the uterine artery in a pregnancy at 12 weeks of gestation (GA). Uterine artery Doppler waveforms have been used for pregnancy risk assessment in some settings. See text for details.

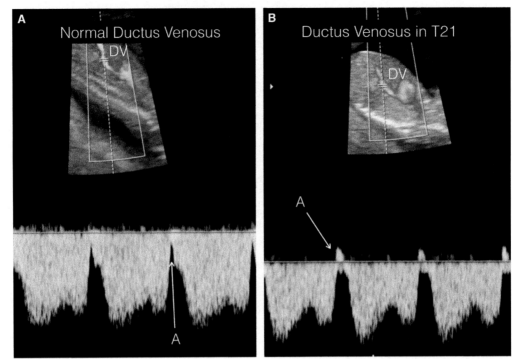

**Figure 3.17:** Color and pulsed Doppler of the ductus venosus (DV) in two fetuses **A** and **B**. Note that the Doppler sample gate is small and is placed within the DV, with an insonation angle of less than 20 to 30 degrees. Normal DV Doppler waveforms show the characteristic biphasic pattern with antegrade flow during the atrial (A) contraction phase as shown in fetus **A**. Note the presence of abnormal reverse flow during the atrial contraction (A) in fetus **B**.

### The Ductus Venosus

The most common use of pulsed Doppler in the first trimester is probably related to the examination of the DV flow velocity waveform. In normal conditions, the DV waveforms are biphasic with low pulsatility and with antegrade flow in the diastolic components (a-wave) throughout the cardiac cycle (Fig. 3.17A). The presence of high pulsatility or a reverse flow of the a-wave in the first trimester (Fig. 3.17B) increases the risk for chromosomal anomalies, cardiac defects, and the occurrence of twin-twin-transfusion syndrome in monochorionic twins.[16–18] There is currently no consensus on whether DV Doppler assessment should be a screening test performed on every fetus or reserved as a second-line assessment in mid- and high-risk fetuses.

### Tricuspid Valve

Color and pulsed Doppler examination across the tricuspid valve is commonly used in the first trimester to assess for the presence of tricuspid valve regurgitation (TR) (Fig. 3.18). The presence of TR in the first trimester (Fig. 3.18B) has been associated with chromosomal abnormalities.[19,20] In the first trimester, TR is found in less than 5% of chromosomally normal fetuses, in more than 65% of fetuses with trisomy 21, and in more than 30% of fetuses with trisomy 18.[19] Interrogation of other cardiac valves with color or pulsed Doppler is reserved for fetuses at risk for valve obstruction or when a cardiac malformation is suspected.

### Other Vessels

In rare situations, clinical indications arise in early gestation for the pulsed Doppler assessment of other fetal vessels such as the hepatic (Fig. 3.19) and middle cerebral arteries. It has been reported that high peak velocities in the hepatic artery are present in the first trimester in fetuses at risk for trisomy 21 (Fig. 3.19B).[21] Furthermore, in rare conditions of suspected fetal anemia in early gestation, such as in pregnancies with serologically confirmed Parvovirus B19 infection, middle cerebral artery Doppler can be of help in assessing for the presence of anemia.

## THREE-DIMENSIONAL ULTRASOUND

3D ultrasound has been associated with a view of the fetal face or the body in surface mode, primarily for keepsake purposes. Beyond its keepsake properties, 3D ultrasound in the first trimester can be accurately used to reconstruct planes and to visualize structures not seen on conventional ultrasound examination. The ability of multiplanar reconstruction of a 3D volume is important, especially during transvaginal ultrasound,

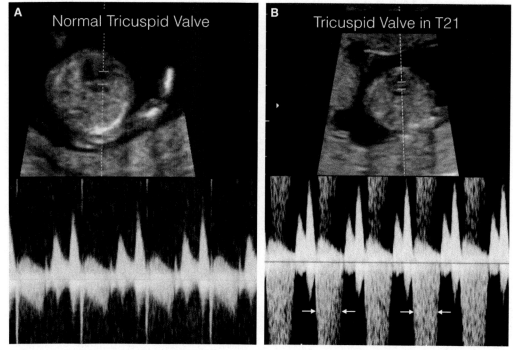

**Figure 3.18:** Doppler velocity waveforms across the tricuspid valve at 12 weeks of gestation in a normal fetus **(A)** and in a fetus **(B)** with trisomy 21 (T21) with severe tricuspid regurgitation (*arrows*).

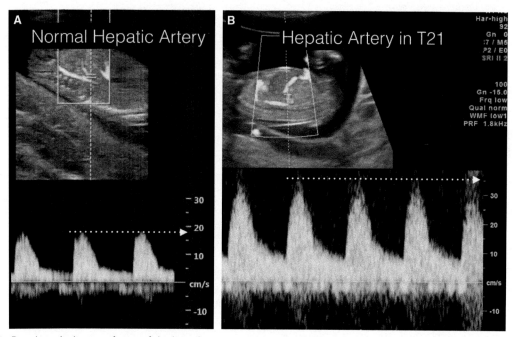

**Figure 3.19:** Doppler velocity waveforms of the hepatic artery at 12 weeks of gestation in a normal fetus **(A)** and in a fetus **(B)** with trisomy 21 (T21). Note the presence of low peak systolic velocities (18 cm per second) in the normal fetus **A**, as compared to high velocities (35 cm per second) in the fetus with trisomy 21 (T21) **(B)**.

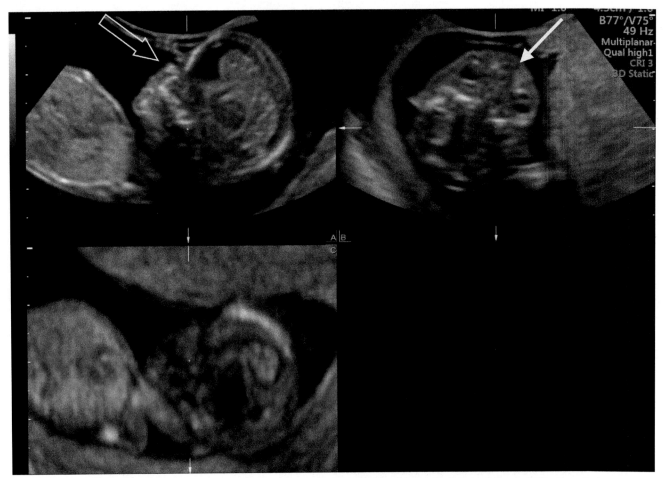

**Figure 3.20:** Transvaginal 3D volume of the fetal face, obtained from an oblique plane of the face (*solid arrow* in **B**), given that a midsagittal plane of the fetal face could not be imaged on 2D ultrasound (*open arrow* in **A**). The volume data are displayed in the multiplanar orthogonal mode showing A, B, and C planes. Compare with Figure 3.21, produced after manipulation of this volume.

where transducer manipulation is limited and the fetus is not in an appropriate position to directly visualize target anatomic regions. For further information on the value of 3D ultrasound, the reader is referred to dedicated monographs and articles on this subject.[22,23]

## Multiplanar Reconstruction

Given that embryos and fetuses rarely present in the first trimester in an ideal position to visualize all of the anatomic structures on 2D ultrasound, the acquisition of static 3D volumes with multiplanar display of reconstructed planes can be of significant help. Using tomographic mode display of a 3D volume, the examiner is able to show in one image several anatomic regions of the fetus. Figures 3.20 and 3.21 show examples of reconstructed fetal profile and NT respectively out of a 3D volume. Figures 3.22 and 3.23 show an example of the fetal head in tomographic mode. Examples of tomographic display of the fetal chest and abdomen are shown in their respective chapters (Chapters 10 and 12). The fetal spine, limbs, profile,

and internal organs such as lungs, diaphragm, and kidneys can be reconstructed in sectional planes from a 3D volume. The brain is probably the best organ to examine starting at 7 weeks of gestation using multiplanar mode. Brain development can be followed from early gestation and into the early second trimester. Careful rotation of the volume along the X, Y and Z-axes, in multiplanar mode, helps to display midline planes of the face (Fig. 3.22), head (Fig. 3.23), lungs, and kidneys. The use of 3D ultrasound in the assessment of fetal anatomy in the first trimester is presented in more detail in Chapters 8 to 15 of this book.

## Three-Dimensional Volume Rendering

The use of surface mode is the most commonly used 3D rendering mode in the first trimester as it allows for optimal visualization of the developing embryo and fetus (Fig. 3.24). Images acquired using 3D surface mode of the embryo and

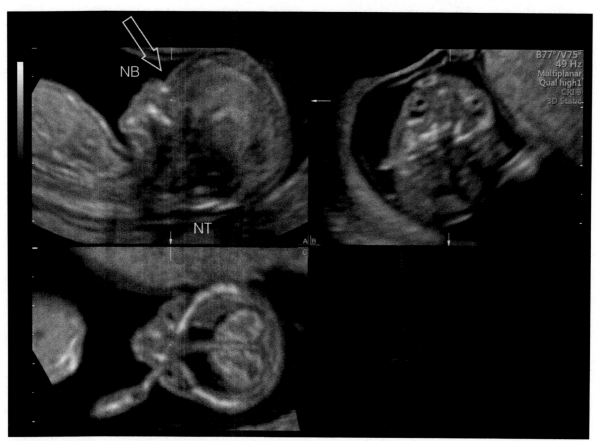

**Figure 3.21:** The result of post-processing of the volume data set displayed in Figure 3.20. Post-processing allowed for the retrieval of the midsagittal plane in the left upper plane (*open arrow* in **A**), with the display of the nasal bone (NB) and nuchal translucency (NT).

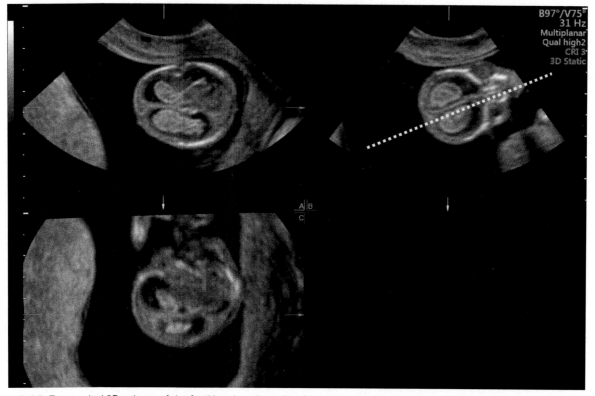

**Figure 3.22:** Transvaginal 3D volume of the fetal head at 12 weeks of gestation displayed in the multiplanar orthogonal mode showing A, B, and C planes. This volume was obtained from an oblique orientation of the fetal head as shown in the upper right image with oblique falx cerebri (*dashed line*). Post-processing of this volume to display important anatomic brain landmarks is shown in Figurve 3.23 and in the surface mode display in Figure 3.28.

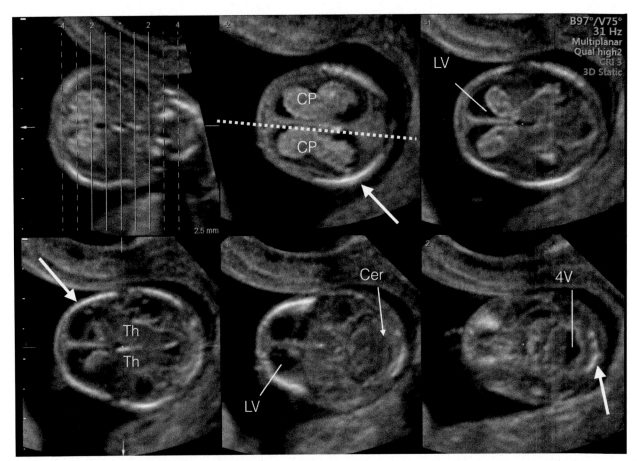

**Figure 3.23:** Post-processing of the 3D volume data set shown in Figure 3.22. Post-processing of the 3D volume included rotations and display in tomographic mode. Five planes are shown at 2.5 mm spacing. Anatomic details of the fetal brain that are shown in these five planes include skull ossifications (*arrows*), the falx cerebri (*dashed line*), the choroid plexuses (CP), the lateral ventricles (LV), the thalami (Th), the developing cerebellum (Cer), and the fourth ventricle (4V).

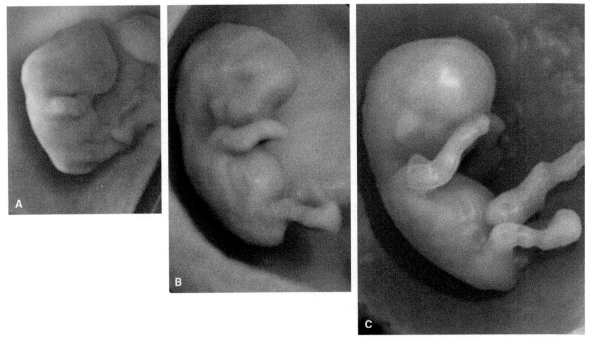

**Figure 3.24:** Surface mode display of 3D volumes of three normal embryos **A**, **B**, and **C** at 8, 9 and 10 weeks, respectively. Note at 8 weeks, the relatively large size of the embryo's head as compared to the body.

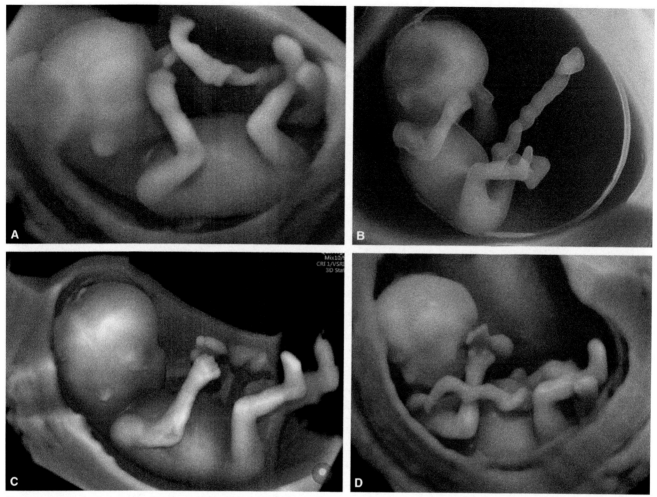

**Figure 3.25:** Surface mode display of 3D volumes of four normal fetuses between 11 **(B)** and 13 weeks of gestation **(A,C,D)**. Note the clear display of surface anatomy and of extremities.

fetus (Fig. 3.24) are similar to images shown in embryology textbooks. As early as the 11th week of gestation, the head, trunk, extremities, and other fetal anatomic details can be reliably demonstrated (Figs. 3.24 to 3.27). On occasions, 3D ultrasound can better display normal internal anatomy of the fetus in the first trimester (Fig. 3.28). Major anomalies affecting the external surface and internal organs of the body can be well recognized in the first trimester in 3D surface mode (Figs. 3.29 and 3.30). In the first trimester fetal anatomy survey, the authors caution about relying on 3D ultrasound only before a detailed evaluation of fetal anatomy is performed on 2D imaging. In addition to 2D ultrasound examination, 3D ultrasound plays an important role in ruling out major fetal malformations in the first trimester in pregnant women with a prior history of severe fetal malformations. In multiple pregnancies, fetuses can be well visualized on 3D ultrasound along with surrounding structures. The diagnosis of chorionicity in multiple pregnancies is best performed on 2D ultrasound. (See Chapter 7 for more details on this subject.)

Other volume rendering modes used in 3D ultrasound include the maximum mode, which is infrequently applied in the first trimester due to the reduced level of ossification in the fetal skeleton, the inversion mode, which is used to visualize intracerebral ventricular system in early gestation, and the silhouette mode (Fig. 3.26C), which has potential for more clinical applications in the future. Combining 3D with color Doppler in glass-body mode highlights internal vasculature. This can be used in the first trimester to visualize the fetal heart, and the arteries and veins inside the abdomen and thorax (Fig. 3.31).

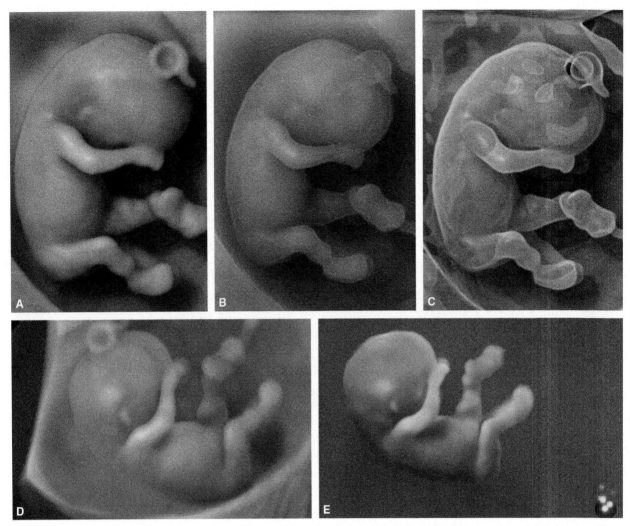

**Figure 3.26:** Three-dimensional volume of a normal fetus at 11 weeks of gestation displayed in surface mode and showing the effect of various post-processing tools. The upper panel **(A–C)** shows the effect of augmenting the transparency effect, with the display of fetal internal anechoic structures. In the lower panel **(D and E)**, adjusting light effects in **D** and digitally erasing surrounding structures in **E** shows the fetus without a background.

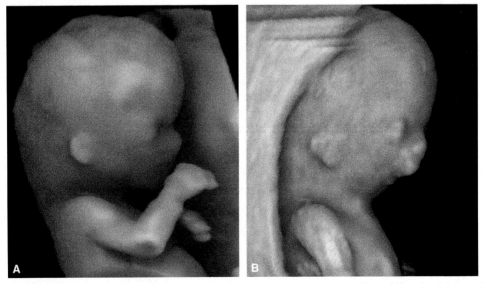

**Figure 3.27:** Three-dimensional volume in surface mode at 12 weeks of gestation in a normal fetus **(A)** and in a fetus with facial dysmorphism with abnormal ears and micrognathia **(B)**.

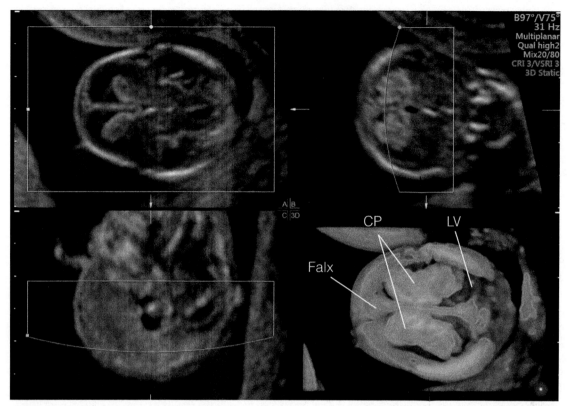

**Figure 3.28:** Transvaginal 3D volume of a fetal head at 12 weeks of gestation displayed in the orthogonal (A,B,C) and surface display mode (3D). This is the same volume shown in Figures 3.22 and 3.23. Rendering of the volume shows in the right lower panel the large choroid plexuses (CP), the falx cerebri (Falx), and the lateral ventricles (LV). Compare with Figure 3.29.

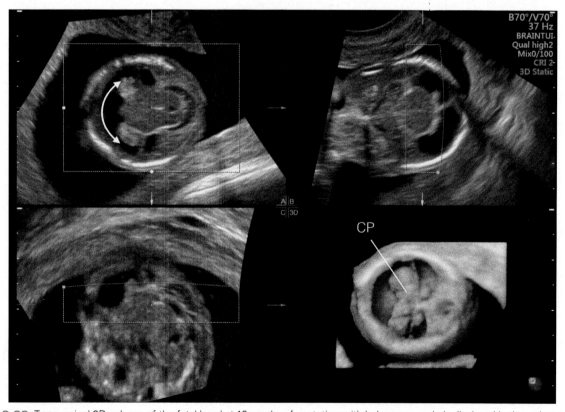

**Figure 3.29:** Transvaginal 3D volume of the fetal head at 12 weeks of gestation with holoprosencephaly displayed in the orthogonal **(A, B, C)** and surface display mode (3D). Rendering of the volume shows in the right lower panel fused choroid plexuses (CP), single ventricle (*double arrow* in **A**), and absent falx cerebri. Compare with normal brain anatomy shown in Figure 3.28.

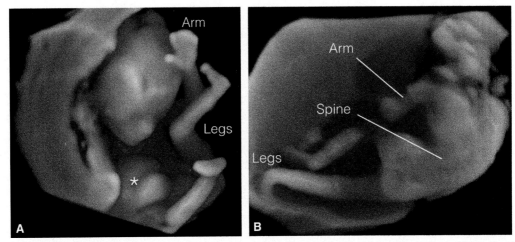

**Figure 3.30:** Three-dimensional (3D) ultrasound images in surface mode in a fetus at 13 weeks of gestation with a body stalk anomaly visualized from the front **(A)** and back **(B)**. The abdominal wall defect is recognized (*asterisk*) and fetal deformities of body and spine are shown in panels **A** and **B**. 3D ultrasound is optimal imaging modality in such cases as it clearly displays the extent of fetal deformities. Compare with normal anatomy in Figure 3.25.

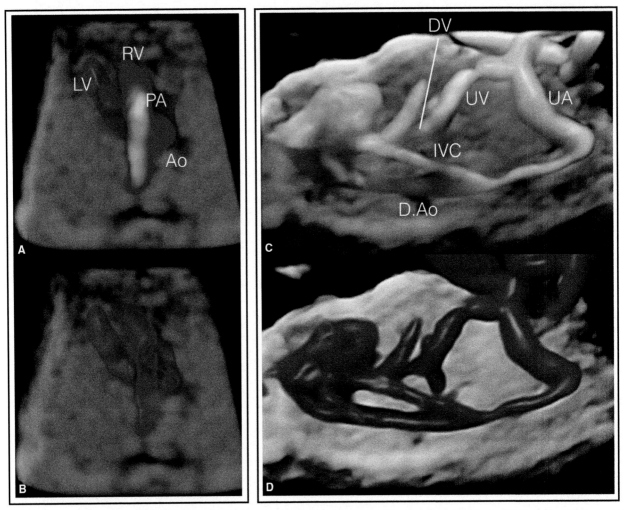

**Figure 3.31:** The left upper panel **(A)** shows a 3D volume of the fetal heart in color Doppler at 12 weeks of gestation. The left lower panel **(B)** shows the same volume as in **A** displayed in glass-body mode with transparency. The right upper panel **(C)** shows a 3D volume of the fetal abdomen in high-definition color Doppler in glass-body mode at 12 weeks of gestation. The right lower panel **(D)** displays the same volume in unidirectional Doppler flow. The right upper **(C)** and lower **(D)** panels show the spatial anatomic relationship of the descending aorta (D.Ao), the umbilical vein (UV), the umbilical artery (UA), the inferior vena cava (IVC), and the ductus venosus (DV). RV, right ventricle; LV, left ventricle; Ao, aorta; PA, pulmonary artery.

# REFERENCES

1. Salomon LJ, Alfirevic Z, Bilardo CM, et al. ISUOG practice guidelines: performance of first-trimester fetal ultrasound scan. *Ultrasound Obstet Gynecol.* 2013;41:102–113.

2. Kaisenberg von C, Chaoui R, Häusler M, et al. Quality Requirements for the early Fetal Ultrasound Assessment at 11-13+6 Weeks of Gestation (DEGUM Levels II and III). *Ultraschall Med.* 2016; 37: 297–302.

3. Persico N, Moratalla J, Lombardi CM, et al. Fetal echocardiography at 11-13 weeks by transabdominal high-frequency ultrasound. *Ultrasound Obstet Gynecol.* 2011;37:296–301.

4. Abuhamad A, Chaoui R. *A Practical Guide to Fetal Echocardiography: Normal and Abnormal Hearts.* 3rd ed. Philadelphia, PA: Wolters Kluwer Health/Lippincott Williams & Wilkins, 2015.

5. Abuhamad AZ, Chaoui R, Jeanty P, et al. Ultrasound in obstetrics and gynecology: a practical approach, 2015. www.openultrasound.com. Accessed March 11, 2017.

6. Chaoui R, McEwing R. Three cross-sectional planes for fetal color Doppler echocardiography. *Ultrasound Obstet Gynecol.* 2003;21:81–93.

7. Wiechec M, Knafel A, Nocun A. Prenatal detection of congenital heart defects at the 11- to 13-week scan using a simple color Doppler protocol including the 4-chamber and 3-vessel and trachea views. *J Ultrasound Med.* 2015;34:585–594.

8. Sinkovskaya E, Klassen A, Abuhamad A. A novel systematic approach to the evaluation of the fetal venous system. *Semin Fetal Neonatal Med.* 2013;18:269–278.

9. Chaoui R, Heling K, Karl K. Ultrasound of the fetal veins. Part 1: the intrahepatic venous system. *Ultraschall Med.* 2014; 35: 208–228.

10. Pati M, Cani C, Bertucci E, et al. Early visualization and measurement of the pericallosal artery: an indirect sign of corpus callosum development. *J Ultrasound Med.* 2012;31:231–237.

11. Díaz-Guerrero L, Giugni-Chalbaud G, Sosa-Olavarría A. Assessment of pericallosal arteries by color Doppler ultrasonography at 11-14 weeks: an early marker of fetal corpus callosum development in normal fetuses and agenesis in cases with chromosomal anomalies. *Fetal Diagn Ther.* 2013;34:85–89.

12. Conturso R, Contro E, Bellussi F, et al. Demonstration of the pericallosal artery at 11-13 weeks of gestation using 3D ultrasound. *Fetal Diagn Ther.* 2015;37:305–309.

13. Karl K, Heling KS, Chaoui R. Ultrasound of the fetal veins. Part 3: the fetal intracerebral venous system. *Ultraschall Med.* 2016;37(1):6–26.

14. Nicolaides KH. Turning the pyramid of prenatal care. *Fetal Diagn Ther.* 2011;29:183–196.

15. Salvesen KÅ, Lees C, Abramowicz J, Brezinka C, Haar Ter G, Maršál K. Safe use of Doppler ultrasound during the 11 to 13 + 6-week scan: is it possible? *Ultrasound Obstet Gynecol.* 2011;37:625–628.

16. Matias A, Gomes C, Flack N, et al. Screening for chromosomal abnormalities at 10-14 weeks: the role of ductus venosus blood flow. *Ultrasound Obstet Gynecol.* 1998;12:380–384.

17. Matias A, Huggon I, Areias JC, et al. Cardiac defects in chromosomally normal fetuses with abnormal ductus venosus blood flow at 10-14 weeks. *Ultrasound Obstet Gynecol.* 1999;14:307–310.

18. Maiz N, Nicolaides KH. Ductus venosus in the first trimester: contribution to screening of chromosomal, cardiac defects and monochorionic twin complications. *Fetal Diagn Ther.* 2010;28:65–71.

19. Falcon O, Faiola S, Huggon I, et al. Fetal tricuspid regurgitation at the 11 + 0 to 13 + 6-week scan: association with chromosomal defects and reproducibility of the method. *Ultrasound Obstet Gynecol.* 2006;27:609–612.

20. Khalil A, Nicolaides KH. Fetal heart defects: potential and pitfalls of first-trimester detection. *Semin Fetal Neonatal Med.* 2013;18:251–260.

21. Zvanca M, Gielchinsky Y, Abdeljawad F, et al. Hepatic artery Doppler in trisomy 21 and euploid fetuses at 11-13 weeks. *Prenat Diagn.* 2011;31:22–27.

22. Abu-Rustum RS. *A Practical Guide to 3D Ultrasound.* London: CRC Press, Taylor & Francis Group; 2014.

23. Chaoui R, Heling K-S. *3D-Ultrasound in Prenatal Diagnosis: A Practical Approach.* 1st ed. Berlin, New York: DeGruyter; 2016.

# CHAPTER 4

# Fetal Biometry and Pregnancy Dating in the First Trimester

## INTRODUCTION

Accurate performance of an ultrasound examination in the first trimester is important given its ability to confirm an intrauterine gestation, assess number and viability of embryos or fetuses, accurately date the pregnancy, and diagnose major fetal malformations. In this chapter, we present the approach and indications to the first trimester ultrasound examination, the parameters of pregnancy dating, and the ultrasound markers of pregnancy failure. Normal fetal anatomy and fetal malformations will be discussed in detail in subsequent chapters.

## APPROACH TO THE FIRST TRIMESTER ULTRASOUND EXAMINATION

The first trimester ultrasound examination can be performed transabdominally or transvaginally. There is general consensus that, with rare exceptions, obstetrical ultrasound examinations at less than 10 weeks of gestation are best performed transvaginally. The transvaginal approach provides for higher resolution than the transabdominal approach and positions the transducer in close proximity to the target anatomic region (gestational sac). Beyond the 12th week of gestation, the transabdominal approach with high-resolution transducers and with optimal imaging can provide sufficient details to allow for systemic assessment of fetal anatomy. In the presence of first trimester suspected fetal malformations, a combined transabdominal and transvaginal approach is recommended.

## INDICATIONS FOR THE FIRST TRIMESTER ULTRASOUND EXAMINATION

There is currently varying opinions on whether the first trimester ultrasound examination is offered routinely to all pregnant women or is indication driven.[1,2] Indications for the first trimester ultrasound are many and most pregnant women in resourced settings receive at least one such ultrasound during their pregnancies. With mounting evidence on the important role of the first trimester ultrasound in pregnancy dating, aneuploidy risk assessment, diagnosis of multiple pregnancies, and in detection of major fetal malformations, the authors believe that ultrasound in early gestation will ultimately be offered routinely to pregnant women. Table 4.1 lists common indications for the first trimester ultrasound examination in pregnancy.

## SONOGRAPHIC LANDMARKS IN THE FIRST TRIMESTER

The normal intrauterine pregnancy undergoes significant and rapid change in the first trimester, from a collection of undifferentiated cells to a fetus within an amniotic sac connected to a placenta and a yolk sac. This significant progression can be seen on ultrasound beginning with the chorionic sac, which

---

**Table 4.1** • Common Indications for Ultrasound examination in the First Trimester

- Amenorrhea
- Pelvic pain
- Vaginal bleeding
- Unknown menstrual dates
- Subjective feeling of pregnancy
- Uterus greater or smaller than dates on clinical evaluation
- Positive pregnancy test
- Aneuploidy risk assessment and nuchal translucency measurement
- Fetal anatomy survey
- Ruling out multiple pregnancies

is the first sonographic evidence of pregnancy and progressing to the embryo and fetus with cardiac activity. Identifying ultrasound landmarks and understanding its normal progression in the first trimester help in confirming a normal pregnancy and in the diagnosis of pregnancy failure.

## Gestational Sac

The gestational sac, also referred to as the chorionic cavity, is the first sonographic evidence of pregnancy. The gestational sac on transvaginal ultrasound is first seen at 4 to 4.5 weeks from the first day of the last menstrual period (LMP) (Fig. 4.1). When the gestational sac has a mean diameter of 2 to 4 mm, its borders appear echogenic, which makes its demonstration easy (Fig. 4.1). The echogenic ring of the gestational sac is an important ultrasound sign, which helps to differentiate it from intrauterine fluid or blood collection (Fig. 4.2). The shape of the gestational sac is first circular but with the appearance of the yolk sac and the embryo it becomes more ellipsoid (Fig. 4.3).

## Yolk Sac

The yolk sac is seen at 5 weeks of gestation (menstrual age) on transvaginal ultrasound, as a small ring within the gestational sac with highly echogenic borders (Figs. 4.3 and 4.4). It has a diameter of around 2 mm at 6 weeks and increases slowly to around 6 mm at 12 weeks. The first detection of the embryo by ultrasound is noted in close proximity to the free wall of the yolk sac, because the yolk sac is connected to the embryo by the vitelline duct. A small yolk sac with a diameter less than 3 mm between 6 and 10 weeks or a diameter of more than 7 mm before 9 weeks is a cause for concern for an abnormal pregnancy and thus this observation requires a follow-up ultrasound examination to assess normalcy of pregnancy (Fig. 4.5A and B).

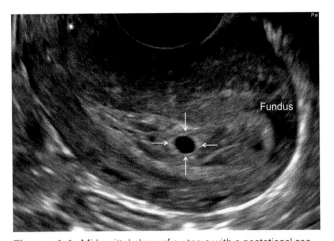

**Figure 4.1:** Midsagittal plane of a uterus with a gestational sac at 4.5 weeks of gestation. Note the echogenic borders (*arrows*) of the gestational sac. The echogenic borders (*ring*) of the gestational sac help to differentiate it from an intrauterine fluid or blood collection. The fundus of the uterus is labeled for orientation.

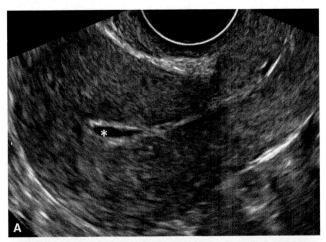

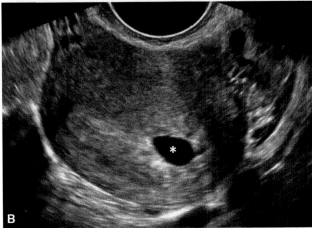

**Figure 4.2:** Midsagittal **(A)** and transverse **(B)** planes of two uteri showing fluid accumulation (*asterisk*) between the decidual layers. This finding should not be confused with an intrauterine gestational sac. See text for details.

## Amnion

The amniotic sac develops as a thin echogenic structure surrounding the embryo (Fig. 4.6). The amniotic sac appears following the appearance of the yolk sac and just before the appearance of the embryo. Whereas the gestational sac shows variations in size and shape, the growth of the amniotic sac is closely related to that of the embryo between 6 and 10 weeks of gestation.

## Embryo

The embryo is first seen on transvaginal ultrasound as a focal thickening on top of the yolk sac, at around the fifth menstrual week (Fig. 4.7). First cardiac activity is typically seen by 6 to 6.5 weeks. The embryo can be recognized by high-resolution transvaginal ultrasound at the 2 to 3 mm length size (Fig. 4.7), but cardiac activity can be consistently seen when the embryo reaches a 5 to 7 mm in length or greater. Embryonic heart rate increases rapidly in early gestation being around 100 to 115 before 6 weeks, rising to 145 to 170 at 8 weeks, and dropping down to a plateau of 137 to 144 after 9 weeks of gestation.

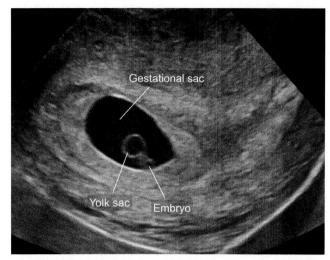

Figure 4.3: Midsagittal plane of a uterus with a gestational sac at 6 weeks of gestation. Note the presence of a yolk sac and a small embryo. The shape of the gestational sac is more ellipsoid than circular.

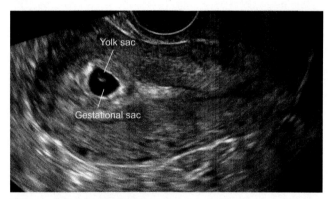

Figure 4.4: Midsagittal plane of a uterus with a gestational sac at 5.5 weeks of gestation. Note the yolk sac seen within the gestational sac with highly echogenic borders.

The size of the embryo increases rapidly by approximately 1 mm per day in length. Note that the embryo develops within the amniotic cavity and is referred to as intraamniotic whereas the yolk sac is outside of the amniotic cavity and is referred to as extraamniotic. The fluid that the yolk sac in embedded within is the extraembryonic coelom.

The appearance of the embryo on ultrasound changes from 6 to 12 weeks of gestation. At 6 weeks of gestation, the embryo appears as a thin cylinder with no discernible body parts, "the grain of rice appearance" (Fig. 4.8). As gestational age advances, the embryo develops body curvature and clear delineation on ultrasound of a head, chest, abdomen, and extremities, "the gummy-bear appearance" (Figs. 4.9 and 4.10). Clear delineation of a head, chest, abdomen, and extremities on gray scale ultrasound is noted at 10 weeks of gestation and beyond (Fig. 4.11). Close observation of anatomic details on transvaginal ultrasound at or beyond 12 weeks of gestation may allow for the diagnosis of major fetal malformations. This will be discussed in detail in Chapters 8 to 14, organized by anatomic organ system.

## FIRST TRIMESTER PREGNANCY DATING

One of the most important aspects of the first trimester obstetric ultrasound is pregnancy dating as this is accomplished by performing few simple biometric measurements: (1) the gestational sac diameter, when no embryo is seen; (2) the length of the embryo, or crown-rump length (CRL); (3) in the late first trimester (12 to 14 weeks), the biparietal diameter (BPD), head circumference (HC), abdominal circumference (AC), and femur length (FL). Obtained biometric values are compared to established reference ranges to provide for accurate dating. With an accurate ultrasound-derived gestational age in

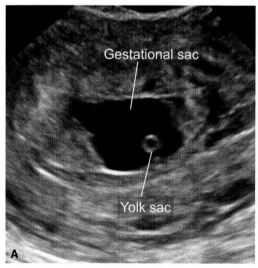

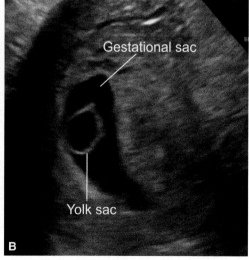

Figure 4.5: **A and B**: Two gestational sacs with abnormal size of yolk sacs: small in **A** and large in **B**. Abnormal size of yolk sacs is a concern for an abnormal pregnancy and follow-up ultrasound is recommended.

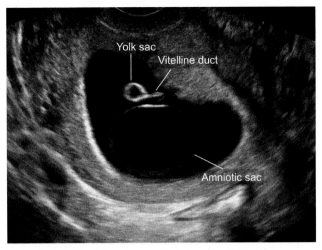

Figure 4.6: Gestational sac at 7 weeks of gestation. The amniotic sac is seen as a thin reflective circular membrane. The yolk sac and vitelline duct are seen as extraamniotic structures.

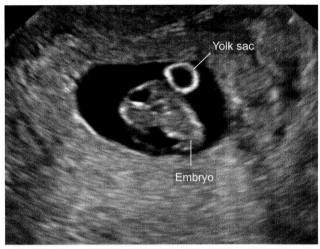

Figure 4.9: Gestational sac with an embryo at 8 weeks. Note the body curvature of the embryo, resembling a "gummy bear" in shape. The yolk sac is seen adjacent to the embryo.

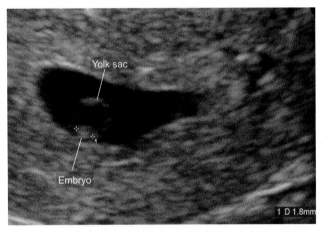

Figure 4.7: Transvaginal ultrasound of a gestational sac with an embryo measuring 1.8 mm in size. Note the proximal location of the yolk sac to the embryo.

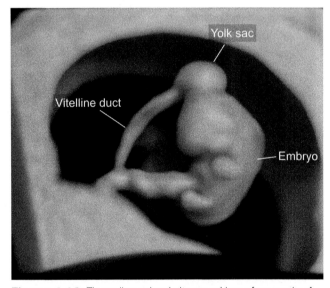

Figure 4.10: Three-dimensional ultrasound in surface mode of a fetus at 8 weeks of gestation showing the body curvature of the embryo, resembling a "gummy bear" in shape. The yolk sac is seen adjacent to the embryo and the vitelline duct is seen connecting the yolk sac to the umbilical cord.

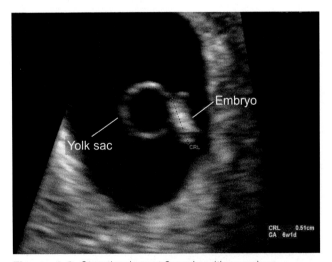

Figure 4.8: Gestational sac at 6 weeks with an embryo measuring 5.1 mm in crown-rump length (CRL). Note the straight shape of the embryo, resembling a "grain of rice." The yolk sac is seen adjacent to the embryo. GA, gestational age.

the first and second trimesters of pregnancy, ultrasound can reliably date a pregnancy with unknown dates and establish an estimated date of delivery with accuracy.

In clinical medicine, the age of an embryo or a fetus is expressed in *weeks of gestation* and not in months, and these weeks are calculated from the first day of the LMP, which corresponds to two additional weeks from the date of conception. Gestational age is therefore calculated from the first day of the LMP and roughly corresponds to the dates of conception plus about 14 days. Ultrasound equipment has an integrated calculator, which calculates the estimated date of delivery as the LMP is entered. Formulas for calculating gestational age from various biometric measurements are also part of the software of ultrasound equipment.

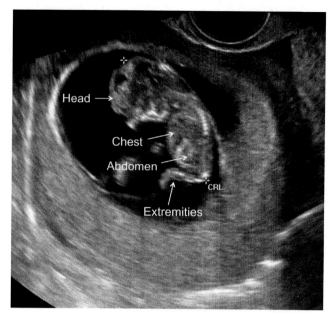

**Figure 4.11:** Gestational sac with an embryo at 10 weeks of gestation. Note the clear delineation of a head, chest, abdomen, and extremities. CRL, crown-rump length.

In estimating gestational age by ultrasound, it is important to remember these critical points:

- Once an established date of delivery is assigned to a pregnancy following an ultrasound examination, irrespective of whether the assigned established dates were those by ultrasound or by menstrual dates, these dates should not be changed later on in pregnancy.
- If a patient reports no menstrual dates, ultrasound in the first or second trimester should date the pregnancy and establish the estimated date of delivery.
- If the ultrasound biometric measurements vary from the menstrual dates by more than 5 to 7 days in the first trimester, then ultrasound should be used to establish the date of delivery.[3]
- Ultrasound dating of pregnancy is most accurate in the first trimester.

# BIOMETRIC MEASUREMENTS IN THE FIRST TRIMESTER

Biometric measurements for first trimester dating include the mean gestational sac diameter (MSD), the CRL and the fetal BPD and HC (greater than 11 weeks). The most accurate and reproducible biometric measurement is the CRL and should be the preferred biometric measurement for pregnancy dating when feasible.

## Mean Sac Diameter

Because the gestational sac is the first evidence of pregnancy on ultrasound and is first visualized within the endometrial cavity at 4 to 4.5 weeks after the LMP, its detection and measurement can be used to confirm and date a pregnancy. The biometric measurement for pregnancy dating uses the MSD, calculated as the arithmetic mean diameters derived from its greatest sagittal, transverse, and coronal planes (Fig. 4.12A and B). The presence of a gestational sac in the endometrial cavity confirms the presence of an intrauterine pregnancy but not the viability of the embryo. The presence of a gestational sac within the endometrial cavity without an embryo, suggests that the pregnancy is at 5 to 6 weeks of gestation. It is not recommended to rely solely on the MSD for estimating the due date, as the CRL is a more precise dating method and should be the preferred choice.

## Crown-Rump Length

The CRL corresponds to the length of the embryo in millimeters. Although the name implies a measurement from the crown to the rump of the embryo, the actual measurement corresponds to the longest "straight line" distance from the top of the head to the rump of the embryo/fetus (Figs. 4.7, 4.8, 4.11, and 4.13), despite the noted body curvature. The CRL measurements are more accurate in the embryo/fetal neutral position and between 11+0 and 13+6

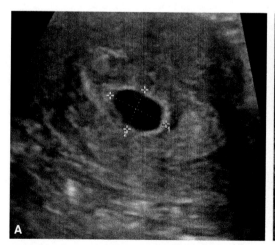
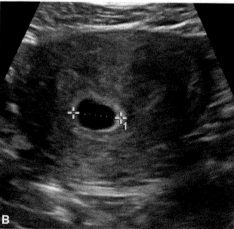

**Figure 4.12: A and B:** Measurements of the mean sac diameter (MSD) of a gestational sac at 5 weeks. The MSD is calculated as the arithmetic mean diameters derived from its greatest sagittal (*1*), transverse (*2*) in **A** and coronal planes (*1*) in **B**.

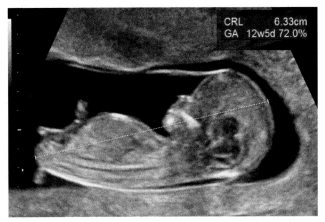

**Figure 4.13:** Crown-rump length (CRL) measurement of a fetus at 12 + 5 weeks of gestation. Note that the CRL measurement corresponds to the longest straight line from the top of the head to the rump region. GA, gestational age.

weeks of gestation. When measuring the CRL, the operator should use the mean of three discrete measurements, obtained in a midsagittal plane of the embryo/fetus. It is recommended to follow these parameters when dating a pregnancy in the first trimester (<14 weeks) by CRL:

- For pregnancies at less than 9 weeks of gestation, a discrepancy of more than 5 days from LMP is an appropriate reason for changing the expected date of delivery (EDD).[3]
- For pregnancies between 9 and 13 6/7 weeks of gestation, a discrepancy of more than 7 days should result in a change in the EDD.[3]

The CRL increases rapidly at a rate of approximately 1.1 mm per day. An approximate formula to calculate gestational age from the CRL is gestational age in days = CRL (mm) + 42; however, this may not be needed because most ultrasound equipment have integrated software, which allows gestational age determination upon measurement of CRL or other biometric data.

## Biparietal Diameter

Measurement of the BPD, HC, AC, and FL in the first trimester is typically performed at 12 to 14 weeks and follows the same anatomic landmarks as those in the second and third trimesters. The BPD is measured in an axial plane of the fetal head at the level of the thalami (Fig. 4.14). Sonographic landmarks identifying the correct BPD plane are listed in Table 4.2. In some settings, the BPD is measured by placing the near and far calipers on the outside of the proximal and distal parietal bones (Fig. 4.14A) and in other settings, the near caliper is placed on the outside of the parietal bone and the far caliper is placed on the inside of the parietal bone (Fig. 4.14B). Readers should conform to their regional standards for BPD measurements.

## Head Circumference

The HC is measured in the trans-thalamic axial view, which is the same plane as that for the BPD measurement (Fig. 4.15). We recommend that you perform the HC measurement following the BPD measurement. This approach allows the operator to utilize the calipers placed for BPD measurement, which expedites the process. It is of note that when the HC is being measured, the lower caliper from the BPD diameter should be moved to the outer bony parietal edge (Fig. 4.15).

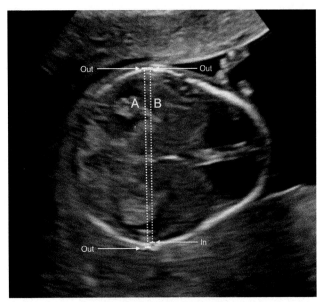

**Figure 4.14:** Biparietal diameter (BPD) measurement of a fetus at 13 weeks of gestation. According to the setting used, the measurement is achieved either outside to outside **(A)** or outside to inside **(B)**. See Table 4.2 for details.

---

**Table 4.2 • Sonographic Landmarks for the Measurement of the Biparietal Diameter (BPD) Plane**

- Focal zone at appropriate level
- Image magnified
- Axial plane of the fetal head
- Symmetric appearance of cerebral hemispheres
- Midline falx imaged
- Thalami imaged
- Cavum septi pellucidi imaged[a]
- Insula imaged[a]
- No cerebellum visualized
- Near caliper on outside edge of bone
- Far caliper on inside/outside edge of bone (see text)
- Measurement at widest diameter
- Measurement perpendicular to falx

---

[a]Not visible in the first trimester

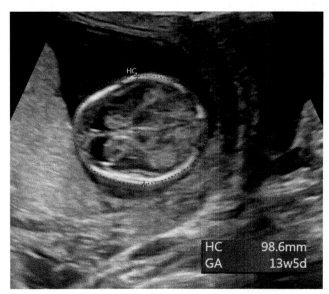

**Figure 4.15:** Head circumference (HC) measurement of a fetus at 13 + 5 weeks of gestation. Note that the calipers are placed outside to outside for HC measurement. GA, gestational age.

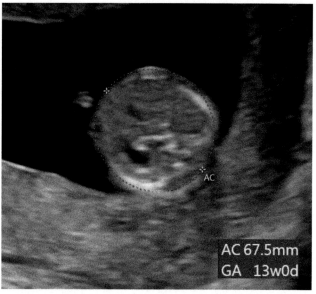

**Figure 4.16:** Abdominal circumference (AC) measurement of a fetus at 13 weeks of gestation. See Table 4.3 for details. GA, gestational age.

## Abdominal Circumference

The AC is measured on a transverse (axial) section of the upper fetal abdomen. Sonographic landmarks identifying the correct plane for the AC measurement are listed in Table 4.3 and Figure 4.16.

## Femur Length

In order to optimize the measurement of the FL, the whole femur diaphysis should be displayed on the screen, and the angle between the insonating beam and the shaft of the femur should be kept in the range of 45 to 90 degrees in order to avoid underestimating the length of the femur due to ultrasound wave deflection (Fig. 4.17). The longest visible diaphysis should be measured by placing each caliper at the end of the diaphysis. Femur measurements can be difficult to perform in early gestation, as the diaphyseal segment of the bone is not fully ossified. Sonographic landmarks identifying the correct plane for the FL measurement are listed in Table 4.4.

---

**Table 4.3 •** Sonographic Landmarks for the Measurement of the Abdominal Circumference (AC) Plane

- Focal zone at appropriate level
- Image magnified
- Axial plane of the abdomen
- Abdomen as circular as possible
- Spine imaged in cross section in 3- or 9-o'clock position if possible
- Stomach bubble imaged
- Intrahepatic portion of the umbilical vein imaged in a short segment[a]
- No more than one rib visible on either side laterally
- Kidneys not to be visualized in the image
- Surrounding skin seen in its entirety if possible[a]
- Measurement of circumference ellipse on outside edge of skin[a]

---

[a]Not clearly visible in the first trimester

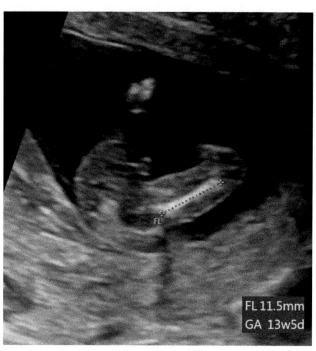

**Figure 4.17:** Femur length (FL) measurement of a fetus at 13 weeks of gestation. See Table 4.4 for details. GA, gestational age.

**Table 4.4 •** Sonographic Landmarks for the Measurement of the Femur Length (FL)

- Focal zone at appropriate level
- Image magnified
- Whole femur diaphysis imaged
- Ultrasound beam perpendicular to long axis of femur
- Calipers placed at end of diaphysis
- Longest visible diaphysis is measured

**Table 4.5 •** Diagnostic Signs of Early Pregnancy Failure in the First Trimester

- Crown-rump length of equal to or greater than 7 mm without cardiac activity
- Mean sac diameter of equal to or greater than 25 mm without an embryo
- Absence of embryo with heartbeat at two or more weeks after an ultrasound that showed a gestational sac without a yolk sac
- Absence of embryo with heartbeat at 11 days or more after an ultrasound that showed a gestational sac with a yolk sac

## ELEMENTS OF PREGNANCY FAILURE

Pregnancy failure can occur in up to 10% to 15% of pregnancies. Suspected pregnancy failure is thus a common indication for ultrasound examination in the first trimester. The diagnosis can often be made by ultrasound, typically before symptoms develop by patients. Depending on the gestational age of pregnancy, several scenarios can be expected:

- Pregnancy confirmed by a positive pregnancy test but no gestational sac is noted in the uterine cavity by ultrasound, suggesting the differential diagnosis of an incomplete miscarriage, an ectopic pregnancy, or an early intrauterine pregnancy that is not yet recognizable by transvaginal ultrasound.
- Gestational sac noted by transvaginal ultrasound, but no signs of embryo or yolk sac within it.
- An embryo visualized on transvaginal ultrasound, but no cardiac activity detected.
- An embryo with cardiac activity detected, but various measurements are out of range (heart rate, size of yolk sac, embryo, amniotic sac, etc.).
- Presence of subchorionic bleeding, with or without clinical signs of bleeding.
- Abnormal anatomic appearance of the embryo.

In many conditions, if the health of the patient is not in danger (bleeding, pain etc.) and an ectopic pregnancy is not in the differential diagnosis, a follow-up ultrasound examination is helpful to assess for change in the ultrasound findings and in confirming the suspected diagnosis. Given that the developing gestational sac undergoes notable significant change on a weekly basis in the first trimester, follow-up ultrasound that fails to show a noticeable change after 1 week or more casts a poor prognostic sign and can confirm the diagnosis of a suspected failed pregnancy. The presence of subchorionic bleeding is generally associated with a good outcome in the absence of other markers of pregnancy failure (see Chapter 15). It is the opinion of the authors that in the absence of specific findings of failed pregnancy, conservative management with follow-up ultrasound examination is helpful in the evaluation of a suspected failed pregnancy in early gestation. Table 4.5 lists specific findings of failed pregnancy in the first trimester, which when noted can establish the diagnosis without a need for a follow-up examination.[4]

## CONCLUSION

The first trimester ultrasound examination is an important step in the evaluation of the pregnancy as it allows for confirmation of an intrauterine gestation, accurate pregnancy dating, and evaluation of fetal anatomy. It is of note that significant change occurs in the first trimester and this change can be detected by transvaginal ultrasound examination. Sequential steps of the normal development of the pregnancy should be known in order to better compare the actual ultrasound findings with the corresponding gestational age. This is the basic knowledge that is needed in order to differentiate a normal from an abnormal gestation. Following chapters in this book provide detailed evaluation for screening and diagnosis of major fetal malformations in the first trimester of pregnancy.

## REFERENCES

1. Reddy UM, Abuhamad AZ, Levine D, Saade GR. Fetal Imaging Executive Summary of a Joint Eunice Kennedy Shriver National Institute of Child Health and Human Development, Society for Maternal-Fetal Medicine, American Institute of Ultrasound in Medicine, American College of Obstetricians and Gynecologists, American College of Radiology, Society for Pediatric Radiology, and Society of Radiologists in Ultrasound Fetal Imaging Workshop. *J Ultrasound Med.* 2014;33:745–757.
2. ISUOG. ISUOG practice guidelines: performance of first trimester fetal ultrasound scan. *Ultrasound Obstet Gynecol.* 2013;41:102–113.
3. ACOG-Committee Opinion No 700: Methods for Estimating the Due Date, *Obstet Gynecol* 2017;129:e150–e154.
4. Doubilet PM, Benson CB, Bourne T, et al. Diagnostic criteria for nonviable pregnancy early in the first trimester. *N Engl J Med.* 2013;369(15):1443–1451.

# The Detailed First Trimester Ultrasound Examination

## INTRODUCTION

The role of the ultrasound examination in the first trimester has changed over the last 30 years with the introduction of nuchal translucency (NT) screening and with significant improvements in ultrasound technology. Ultrasound in early gestation, ranging from 6 to 16 weeks, was primarily performed to confirm cardiac activity, location of gestational sac, pregnancy dating, number of fetuses, and to assess the adnexal regions. In addition, ultrasound was used to guide invasive procedures such as chorionic villus sampling and amniocentesis. With the widespread use of the first trimester NT screening, the assessment of fetal anatomy became part of the early gestation ultrasound and many fetal malformations that were detected in the second and third trimesters of pregnancy are now detected in the first trimester. Major fetal anomalies such as fetal hydrops, anencephaly, body stalk anomaly, large anterior abdominal wall defects, megacystis, and others (see Table 5.1) are now almost universally detected in the first trimester.[1] With accumulating knowledge and expanding expertise, the approach to the first trimester ultrasound has changed over time. The current goal of the first trimester ultrasound includes an element of fetal anatomic assessment and in experts' hands, detailed evaluation of fetal anatomy is achievable and detection of several major fetal malformations is now possible with consistency. Advantages of the fetal anatomic survey in the first trimester include the ability to image the fetus in its entirety in one view, lack of bone ossification which obstructs view later in gestation, increased fetal mobility, which allows imaging from many different angles, and the availability of high-resolution transvaginal ultrasound, which brings the ultrasound transducer in proximity to fetal organs. Challenges of the first trimester anatomic survey however include the need to combine the abdominal and transvaginal approach in some cases, the small size of fetal organs, and the lack of some sonographic markers of fetal abnormalities that are commonly seen in the second trimester of pregnancy. In our experience, the performance of the fetal anatomic survey in the first trimester is enhanced if a systematic approach is employed.

In this chapter, we report on our systematic approach to the detailed fetal anatomic survey in the first trimester, defined at 11 to 14 weeks of gestation. We coined the term *detailed* to reflect on the comprehensive nature of this approach to fetal anatomy in the first trimester. This *systematic* approach is modeled along the "morphology/anatomy" ultrasound examination in the second trimester. It is important to emphasize that the performance of the detailed first trimester ultrasound examination requires substantial operator expertise in obstetric sonography, high-resolution ultrasound equipment, and knowledge of the current literature on this subject. Optimizing the first trimester ultrasound examination as described in Chapter 3 of this book, along with the use of the transvaginal approach with color Doppler and three-dimensional (3D) ultrasound when clinically indicated, will enhance its accuracy. In Chapter 1, we listed existing national and international guidelines for the performance of the first trimester ultrasound examination. The systematic approach that is proposed in this chapter expands on existing guidelines and is geared toward a detailed evaluation of fetal anatomy in early gestation. We have developed this approach to the detailed first trimester ultrasound over several years and have found it to be effective in screening for

**Table 5.1 • Major Fetal Abnormalities That can Potentially be Easily Identified on First Trimester Ultrasound**

Early hydrops
Anencephaly
Alobar holoprosencephaly
Body stalk anomaly
Ectopia cordis
Large omphalocele
Large gastroschisis
Megacystis
Molar placenta

fetal malformations in early gestation. Undoubtedly, as new information comes about and with technological advances in ultrasound imaging, the approach to the detailed first trimester ultrasound examination will evolve over time.

# DETECTION OF FETAL MALFORMATIONS IN THE FIRST TRIMESTER

Over the past 25 years, several studies reported on the feasibility of ultrasound for the detection of fetal malformations in early gestation.[2-14] Studies on this subject varied with some reporting high detection rates of fetal anomaly by ultrasound in early gestation performed in specialized centers with significant expertise.[9,12,15-18] Only few studies reported on the early gestation detection of fetal malformations in large screening populations with ultrasound examinations performed by several examiners with various level of expertise.[1] Furthermore, the gestational age window varied between studies, with some reporting detection rates up to 16 weeks of gestation as part of the "early gestation ultrasound" whereas others have limited the ultrasound examination to the 11 to 14 weeks of gestation. Of particular interest is the comprehensive study of Syngelaki et al.,[1] which reported on the detection of fetal anomalies during the 11- to 13-week scan in a population of 44,859 patients after excluding 332 detected aneuploidies.[1] The authors classified the type of first trimester fetal malformations into four main groups: always detectable, occasionally detectable, rarely detectable and non-detectable.[1] Table 5.2 summarizes the results of this study.[1]

**Table 5.2 • Diagnosis of Fetal Anomalies at 11 to 13 Weeks Scan, after Excluding Detected Aneuploidies (N = 44,859)**

| Fetal Abnormality | Diagnosis at 11–13 Weeks in Relation to all Present[a] |
|---|---|
| **Neural Tube, Brain, Face**[b] | |
| Acrania/iniencephaly | 29/29 (100%) |
| Open spina bifida | 3/21 (14.3%) |
| Ventriculomegaly | 1/11 (9.1%) |
| Alobar holoprosencephaly | 2/2 (100%) |
| Facial clefts | 1/20 (5%) |
| **Lungs, Heart**[c] | |
| Diaphragmatic hernia | 4/8 (50%) |
| Cardiac anomalies (all) | 28/106 (26.4%) |
| **Abdomen, Renal**[d] | |
| Omphalocele | 60/60 (100%) |
| Gastroschisis | 19/19 (100%) |
| Megacystis | 29/29 (100%) |
| Infantile polycystic kidneys | 2/6 (33.3%) |
| **Skeleton**[e] | |
| Lethal skeletal dysplasia | 3/6 (50%) |
| Short long bones unilateral | 2/4 (50%) |
| Absent hand/or foot | 7/9 (77.8%) |
| Polydactyly | 12/20 (60%) |
| **Others and Multiple Anomalies** | |
| Body stalk anomaly | 5/5 (100%) |
| Cloacal defect | 1/1 (100%) |
| Multiple anomalies | 8/8 (100%) |

[a] In cases not diagnosed, absolute number are reported.
[b] None diagnosed at 11–13 weeks: Hemivertebra (1), microcephaly (1), craniosynostosis (1), agenesis corpus callosum (10), semilobar holoprosencephaly (1), cerebellar hypoplasia (1), vermian agenesis (1), nasopharyngeal teratoma (1), retrognathia (1).
[c] None diagnosed at 11–13 weeks: Cystic adenomatoid malformation (4), extralobar sequestration (2), isolated ventricular septal defect (10), cardiac tumors (4).
[d] None diagnosed at 11–13 weeks: Bladder exstrophy (1), duodenal atresia (2), bowel obstruction (1), renal agenesis unilateral (6), renal agenesis bilateral (1), renal agenesis and multicystic (3), hydronephrosis unilateral and bilateral (11), multicystic unilateral and bilateral (17), duplex kidneys (12).
[e] None diagnosed at 11–13 weeks: Arthrogryposis (1), talipes unilateral and bilateral (38), ectrodactyly (1).

Modified from Syngelaki A, Chelemen T, Dagklis T, et al. Challenges in the diagnosis of fetal non-chromosomal abnormalities at 11–13 weeks. *Prenat Diagn.* 2011;31:90–102; copyright John Wiley & Sons, Ltd., with permission.

In our experience, there are four main pathways that result in the prenatal diagnosis of fetal malformations in the first trimester:

1. **Major Malformation, Clearly Visible:** The malformation is easily recognized during a routine first trimester ultrasound or an ultrasound performed for NT measurement, even with limited skills of the examiner.[1,13] **Table 5.1** summarizes some of the major anomalies that are clearly visible in the first trimester.

2. **Thickened Nuchal Translucency:** Many fetal malformations have been reported in association with thickened NT in the presence or absence of chromosomal aneuploidy. When a thickened NT is encountered, invasive genetic testing is typically offered along with an ultrasound examination of the fetus. This approach has led to the first trimester diagnosis of complex cardiac, brain, skeletal, gastrointestinal, and genitourinary anomalies as presented in various chapters in this book. On occasions, the associated fetal malformation is not seen in the first trimester but rather detected in the second trimester or even after birth and the relationship with an increased NT is thus assumed. Table 9.3 in Chapter 9 summarizes fetal malformations that are known to be associated with thickened NT.

3. **Pregnancies at High Risk for Fetal Malformations:** When the pregnancy is at high risk for fetal anomaly due to a prior history of an affected child or due to a known inheritance pattern of a specific malformation, a detailed ultrasound in the first trimester can identify the fetal malformation. Examples include a pregnancy with prior spina bifida, an autosomal recessive inheritance pattern identified in a prior pregnancy, or an autosomal dominant inheritance pattern present in one of the parents. The presence of subtle findings in the first trimester ultrasound can be of significance in such cases such as the presence of abnormal intracranial translucency, polydactyly, echogenic kidneys, skeletal abnormalities, and cleft lip and palate, among others. Several of these subtle findings are discussed in detail in various chapters in this book.

4. **Detailed First Trimester Ultrasound in Low-Risk Pregnancies:** The detection of fetal malformations in the first trimester can also be the result of a detailed ultrasound examination that is routinely performed beyond the 11th week of gestation.[11,13,19] With increasing skills and expertise in the detailed first trimester ultrasound, sonographers and sonologists may decide to apply this approach to all first trimester pregnancies beyond the 11th week of gestation for fetal anomaly screening. The detailed first trimester ultrasound will thus be an adjunct to the second trimester ultrasound examination. It is important to note however that several limitations currently exist to the detailed first trimester ultrasound examination and it is thus important to list these limitations before its introduction.

# LIMITATIONS OF THE DETAILED FIRST TRIMESTER ULTRASOUND

## Maternal Aspects

One of the main limitations of the detailed first trimester ultrasound examination is related to the accessibility of the relatively small gestational sac by ultrasound when maternal body habitus is increased, in the presence of prior abdominal surgery with scarring, and/or in the presence of large leiomyomas with posterior shadowing. In such conditions, the use of the transvaginal approach or a repeat ultrasound examination at 16 weeks of gestation either with a transabdominal high-resolution linear probe or with the transvaginal approach, if feasible, may provide sufficient access to assess fetal anatomy in detail. Occasionally, however, transient maternal contractions may trap the fetus in one area of the uterus and limit ultrasound accessibility. In our experience, rescanning the patient 15 to 30 minutes later provides for a better access, because in most cases the uterine contractions will have resolved (Fig. 5.1).

## Indirect Signs of Fetal Malformations

Another limitation of the detailed first trimester ultrasound examination is the absence of classic, indirect signs of fetal malformations that are commonly seen in the second trimester.

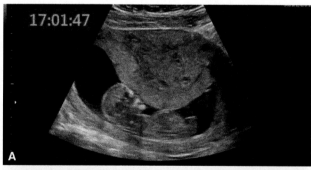

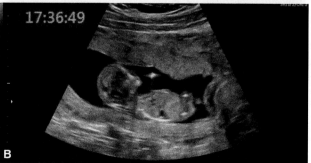

**Figure 5.1: A:** A transabdominal ultrasound examination in the first trimester showing a mid-uterine contraction, which is trapping the fetus in the midsection of the cavity. We were not able to complete the ultrasound examination despite an attempt by the transvaginal approach. The ultrasound examination was repeated 35 minutes later **(B)**, which showed resolution of the contraction, optimization of imaging, and the fetus moving freely within the uterine cavity.

For instance, unlike in the second trimester, bilateral renal agenesis is commonly associated with normal amniotic fluid volume in early gestation and open spina bifida does not typically display a lemon or banana sign in the first trimester as is very often seen in the second trimester of pregnancy. Other examples include the absence of hyperechogenicity or cystic changes in lung lesions in the first trimester and the lack of reliance on the abnormal cavum septi pellucidi in several central nervous system (CNS) lesions as commonly used in the second trimester ultrasound. Furthermore, fetal biometric changes and growth restriction that are commonly associated with fetal malformations do not manifest in early gestation and cannot be used as clues to the presence of associated malformations. It is important to note for all these reasons and others that the detailed first trimester ultrasound examination for fetal anatomy survey does not replace the traditional second trimester ultrasound but rather is complementary to it, especially in a high-risk pregnancy. Pregnant women should be informed of these limitations.

## Time in Gestation of Development of Certain Malformations

It is important to note that a major limitation of the detailed first trimester ultrasound examination for fetal anatomy survey is that some ultrasound findings that are seen in early gestation may disappear upon follow-up into the second trimester of pregnancy. Examples include some cases of thickened NT, tricuspid regurgitation, cardiac ventricular disproportion, early fetal hydrops, and intraabdominal cystic lesions among others. On the other hand, some malformations that are traditionally visible in the second trimester, such as cystic lesions of lungs and kidneys, cardiac valvular stenosis, cortical brain abnormalities, cerebellar vermis dysgenesis, agenesis of corpus callosum, gastrointestinal atresias, and others are commonly associated with normal ultrasound findings in early gestation. It is therefore important for the sonographers and sonologists to be familiar with the natural course of congenital malformations and counsel patients regarding limitations of the first trimester ultrasound examination in that regard.

## Safety Aspects

The detailed first trimester ultrasound examination is performed during a period of development and rapid growth of fetal organs. It is thus critical to minimize ultrasound exposure to the fetus, especially the use of pulsed Doppler, given its associated high energy. As discussed in detail in Chapter 2, the ALARA (as low as reasonably achievable) principle should always be followed and the operator should ensure that the thermal and mechanical indices levels always comply with safe practices. The risk of fetal exposure to ultrasound energy should always be balanced against the benefit of the ultrasound examination in early gestation. Refer to Chapter 2 of this book for a comprehensive discussion on ultrasound bioeffects and safety.

# THE DETAILED FIRST TRIMESTER ULTRASOUND

In this section, we define our approach to the detailed first trimester ultrasound for fetal anatomy survey and describe the components of this ultrasound examination. As stated in the Introduction section of this chapter, the detailed first trimester ultrasound is performed at 11 to 14 weeks of gestation. Components of the detailed first trimester ultrasound examination include general overview and fetal biometry, comprehensive evaluation of fetal anatomy, and an assessment of the uterus and adnexal regions. This detailed first trimester ultrasound examination is not intended to replace the traditional second trimester ultrasound but rather to complement it, and in the majority of pregnancies to provide early reassurance of normalcy. The three components of the detailed first trimester ultrasound are described in the following sections of this chapter.

## General Overview and Fetal Biometry

Initial aspects of the first trimester ultrasound include the confirmation of the location of the gestational sac within the endometrial cavity, the presence of cardiac activity, and the number of fetuses. This can be easily accomplished by the abdominal ultrasound, but on occasions may require the transvaginal approach. The position of the placenta in relation to the internal cervical os (Fig. 5.2) should be noted, keeping in mind that most placenta previas that are diagnosed in early gestation are of no clinical significance and will resolve upon follow-up ultrasound examination in the third trimester of pregnancy (see Chapter 15). In pregnancies with prior cesarean sections,

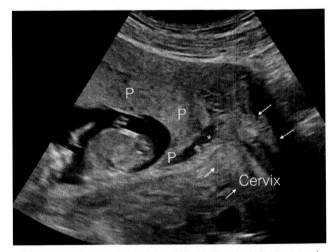

**Figure 5.2:** The position of the placenta (P) should be assessed in relation to the cervix (*arrows*) in the first trimester of pregnancy. This is often performed by the transabdominal ultrasound. Note that the placenta (P) is a previa in this pregnancy as it is shown to cover the internal cervical os (*asterisk*). The presence of placenta previa in the first trimester is of little clinical significance and should be followed up in the second trimester of pregnancy.

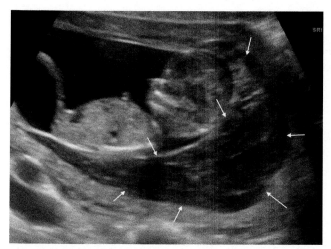

**Figure 5.3:** Subchorionic hematoma (*arrows*) in a pregnancy at 12 weeks of gestation in a patient presenting with vaginal bleeding. See text for details.

Biometric measurements for pregnancy dating are an integral part of the first trimester ultrasound and include the measurement of the crown-rump length, the biparietal diameter, head circumference, abdominal circumference (AC), and femur length (FL) (Fig. 5.4). Any significant discrepancy in biometric measurements should alert for the possible presence of anatomic abnormalities or genetic malformations. First trimester fetal biometry and pregnancy dating are discussed in detail in Chapter 4. Table 5.3 lists the components of the general overview and fetal biometry of the detailed first trimester ultrasound.

## Comprehensive Assessment of Fetal Anatomy

The comprehensive assessment of fetal anatomy is an important component of the detailed first trimester ultrasound. This approach to fetal anatomy in early gestation involves multiple sagittal, axial, and coronal planes of the fetus. Acquiring the technical skills required for the display of the corresponding anatomic planes and an in-depth knowledge of the current literature on this subject are prerequisites for the performance of the detailed first trimester ultrasound examination. In this section, we present our systematic approach to the assessment of fetal anatomy in the detailed first trimester ultrasound examination.

### General Anatomic Assessment

The initial step of the fetal anatomy survey in the first trimester involves obtaining an anterior midsagittal plane of the fetus when technically feasible. This midsagittal plane allows for

the scar is ideally assessed by transvaginal ultrasound.[20] In these pregnancies the location of the gestational sac within the endometrial cavity should be noted and implantations in the lower uterine segment should raise suspicion for increased risk for placenta accreta[21,22] (see Chapter 15). Furthermore, implantation of the gestational sac in the cesarean scar (cesarean scar implantation) is of significant importance given its association with placenta accreta and serious pregnancy complications.[22,23] In the presence of twins or higher order multiple pregnancy, determining the chorionicity and amnionicity in the first trimester is of paramount importance. The presence and size of any significant subchorionic bleed (Fig. 5.3) should also be reported.

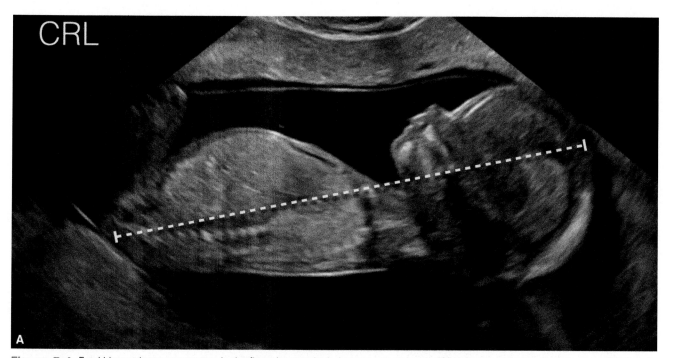

**Figure 5.4:** Fetal biometric measurements in the first trimester include crown-rump length (CRL) shown in **A**, biparietal diameter (BPD) and head circumference (HC) shown in **B**, abdominal circumference (AC) shown in **C**, and femur length (FL) shown in **D**.

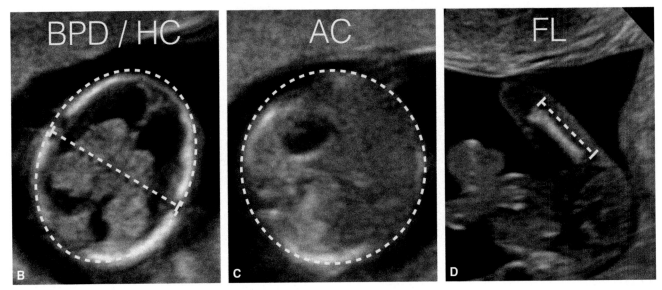

**Figure 5.4:** (continued)

**Table 5.3 •** General Overview and Fetal Biometry of the Detailed First Trimester Ultrasound

Location of gestational sac
Cardiac activity
Number of fetuses
Placental location in relation to cervix
Presence of subchorionic bleed
Fetal biometry

a general anatomic assessment, given that the whole fetus is commonly included in this plane (Fig. 5.5). This midsagittal plane displays several important anatomic landmarks, which are listed in Table 5.4. In this midsagittal plane, the size and proportions of the fetal head, chest, and body are subjectively assessed and the following anatomic regions are recognized: fetal facial profile and midline intracranial structures, the anterior abdominal wall, the fetal stomach, and bladder. By slightly tilting the transducer from the midline to the left and right parasagittal planes, the arms and legs can be visualized. Many of the severe fetal malformations that can be detected in the first trimester (Table 5.1) will show abnormalities in the midsagittal

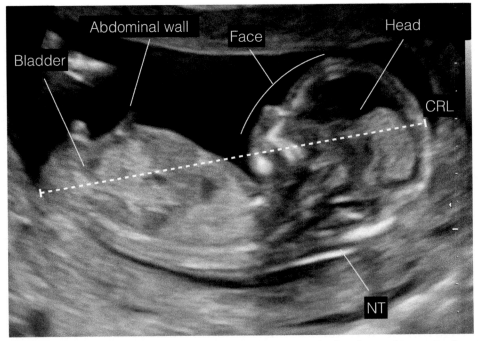

**Figure 5.5:** Midsagittal plane of the fetus in dorsoposterior position allows for an evaluation of several key anatomic regions such as the head, face, nuchal translucency (NT), abdominal wall, and bladder. See Table 5.4 and text for more details. CRL, crown-rump length.

**Table 5.4 •** Midsagittal Plane of the Fetus

| Anatomic Region | What to Look for |
|---|---|
| Head and facial profile | Forehead to chin with normal physiologic bossing of forehead. Normal nose, mouth, and intracerebral structures |
| Head and body | Normal proportion of head to body with head slightly more prominent. CRL within the normal range |
| Thorax | Heart activity confirmed. Normal lungs and diaphragm |
| Abdomen and pelvis | Normal cord insertion, slightly large abdomen, normal stomach and bladder, absence of abnormal cystic structures and echogenic abnormal lesions |

CRL, crown-rump length.

plane and an in-depth evaluation of fetal anatomic regions, as described in the following sections, will help to confirm the presence or absence of other fetal abnormalities. When clinically indicated, color and pulsed Doppler interrogation of the ductus venosus is also best assessed in this midsagittal plane.

### The Fetal Head and Neck

Evaluation of the anatomy of the fetal head and neck in the first trimester requires imaging from the midsagittal, axial, and coronal planes.

### Midsagittal Plane

The magnified midsagittal plane of the head and neck enables the assessment of many anatomic regions to include NT, facial profile with nasal bone and posterior fossa. Normal anatomic features of the midsagittal plane of the head and neck are shown in Figure 5.6.

- **Nuchal Translucency:** The quantitative assessment of the NT in the midsagittal plane of the head and neck is

important, as a thickened NT is associated with a large number of fetal anatomic and genetic abnormalities. The actual measurement of a thickened NT is also important as the thickness correlates with pregnancy outcome (see Chapter 9).

- **Facial Profile:** The facial profile is assessed in its entirety to include the forehead, nasal bridge, nasal bone, maxilla, and mandible (Fig. 5.6). Table 5.5 is a checklist of the anatomic evaluation of the magnified midsagittal plane of the fetal face in the first trimester. Abnormalities that can be detected in this plane include anencephaly, holoprosencephaly, anterior cephalocele, proboscis, absent nasal bone, maxillary gap or protrusion (associated with cleft palate), epignathus, retrognathia, and others. Abnormalities that can be detected in the midsagittal plane of the facial profile are described and illustrated in Chapter 9.

- **Posterior Fossa:** In the midsagittal plane, the anatomy of the posterior fossa can be thoroughly examined (Fig. 5.6) and include the following landmarks: hypoechoic brainstem with echogenic posterior border, anechoic fourth ventricle,

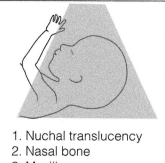

1. Nuchal translucency
2. Nasal bone
3. Maxilla
4. Mandible
5. Thalamus
6. Brain stem
7. Fourth ventricle (IT)
8. Choroid plexus
9. Cisterna magna

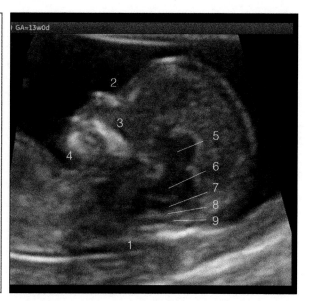

**Figure 5.6:** Midsagittal plane of the fetal head showing a checklist for the anatomic regions for a comprehensive assessment of the face and brain. See Tables 5.5 and 5.6 and text for more details. IT, intracranial translucency.

**Table 5.5 • Midsagittal and Coronal Planes of the Fetal Face**

| Anatomic Region | What to Look for |
| --- | --- |
| Forehead | Normal shape: not too flat, no excessive bossing. No structure protruding |
| Nasal region | Nose present and nasal bone ossified |
| Maxilla | No maxillary gap, no protrusion |
| Mouth | Upper and lower lips appear normal |
| Mandible | Normal appearance, no retrognathia |
| Both eyes | In coronal plane, eyes seen with the nose between |
| Retronasal triangle | In coronal plane, no cleft and normal mandibular gap |

described as intracranial translucency, posterior echogenic choroid plexus of the fourth ventricle, and the anechoic cisterna magna, posterior to the fourth ventricle and anterior to the echogenic occipital bone. **Table 5.6** is a checklist of the anatomic evaluation of the midsagittal plane of the posterior fossa in the first trimester. Abnormalities that can be detected in this plane include open spina bifida with thickened brainstem and reduced fluid, increased fluid in the fourth ventricle seen in aneuploidies, Blakes' pouch cyst, Dandy–Walker malformation, posterior cephaloceles, and other conditions. Abnormalities that can be detected by the midsagittal plane of the posterior fossa are presented and illustrated in Chapter 8.

## Axial Planes

From the midsagittal plane, the transducer is rotated 90 degrees to get the axial planes of the fetal head, ideally imaged from the

**Table 5.6 • Magnified Midsagittal Plane of the Fetal Brain**

| Anatomic Region | What to Look for |
| --- | --- |
| Thalamus | Visualized as midline structure |
| Brainstem | Visualized with posterior echogenic border, normal shape, not thickened, not kinked, and not thin |
| Intracranial translucency (Fourth ventricle) | Typical fluid space and echogenic lines, choroid plexus of fourth ventricle and cisterna magna visualized |
| Occipital bone | Visualized and intact |

lateral aspects. Similar to the approach in the second trimester, four axial planes of the fetal head in the first trimester allow for a comprehensive evaluation of CNS anatomy. These planes include the axial plane at the level of the lateral ventricles, the axial plane at the level of the thalami, the axial-oblique plane at the level of the cerebellum and posterior fossa, and the axial plane at the level of the orbits. Normal anatomic features of these four axial planes of the fetal head are shown in **Figures 5.7, 5.8, and 5.9**. **Table 5.7** is a checklist of the anatomic evaluation of the axial planes of the fetal head in the first trimester.

The assessment of the normal oval head shape, the continuity of the head contour, the variable ossification of cranial bones, and the presence of a falx cerebri dividing the hemispheres into two equal portions can be seen in the first three axial planes (**Figs. 5.7 and 5.8**). The axial plane at the level of the lateral ventricles (**Fig. 5.7**, plane 1) shows two large hyperechoic choroid plexuses that fill significant portions of the lateral ventricles with a thin peripheral cortex. The choroid plexuses are often asymmetrical and touch the lateral and medial borders of the ventricles and their area is between 50% and 75% of the areas of the ventricles (**Fig. 5.7**, plane 1). The plane at the level of the thalami (**Fig. 5.7**, plane 2) is used to demonstrate the presence of two separated thalami and posterior to them the cerebral peduncles with the cerebral

**Table 5.7 • Axial Planes (1 to 4) of the Fetal Head in the First Trimester**

| Anatomic Region | What to Look for |
| --- | --- |
| Head (planes 1–3) | Oval shape, normal contour, and ossification |
| Biparietal diameter/ head circumference (plane 2) | Values within the normal range |
| Falx cerebri (planes 1–3) | Visualized, separating two hemispheres |
| Choroid plexuses of lateral ventricles (plane 1) | Two echogenic separated plexuses visualized often of unequal size and filling more than half of the lateral ventricles |
| Thalami (planes 2 and 3) | Two separated thalami visualized, with third ventricle in between |
| Cerebral peduncles (plane 2) | Visualized with aqueduct of Sylvius in between. The aqueduct is not stuck to the occipital bone |
| Fourth ventricle (plane 3) | Visualized with choroid plexus of fourth ventricle, hourglass shape |
| Eyes (plane 4) | In anterior axial planes, two orbits with eyes are visualized with the nose arising between |

Some details are better seen on transvaginal ultrasound.

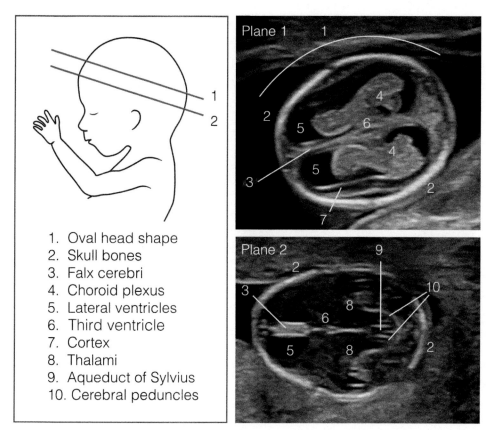

1. Oval head shape
2. Skull bones
3. Falx cerebri
4. Choroid plexus
5. Lateral ventricles
6. Third ventricle
7. Cortex
8. Thalami
9. Aqueduct of Sylvius
10. Cerebral peduncles

**Figure 5.7:** Planes 1 and 2 of four axial planes for the anatomic assessment of the head: Plane 1 corresponds to the transventricular plane and plane 2 corresponds to the transthalamic plane. See Table 5.7 and text for more details. Planes 1 and 2 are obtained from fetuses at 13 weeks of gestation and examined by the transabdominal linear probe. See Figures 5.8 and 5.9 for planes 3 and 4, respectively.

aqueduct. The axial-oblique plane at the level of the posterior fossa (Fig. 5.8) can be used to visualize the developing cerebellum and is best shown in transvaginal ultrasound. In this plane, the hourglass shape of the fourth ventricle and its choroid plexus is best visualized along with the developing cisterna magna (Fig. 5.8). The fourth plane at the level of the orbits (Fig. 5.9) demonstrates both eyes with the nose arising between them. Abnormalities that can be detected by

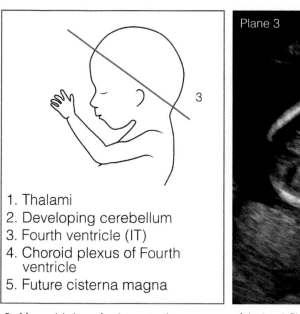

1. Thalami
2. Developing cerebellum
3. Fourth ventricle (IT)
4. Choroid plexus of Fourth ventricle
5. Future cisterna magna

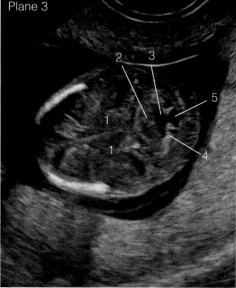

**Figure 5.8:** Plane 3 of four axial planes for the anatomic assessment of the head: Plane 3 is a slightly oblique plane at the level of the posterior fossa, demonstrating the developing cerebellum and fourth ventricle as intracranial translucency (IT). The posterior fossa is easily assessed in the midsagittal view shown in Figure 5.6. Plane 3 is best assessed by the transvaginal route. See Table 5.7 and text for more details.

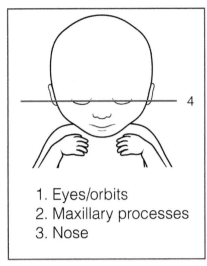
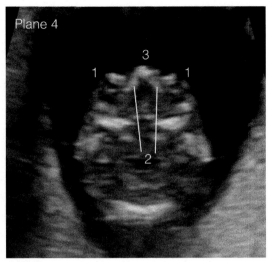

1. Eyes/orbits
2. Maxillary processes
3. Nose

**Figure 5.9:** Plane 4 of four axial planes for the anatomic assessment of the head: Plane 4 is an axial plane obtained at the level of the orbits demonstrating two orbits, the eyes, and the nose in between. See text for more details.

these axial planes of the fetal head include anencephaly, holoprosencephaly, ventriculomegaly, encephalocele, open spina bifida, and some severe eyes and face anomalies as described and illustrated in Chapters 8 and 9.

### Coronal Plane

In an oblique coronal plane of the face, the eyes, orbits, and the retronasal triangle consisting of the nasal bones, the maxillary processes, and the anterior maxilla with the alveolar ridge can be recognized (Fig. 5.10) (Table 5.5). The mandibular gap is also seen in this plane (Fig. 5.10). The coronal plane of the face is helpful in the detection of severe anomalies of the eyes, large facial clefts, and retrognathia/micrognathia. A more comprehensive discussion of the normal and abnormal facial anatomy is presented in Chapter 9.

### The Fetal Chest and Heart

The detailed first trimester ultrasound examination of the fetal chest is best performed by two axial planes and one coronal plane. The two axial planes are most informative when the

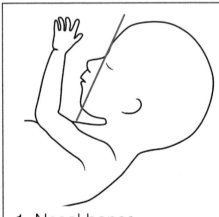
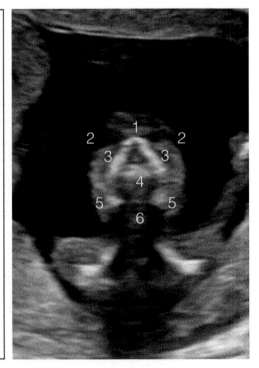

1. Nasal bones
2. Orbits/eyes
3. Maxillary processes
4. Maxilla-alveolar ridge
5. Mandible
6. Mandibular gap

**Figure 5.10:** The comprehensive assessment of facial anatomy involves imaging the face from two planes: the midsagittal plane as shown in Figure 5.6 and the coronal plane shown here. This coronal plane demonstrates both eyes and the retronasal triangle. See text for more details.

**Table 5.8 • Axial Planes (1 and 2) of the Fetal Chest in the First Trimester**

| Anatomic Region | What to Look for |
| --- | --- |
| Lungs (plane 1) | Both lungs visualized with no pleural effusion |
| Ribs (plane 1) | Ribs visualized, normal shape and length, no irregularity |
| Cardiac axis (plane 1) | Left cardiac axis around 45 degrees +/− 15-20 degrees |
| Four-chamber view (plane 1) | Two almost equal ventricles, two atrioventricular valves, no pericardial effusion, antegrade filling of two distinct ventricles on color Doppler, no valve regurgitation |
| Three-vessel trachea view (plane 2) | V-shaped aorta and pulmonary artery on color Doppler with antegrade flow, and course to the left of trachea |

fetus is in a dorsoposterior position in the uterus and the coronal plane is primarily for the assessment of the diaphragm.

## Axial Planes

The two axial planes for the anatomic assessment of the chest and heart include the plane at the level of the four-chamber view (4CV) and the plane at the level of the three-vessel trachea view (3VT). Normal anatomic features of the 4CV and 3VT view are shown in Figures 5.11 and 5.12 and in Table 5.8.

In the 4CV plane, ribs, lungs, and cardiac position in the chest are assessed, with the cardiac axis pointing to the left (Fig. 5.11, plane 1). Color Doppler helps to confirm the presence of two distinct ventricles with separate filling in diastole and the absence of significant atrioventricular valve regurgitation (Fig. 5.11). When indicated, pulsed Doppler can assess for the presence or absence of tricuspid valve regurgitation. Color Doppler at the 4CV also helps in the accurate measurement of the cardiac axis (Fig. 5.11) when an abnormal cardiac axis is suspected. An abnormal cardiac axis or abnormal cardiac position in the chest is associated with cardiac malformations[24] or a diaphragmatic hernia. Abnormalities that can be detected in this plane include hypoplastic left or right ventricle, single ventricle, ventricular disproportion, large septal defects, arrhythmias, pericardial effusion, diaphragmatic hernia, and others.

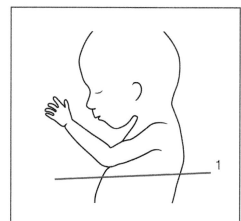

1. Lungs
2. Ribs
3. Thoracic aorta
4. Right ventricle
5. Left ventricle
6. Cardiac axis
7. Diastolic ventricular filling

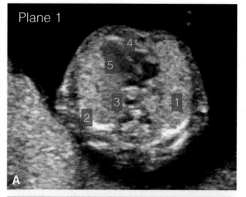

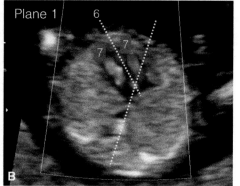

**Figure 5.11:** The fetal chest is assessed in two planes: axial plane at the level of the four-chamber view and axial plane at the level of the three-vessel trachea view. This figure shows plane 1, at the level of the four-chamber view. This plane is for the anatomic assessment of the heart, lungs, and the rib cage. Plane 1 is best assessed in gray scale **(A)** and color Doppler **(B)** as shown here. Cardiac axis can also be measured in this plane and adding color Doppler facilitates its measurement **(B)**. See Table 5.8 and text for more details.

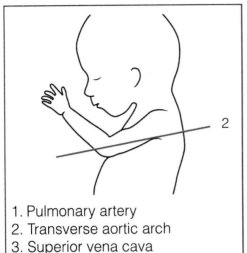

1. Pulmonary artery
2. Transverse aortic arch
3. Superior vena cava
4. Trachea
5. Systolic flow in great vessels

Plane 2

**Figure 5.12:** The fetal chest is assessed in two planes: axial plane at the level of the four-chamber view (plane 1, shown in Fig. 5.11) and axial plane at the level of the three-vessel trachea view (plane 2) shown here. Plane 2 is best obtained in color Doppler showing the pulmonary artery, the aorta, the superior vena cava, and the trachea. This plane allows for the detection of complex cardiac anomalies in the first trimester. See Table 5.8, text, and Chapter 11 for more details.

Given the technical difficulty involved in obtaining the left and right outflow tract views in the first trimester, we recommend examination of the great vessels in the 3VT view in color Doppler (Fig. 5.12, plane 2). In the 3VT view, the size of great vessels, anatomic relationships, and directions of blood flow can be assessed, and the continuity of the ductal and aortic arches demonstrated (Fig. 5.12, plane 2). The V-shape of the great vessels with a course left to the echogenic trachea can be recognized (Fig. 5.12, plane 2). If needed, this plane can also be used to demonstrate the normal or aberrant course of the right subclavian artery by applying color Doppler at low velocity scale. Abnormalities that can be detected in the 3VT plane include most conotruncal anomalies, severe right and left ventricular outflow tract obstructions, right or double aortic arches, and others. A more comprehensive discussion of the normal and abnormal cardiac anatomy is presented in Chapter 11.

### Coronal Plane

If a diaphragmatic hernia is suspected in the axial plane or has to be ruled out, the lungs and diaphragm are better imaged in a coronal plane slightly anterior to the spine and ribs (Fig. 5.13). In this plane, the relationship of the stomach, diaphragm, and lungs can be easily evaluated. A more comprehensive discussion of the normal and abnormal chest anatomy is presented in Chapter 10.

### *The Fetal Abdomen and Pelvis*

Ultrasound evaluation of the fetal abdomen and pelvis in the first trimester is performed by three axial planes and one coronal plane. The three axial planes are most informative when the fetus is in a dorsoposterior position in the uterus.

### Axial Planes

The three axial planes are in almost parallel orientation and include the axial plane in the upper abdomen, the axial plane in the mid-abdomen, and the axial plane in the pelvis. Normal anatomic features of the three axial planes in the abdomen and pelvis are shown in Figure 5.14 and in Table 5.9. The upper abdomen plane corresponds to the AC plane and demonstrates the stomach on the left side and the liver filling the right abdomen (Fig. 5.14, plane 1). The liver is slightly less echogenic than the lungs in early gestation. With high

**Table 5.9 •** Axial Planes (1 to 3) of the Fetal Abdomen and Pelvis in the First Trimester

| Anatomic Region | What to Look for |
| --- | --- |
| Upper abdomen (plane 1) | Left-sided filled stomach and right-sided liver |
|  | Descending aorta and inferior vena cava. Umbilical vein with ductus venosus. |
| Middle abdomen (plane 2) | Normal cord insertion, intact anterior abdominal wall, and no fluid in abdomen |
| Lower abdomen and pelvis (plane 3) | Bladder filled, with length <7 mm. Two umbilical arteries in color Doppler bordering the bladder |

Some details are better seen on transvaginal ultrasound and on color Doppler.

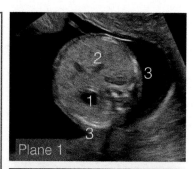

Figure 5.13: Coronal plane of the fetal chest and abdomen for the assessment of the diaphragm when there is a suspicion of diaphragmatic hernia. This plane shows both lungs at the same level and the stomach and liver in abdomen. See text and Chapter 11 for more details.

1. Lungs at same level
2. Stomach in abdomen
3. Ribs

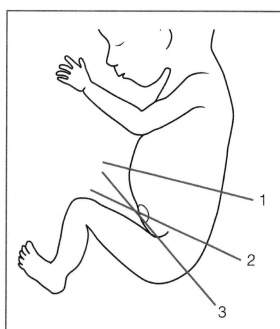

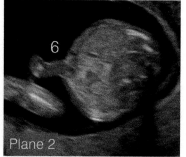

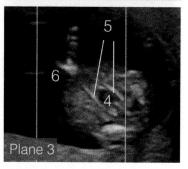

Figure 5.14: Three axial planes (planes 1–3) for the anatomic evaluation of the fetal abdomen. Plane 1 is at the level of the stomach and demonstrates the normal position of the stomach and liver. Plane 2 is at the level of the cord insertion in the abdomen and demonstrates an intact anterior abdominal wall and plane 3 is in color Doppler at the level of the bladder confirming its presence along with the presence of two umbilical arteries. See Table 5.9 and text for more details.

1. Stomach left-sided and filled
2. Liver
3. Ribs
4. Bladder, filled
5. Umbilical arteries
6. Abdominal wall

resolution, the normal course of the umbilical vein and ductus venosus, along with the inferior vena cava (IVC), can be demonstrated. The location of the IVC in the right anterior abdomen is seen compared to the posterior location of the descending aorta to the left of the spine.

The second plane, the mid-abdomen plane, is obtained at the level of the cord insertion into the abdomen in order to confirm integrity of the anterior abdominal wall (Fig. 5.14, plane 2). In this view, the bowels fill the abdomen and are slightly more echogenic than the liver (Fig. 5.14, plane 2). It is important to note the absence of any abnormal hyperechoic or anechoic structures in the abdomen and pelvis as this may suggest the presence of fetal malformations. The kidneys can be occasionally seen in the posterior abdomen due to their increased echogenicity and due to the anechoic renal pelvis. It is often difficult however to see the kidneys in the first trimester on the transabdominal axial plane. Demonstration of the fetal kidneys is best performed in the coronal plane as discussed later in this section.

The third plane is obtained in the pelvis and demonstrates a normally filled urinary bladder (Fig. 5.14, plane 3). The length of the filled bladder (obtained in sagittal length) should be less than 7 mm. Color Doppler is added to this plane to demonstrate the two umbilical arteries surrounding the bladder (Fig. 5.14, plane 3) and this is performed for three purposes: (1) to confirm that the anechoic structure is the bladder, especially if the bladder is mildly filled; (2) to confirm with color Doppler the closed anterior abdominal wall; and (3) to rule out a single umbilical artery, which can be associated with other fetal malformations.

## Coronal Plane

A coronal oblique plane of the mid-abdomen and pelvis is obtained to demonstrate the right and left kidneys. This is achieved by turning the transducer 90 degrees from the axial plane at the level of the mid-abdomen and sliding obliquely to display both kidneys in the same view (Fig. 5.15). Color Doppler may be added to demonstrate both renal arteries, thus confirming the presence of both kidneys. This step is not necessary however, especially when the kidneys are easily demonstrated on gray scale ultrasound.

Abnormalities that can be detected by the axial and coronal planes of the fetal abdomen and pelvis include abdominal wall defects, abnormal situs, urogenital anomalies with or without megacystis, intraabdominal cystic structures, bowel dilation, single umbilical artery, and others. A more comprehensive discussion of the normal and abnormal fetal abdomen and pelvis is presented in Chapters 12 and 13.

### The Fetal Skeletal System

Examination of the fetal skeletal system in the first trimester includes the upper and lower extremities and the spine. Given the small size of the fetus and the relatively fixed positions of the extremities in early gestation, we believe that ultrasound evaluation of the fetal extremities in the first trimester is easier to perform than in the second or third trimester of pregnancy when fetal crowding obscures visualization. The fetal spine can also be assessed from various angles and gross abnormalities can be identified.

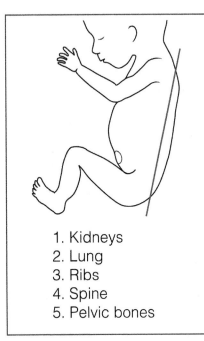

1. Kidneys
2. Lung
3. Ribs
4. Spine
5. Pelvic bones

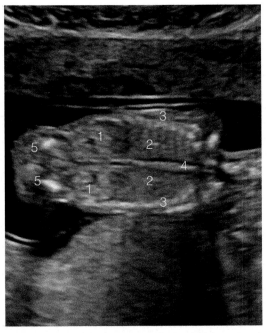

**Figure 5.15:** When the fetal kidneys are not clearly visualized on axial planes, a coronal view at the level of the posterior abdomen allows for the best visualization of the slightly hyperechogenic kidneys.

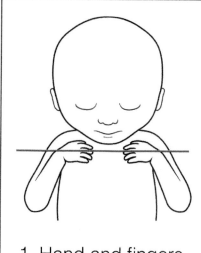
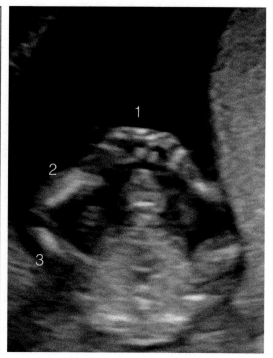

1. Hand and fingers
2. Lower arm
3. Upper arm

Figure 5.16: The upper extremities in the first trimester can be demonstrated in an axial view at the level of the face, thorax, or upper abdomen as shown here. This view shows both arms and hands. Both hands are typically touching in the first trimester. See Table 5.10 and text for more details.

## Axial-Oblique Planes of Fetal Extremities

The approach to the evaluation of the extremities in the first trimester initially involves two axial-oblique planes: an axial-oblique plane at the level of the chest for the upper extremities (Fig. 5.16) and an axial-oblique plane at the level of the pelvis for the lower extremities (Fig. 5.17).

## Left and Right Parasagittal Planes of Fetal Extremities

Following the initial approach with the axial-oblique planes and for more detailed evaluation of the extremities, we recommend tilting the transducer from the midsagittal plane to left and right parasagittal planes to visualize the left and

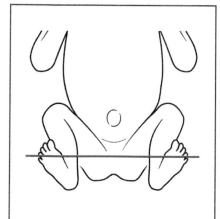
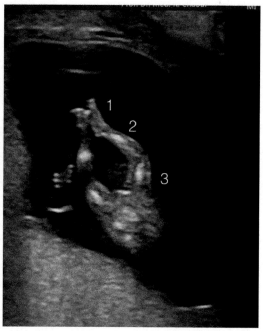

1. Foot
2. Lower leg
3. Upper leg

Figure 5.17: The lower extremities in the first trimester can be demonstrated in an axial view at the level of the pelvis as shown here. This view shows both legs and feet. Both feet are typically touching in the first trimester. See Table 5.10 and text for more details.

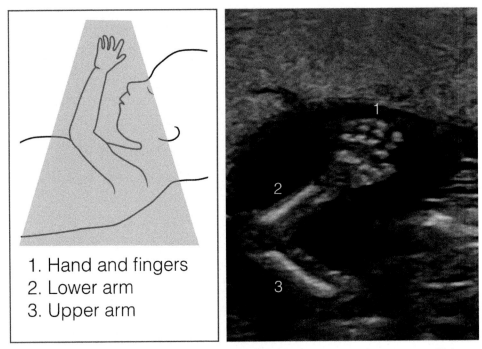

**Figure 5.18:** Parasagittal oblique plane demonstrating the three segments of an upper extremity: upper arm (*3*), lower arm (*2*), and hand with fingers (*1*). The hands with fingers are often better seen in the first trimester than later on in gestation.

right arms and legs respectively (**Figs. 5.18 and 5.19**). In this approach, with image magnification and with the use of high-resolution transducers, evaluation of all segments of the extremities can be performed including upper and lower arms and legs with hands and feet. When technically feasible we attempt to demonstrate a frontal view of the hands and feet to visualize the fingers and toes (**Figs. 5.20 and 5.21**). In our experience, gross anomalies of the limbs, such as transverse limb defects and other severe deformities, can be detected in the detailed first trimester ultrasound. The presence of other subtle abnormalities like polydactyly or clubfeet may escape detection in early gestation. **Table 5.10** is a checklist of the

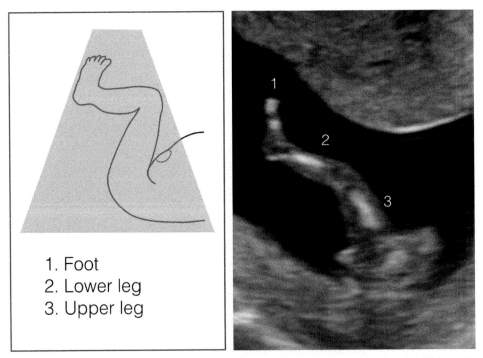

**Figure 5.19:** Parasagittal oblique plane demonstrating the three segments of a lower extremity: upper leg (*3*), lower leg (*2*), and foot with toes (*1*). The feet with toes are often better seen in the first trimester than later on in gestation.

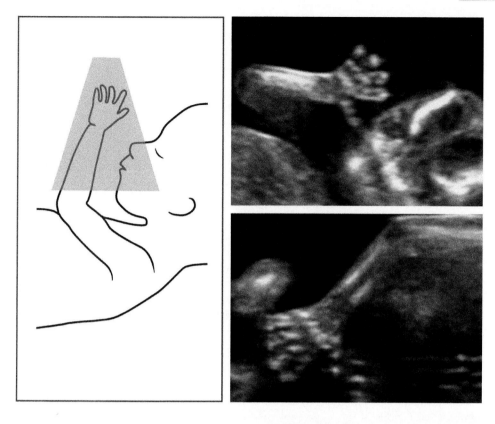

Figure 5.20: Once the upper extremity is demonstrated in the parasagittal oblique plane (Fig. 5.18), the transducer is slightly rotated and the image magnified to display the hand and fingers as shown here. This approach allows for the anatomic assessment of the lower arm, hand, and fingers.

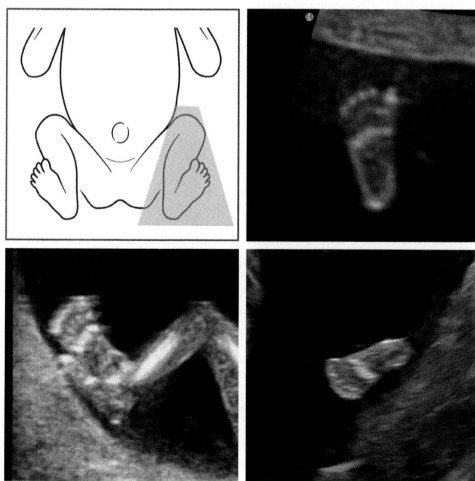

Figure 5.21: Once the lower extremity is demonstrated in the parasagittal oblique plane (Fig. 5.19), the transducer is slightly rotated and the image magnified to display the foot and toes as shown here. This approach allows for the anatomic assessment of the lower leg, foot, and toes.

**Table 5.10 •** Axial-Oblique and Parasagittal planes of the Fetal Extremities in the First Trimester

| Anatomic Region | What to Look for |
| --- | --- |
| Upper limbs | Three segments: Humerus, radius, ulna, and hand visualized on both sides |
| Lower limbs | Three segments: Femur, tibia, fibula, and foot visualized on both sides |

anatomic evaluation of the axial-oblique and parasagittal planes of the fetal extremities in the first trimester. A more comprehensive discussion of normal and abnormal extremities is presented in Chapter 14 on the skeletal system.

## Midsagittal, Coronal, and Axial Planes of the Spine

The spine is ideally examined by ultrasound in the first trimester in a midsagittal and coronal plane, preferably with the fetus in the dorsoanterior position. Where possible we also attempt to obtain the axial views at the cervical, thoracic, and lumbosacral regions of the spine (Fig. 14.14), but in our experience, these axial planes are less informative in the first trimester. The midsagittal view demonstrates the spine in its entirety (Fig. 5.22) and the coronal view is helpful for the demonstration of spinal deformities (Fig. 5.23). Table 5.11 is a checklist of the anatomic evaluation of the sagittal and coronal planes of the fetal spine in the first trimester. Interruption of the spine, such as in sacral agenesis, is recognized in the midsagittal view, by the short size of the body of the fetus in comparison with the size of the head. Major spinal defects, such as body stalk anomaly, are easily recognized in early gestation. More subtle defects like hemivertebrae, spina bifida, or early sacrococcygeal teratoma are often difficult to detect when isolated. While open spina bifida can be suspected if the posterior brain structures appears abnormal and confirmed by the targeted visualization of the spine with high-resolution transvaginal ultrasound, isolated closed spina bifida often escape early detection. For more details, refer to Chapter 8 on CNS and Chapter 14 on spinal anomalies.

## Three-Dimensional Ultrasound

We encourage the use of 3D ultrasound in surface mode for the display of all four extremities in one view (Fig. 5.24A) and if the fetus is in a dorsoposterior position, 3D ultrasound allows for the visualization of the back, in order to demonstrate intact skin and spine (Fig. 5.24B).[25]

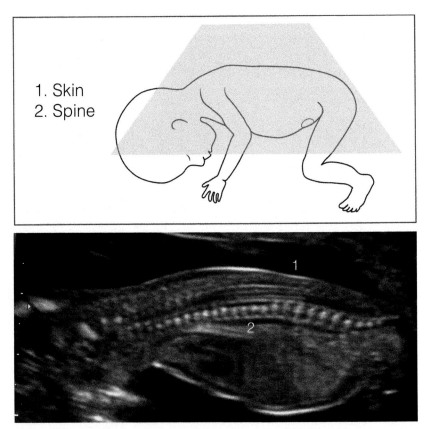

1. Skin
2. Spine

**Figure 5.22:** Midsagittal view of the fetus in a dorsoposterior position demonstrating the fetal spine. Note the beginning of ossification of vertebral bodies and the intact skin covering the back. See Table 5.11 and text for more details.

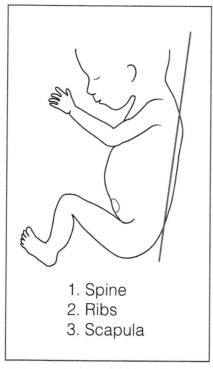
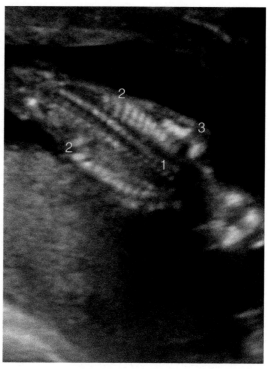

1. Spine
2. Ribs
3. Scapula

**Figure 5.23:** Posterior coronal plane of the fetus demonstrating the spine, scapula, and ribcage. This plane is helpful when spinal deformities are suspected. See Table 5.11 and text for more details.

**Table 5.11 • Midsagittal and Coronal Planes of the Fetal Spine in the First Trimester**

| Anatomic Region | What to Look for |
| --- | --- |
| Spine, vertebral body | Spine completely seen in one view, no interruption, no deformities, vertebral bodies ossified after 12 weeks |
| Ribs, scapulae | Ribs visualized, symmetrical, scapulae visualized |
| Skin over the spine | Intact skin covering the spine, no irregular shape |

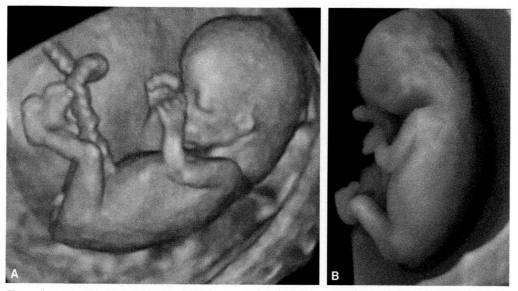

**Figure 5.24:** Three-dimensional (3D) ultrasound in surface mode in two fetuses **(A and B)** in the first trimester. In fetus **A**, the 3D is obtained from the lateral aspect and demonstrates both upper and lower extremities. In fetus **B**, the 3D ultrasound is obtained from the posterior aspect of the fetus and shows an intact back. We encourage the use of 3D ultrasound in the first trimester, which allows for the demonstration of both arms and legs **(A)** and back **(B)**.

**Table 5.12 •** Assessment of Uterus and Adnexa

| Anatomic Region | What to Look for |
|---|---|
| Uterus | Normal shape with absence of Mullerian malformations and leiomyomas |
| Adnexae | Absence of abnormal adnexal masses |
| Uterine arteries | Doppler interrogation of left and right uterine arteries when indicated |

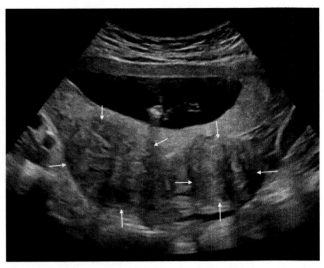

**Figure 5.25:** Two intramural leiomyomas (*arrows*) located within the posterior uterine wall in a pregnancy at 12 weeks of gestation. Location of these leiomyomas will probably have little impact on the pregnancy. Compare with Figure 5.26.

## Assessment of Uterus and Adnexae

Examination of the uterus and adnexal regions is an important part of the detailed first trimester ultrasound (Table 5.12). The presence, size, and location of any leiomyoma should be reported (Figs. 5.25 and 5.26). Follow-up ultrasound examinations closer to term should be considered for leiomyomas in the lower uterine segment in order to assess for obstruction of the birth canal. The presence of a significant amount of peritoneal fluid should also be noted. The adnexal regions should be evaluated for the presence of any abnormal ovarian masses. Often the corpus luteum can still be seen and enlarged multicystic ovaries can be demonstrated in pregnancies of assisted reproduction. Evaluation of the adnexa is commonly performed by the transabdominal approach as the ovaries in the late first trimester are lifted toward the upper pelvis by the enlarging uterus. The presence of any suspected adnexal masses should be evaluated by transvaginal ultrasound if

feasible as this allows for more detailed assessment. Adding color Doppler helps to evaluate the vascularity of adnexal masses. Common adnexal masses in pregnancy include hemorrhagic cysts, endometriomas, dermoid cysts, and pedunculated leiomyomas (Fig. 5.27). It is important to note that endometriomas can be decidualized in pregnancy and this appearance may mimic a cancerous tumor (Fig. 5.28). Follow-up ultrasound examination into the second and third trimesters of pregnancy can help differentiate a decidualized leiomyoma from a malignant tumor. In patients with Mullerian uterine anomalies, such as bicornuate or septate uterus,

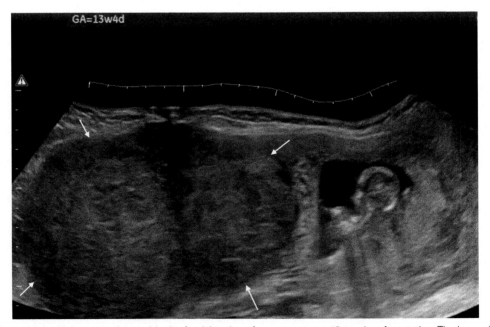

**Figure 5.26:** Large bilobed leiomyoma (*arrows*) in the fundal region of a pregnancy at 13 weeks of gestation. The large size of the leiomyoma reduces the gestational sac. The leiomyoma was too large to be visualized in one image and panorama view was used.

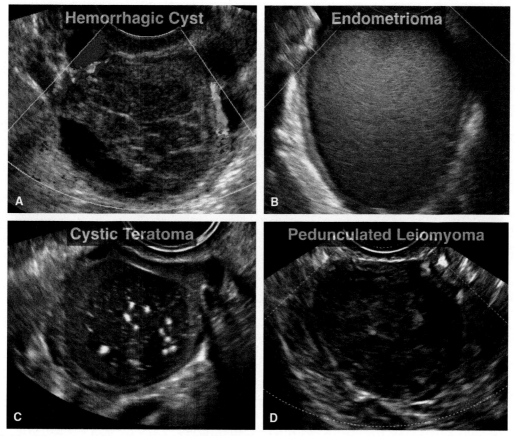

**Figure 5.27:** Adnexal masses commonly seen in the first trimester of pregnancy. Hemorrhagic cyst **(A)** is shown with characteristic reticular pattern and fluid level, endometrioma **(B)** is shown with unilocular ground-glass appearance, cystic teratoma **(C)** with echogenic foci from the fat emulsion, and a pedunculated leiomyoma **(D)** with solid appearance and minimal vascularity on color Doppler. Color Doppler shows no vascular signals within the hemorrhagic cyst and endometrioma.

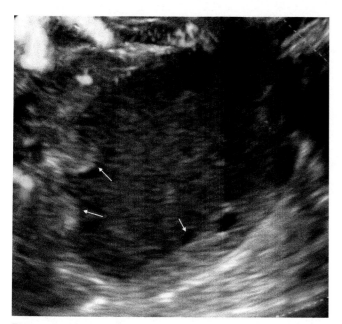

**Figure 5.28:** Decidualized endometrioma shown in a first trimester pregnancy. Note the presence of capsular thickening (*arrows*). Decidualized endometriomas can be mistaken for a malignant tumor with papillary projections.

the localization of the pregnancy and the placenta is easier to demonstrate in the first trimester ultrasound.

## Pregnancy Risk Assessment

Findings from the first trimester ultrasound are currently used in some settings to provide for pregnancy risk assessment in order to predict pregnancy complications such as preeclampsia, fetal growth restriction, and preterm delivery. In general, algorithms combining maternal history, biochemical markers, and first trimester ultrasound parameters are used to generate individualized pregnancy risk assessment, which allows for the identification of high-risk pregnancies and for optimization of pregnancy care. This first trimester risk assessment is incorporated into the concept of "turning the pyramid of pregnancy care,"[26,27] which stratifies pregnancy risk from early gestation and coordinates prenatal care according to risk.

A main component of the first trimester risk assessment includes Doppler of the uterine arteries. The uterine arteries are easily identified in the first trimester on a parasagittal plane of the uterus in color Doppler. The uterine arteries are typically seen to cross over the hypogastric vessels

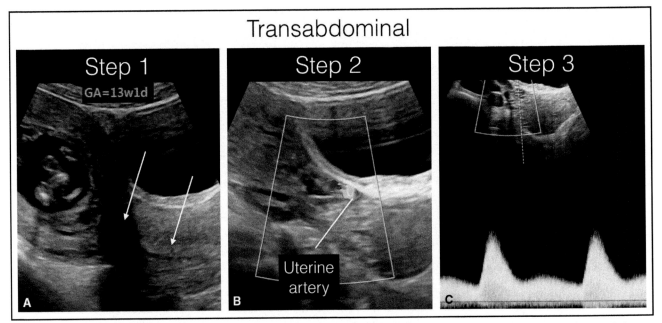

**Figure 5.29:** Steps for obtaining Doppler waveforms of the uterine artery by the transabdominal route. Step 1: Visualize the cervix in a sagittal view on 2D ultrasound (*arrows*). Step 2: Activate color Doppler and tilt the transducer to left or right in a parasagittal plane until visualizing the left or right uterine artery, respectively. The uterine artery is seen crossing over the hypogastric vessels. Step 3: Sample the uterine artery with pulsed Doppler.

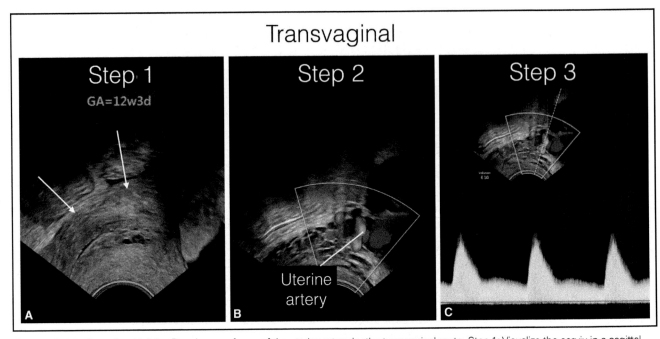

**Figure 5.30:** Steps for obtaining Doppler waveforms of the uterine artery by the transvaginal route. Step 1: Visualize the cervix in a sagittal view on 2D ultrasound (*arrows*). Step 2: Activate color Doppler and tilt the transducer to left or right in a parasagittal plane until visualizing the left or right uterine artery, respectively. The uterine artery is seen crossing over the hypogastric vessels. Step 3: Sample the uterine artery with pulsed Doppler. The image is inverted here from Figure 5.29 as this is the traditional display of gynecologic imaging in some settings.

(Figs. 5.29 and 5.30). The application of uterine artery pulsed Doppler is considered safe in the first trimester, as the Doppler sample volume is applied outside of the gestational sac.[28,29] Figures 5.29 and 5.30 show the steps required for the display of the uterine artery for appropriate Doppler sampling.

Details on the use of uterine artery pulsed Doppler along with other first trimester markers for pregnancy risk assessment are beyond the scope of this book. Interested readers are advised to refer to the literature on this subject, especially that this knowledge is advancing rapidly.

# REFERENCES

1. Syngelaki A, Chelemen T, Dagklis T, et al. Challenges in the diagnosis of fetal non-chromosomal abnormalities at 11-13 weeks. *Prenat Diagn.* 2011;31:90–102.

2. Achiron R, Achiron A. Transvaginal ultrasonic assessment of the early fetal brain. *Ultrasound Obstet Gynecol.* 1991;1:336–344.

3. Achiron R, Tadmor O. Screening for fetal anomalies during the first trimester of pregnancy: transvaginal versus transabdominal sonography. *Ultrasound Obstet Gynecol.* 1991;1:186–191.

4. Blaas HG, Eik-Nes SH, Kiserud T, et al. Early development of the forebrain and midbrain: a longitudinal ultrasound study from 7 to 12 weeks of gestation. *Ultrasound Obstet Gynecol.* 1994;4:183–192.

5. Bronshtein M, Blumenfeld Z. Transvaginal sonography-detection of findings suggestive of fetal chromosomal anomalies in the first and early second trimesters. *Prenat Diagn.* 1992;12:587–593.

6. Bronshtein M, Siegler E, Eshcoli Z, et al. Transvaginal ultrasound measurements of the fetal heart at 11 to 17 weeks of gestation. *Am J Perinatol.* 1992;9:38–42.

7. Gembruch U, Knopfle G, Chatterjee M, et al. First-trimester diagnosis of fetal congenital heart disease by transvaginal two-dimensional and Doppler echocardiography. *Obstet Gynecol.* 1990;75:496–498.

8. Rottem S, Bronshtein M. Transvaginal sonographic diagnosis of congenital anomalies between 9 weeks and 16 weeks, menstrual age. *J Clin Ultrasound* 1990;18:307–314.

9. Becker R, Wegner RD. Detailed screening for fetal anomalies and cardiac defects at the 11–13-week scan. *Ultrasound Obstet Gynecol.* 2006;27:613–618.

10. Abu-Rustum RS, Daou L, Abu-Rustum SE. Role of first-trimester sonography in the diagnosis of aneuploidy and structural fetal anomalies. *J Ultrasound Med.* 2010;29:1445–1452.

11. Iliescu D, Tudorache S, Comănescu A, et al. Improved detection rate of structural abnormalities in the first trimester using an extended examination protocol. *Ultrasound Obstet Gynecol.* 2013;42:300–309.

12. Wiechec M, Knafel A, Nocun A. Prenatal detection of congenital heart defects at the 11- to 13-week scan using a simple color Doppler protocol including the 4-chamber and 3-vessel and trachea views. *J Ultrasound Med.* 2015;34:585–594.

13. Van Mieghem T, Hindryckx A, Van Calsteren K. Early fetal anatomy screening: who, what, when and why? *Curr Opin Obstet Gynecol.* 2015;27:143–150.

14. Karim JN, Roberts NW, Salomon LJ, et al. Systematic review of first trimester ultrasound screening in detecting fetal structural anomalies and factors affecting screening performance. *Ultrasound Obstet Gynecol.* 2016. doi:10.1002/uog.17246.

15. Blaas HG, Eik-Nes SH. Sonoembryology and early prenatal diagnosis of neural anomalies. *Prenat Diagn.* 2009;29:312–325.

16. Grande M, Arigita M, Borobio V, et al. First-trimester detection of structural abnormalities and the role of aneuploidy markers. *Ultrasound Obstet Gynecol.* 2012;39:157–163.

17. Chen F, Gerhardt J, Entezami M, et al. Detection of spina bifida by first trimester screening—results of the prospective multicenter Berlin IT-Study. *Ultraschall Med.* 2017;38:151–157.

18. Colosi E, Musone R, Filardi G, et al. First trimester fetal anatomy study and identification of major anomalies using 10 standardized scans. *J Prenat Med.* 2015;9:24–28.

19. Kaisenberg von CS, Kuhling-von Kaisenberg H, Fritzer E, et al. Fetal transabdominal anatomy scanning using standard views at 11 to 14 weeks' gestation. *Am J Obstet Gynecol.* 2005;192:535–542.

20. Stirnemann JJ, Chalouhi GE, Forner S, et al. First-trimester uterine scar assessment by transvaginal ultrasound. *Am J Obstet Gynecol.* 2011;205:551. e1–551.e6.

21. Comstock CH, Lee W, Vettraino IM, et al. The early sonographic appearance of placenta accreta. *J Ultrasound Med.* 2003;22:19–23–quiz24–26.

22. Stirnemann JJ, Mousty E, Chalouhi G, et al. Screening for placenta accreta at 11–14 weeks of gestation. *Am J Obstet Gynecol.* 2011;205:547.e1–547.e6.

23. Timor-Tritsch IE, Monteagudo A, Cali G, et al. Cesarean scar pregnancy and early placenta accreta share common histology. *Ultrasound Obstet Gynecol.* 2014;43:383–395.

24. Sinkovskaya ES, Chaoui R, Karl K, et al. Fetal cardiac axis and congenital heart defects in early gestation. *Obstet Gynecol.* 2015;125:453–460.

25. Chaoui R, Heling K-S. *3D-Ultrasound in Prenatal Diagnosis: A Practical Approach.* 1st ed. Berlin, New York: DeGruyter; 2016.

26. Nicolaides KH. A model for a new pyramid of prenatal care based on the 11 to 13 weeks' assessment. *Prenat Diagn.* 2011;31:3–6.

27. Nicolaides KH. Turning the pyramid of prenatal care. *Fetal Diagn Ther.* 2011;29:183–196.

28. Salvesen KÅ, Lees C, Abramowicz J, et al. Safe use of Doppler ultrasound during the 11 to 13 + 6-week scan: is it possible? *Ultrasound Obstet Gynecol.* 2011;37:625–628.

29. Salomon LJ, Alfirevic Z, Bilardo CM, et al. ISUOG practice guidelines: performance of first-trimester fetal ultrasound scan. *Ultrasound Obstet Gynecol.* 2013;41:102–113.

# CHAPTER 6

# First Trimester Screening for Chromosomal Aneuploidies

## INTRODUCTION

The incidence of fetal numerical chromosomal aneuploidies such as trisomy 21 (T21; Down syndrome), trisomy 18 (T18; Edwards syndrome), and trisomy 13 (T13; Patau syndrome) increases with advancing maternal age. The presence of fetal chromosomal aneuploidies has been associated with significant pregnancy complications such as multiple malformations, growth restriction, and perinatal deaths. Prenatal screening for chromosomal aneuploidies has received significant attention over the past 30 years and is now considered an integral part of prenatal care. Several major developments impacted prenatal screening for chromosomal abnormalities, such as the identification of ultrasound markers for aneuploidy, the introduction of the second trimester biochemical screen, the introduction of the first trimester screen with nuchal translucency (NT), and recently fetal cell-free DNA in maternal plasma. Advancement in aneuploidy screening has currently led to the prenatal identification of most fetuses with chromosomal abnormalities. The largest study to date on the first trimester role of thickened NT and major malformations in the detection of chromosomal aneuploidies was recently published[1] and included a total of 108,982 fetuses with 654 cases of trisomies 21, 18, or 13. The presence of at least one of the following findings: thickened NT (>3.5 mm), holoprosencephaly, omphalocele, or megacystis had the potential to detect 57% of all aneuploidies. Interestingly, one or more of these four findings was found in 53% of all T21, in 72% of all T18, and 86% of all T13 fetuses.[1] In this chapter, we present detailed first trimester sonographic features of aneuploidies in addition to aspects of other genetic diseases and syndromes.

## FIRST TRIMESTER ULTRASOUND AND MATERNAL BIOCHEMICAL MARKERS IN ANEUPLOIDY

### Trisomy 21

The association in the first trimester fetus of increased nuchal fluid and aneuploidy was first described more than two decades ago,[2–4] and this finding has led to the establishment of first trimester aneuploidy screening with NT and biochemical markers. A thickened NT has been correlated with the presence of trisomy 21 (T21) and T21 fetuses have a mean NT thickness of 3.4 mm.[5] In a study involving 654 fetuses with T21, more than half were shown to have an NT ≥3.5 mm.[1] The NT in the normal fetus increases with increasing crown-rump length (CRL) measurement and NT screening has been successfully used to adjust the pregnancy's aneuploidy a priori risk established by maternal age. This has been one of the most important elements of aneuploidy screening as it resulted in a significant reduction in unnecessary invasive testing on pregnant women with advanced maternal age.

In pregnancies with T21 fetuses, the maternal serum concentration of free β-human chorionic gonadotropin (β-hCG) is about twice as high and pregnancy-associated plasma protein A (PAPP-A) is reduced to half compared to euploid pregnancies (Table 6.1). Although NT measurement alone identifies about 75% to 80% of T21 fetuses, the combination of NT with maternal biomarkers in the first trimester increases the T21 detection rate to 85% to 95%, while keeping the false-positive rate at 5%.[5,6] Indeed, in a recent prospective validation study of screening for trisomies 21, 18 and 13 by a combination of maternal age, fetal NT, fetal heart rate and serum free β-hCG

**Table 6.1** • Biochemical and Sonographic Features of Trisomies 21, 18, and 13

| NT Mixture Model | Euploid | Trisomy 21 | Trisomy 18 | Trisomy 13 |
|---|---|---|---|---|
| CRL-independent distribution, % | 5 | 95 | 70 | 85 |
| Median CRL-independent NT, mm | 2.0 | 3.4 | 5.5 | 4.4 |
| Median serum free β-hCG, MoM | 1.0 | 2.0 | 0.2 | 0.5 |
| Median serum PAPP-A, MoM | 1.0 | 0.5 | 0.2 | 0.3 |
| Absent nasal bone, % | 2.5 | 60 | 53 | 45 |
| Tricuspid regurgitation, % | 1.0 | 55 | 33 | 30 |
| Ductus venosus reversed A-wave, % | 3.0 | 66 | 58 | 55 |

NT, nuchal translucency; CRL, crown-rump length; β-hCG, β-human chorionic gonadotropin; MoM, multiple of the median; PAPP-A, pregnancy-associated plasma protein A.

From Nicolaides KH. Screening for fetal aneuploidies at 11 to 13 weeks. *Prenat Diagn.* 2011;31:7–15; copyright John Wiley & Sons, with permission.

and PAPP-A at 11+0 to 13+6 weeks of gestation in 108,982 singleton pregnancies, T21, 18, and 13 were detected in 90%, 97%, and 92% respectively with a false-positive rate of 4%.[6] Monosomy X was also detected in more than 90% of cases along with more than 85% of triploidies and more than 30% of other chromosomal abnormalities.[6] In addition to NT, other sensitive first trimester ultrasound markers of T21 include absence or hypoplasia of the nasal bone (Fig. 6.1), cardiac malformations (atrioventricular septal defect) with or without generalized edema (Figs. 6.2 and 6.3), tricuspid regurgitation (Fig. 6.4A), aberrant right subclavian artery (Fig. 6.4B), echogenic intracardiac focus (Fig. 6.4C), and increased impedance

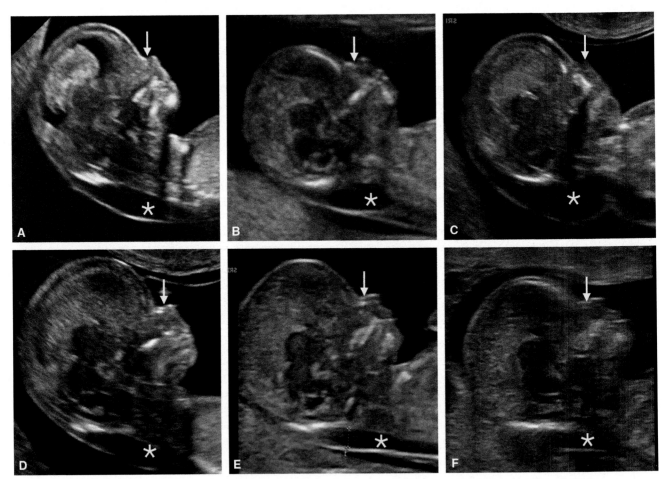

**Figure 6.1:** Midsagittal view of the face in six fetuses with trisomy 21 between 11 and 13 weeks of gestation. Note the various thicknesses of the nuchal translucency (*asterisk*) and the absence (**A, C, F**) or poor ossification (**B, D, E**) of the nasal bone (*arrows*).

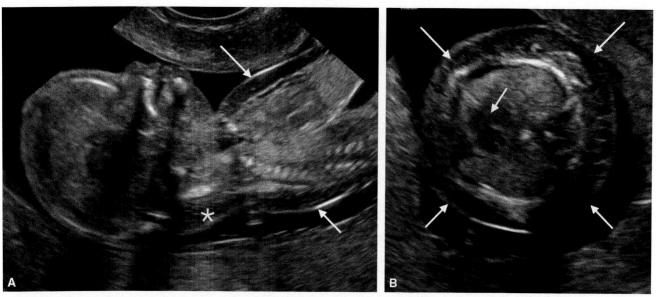

**Figure 6.2:** Sagittal view of the fetal head and chest **(A)** and transverse view of the chest **(B)** in a fetus with trisomy 21 at 13 weeks of gestation. Note the presence of early hydrops with body skin edema (*white arrows* in **A** and **B**) and a thickened nuchal translucency (*asterisk* in **A**). Note also the presence of an atrioventricular septal defect (*yellow arrow*) in **B**.

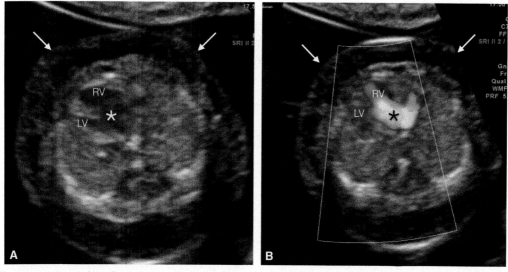

**Figure 6.3:** Transverse views of the fetal chest at the level of the four-chamber view in gray scale **(A)** and color Doppler **(B)** in a fetus with trisomy 21 at 12 weeks of gestation. Note the presence of an atrioventricular septal defect (*asterisk*) in **A** and **B**, which represents the typical cardiac anomaly of this syndrome. Also note the associated body edema (*arrows*), which resolved at 16 weeks upon follow-up. See Figure 6.4 for additional sonographic markers of trisomy 21 in the first trimester. LV, left ventricle; RV, right ventricle.

to flow in the ductus venosus (Fig. 6.5). First trimester features of fetuses with T21 are listed in **Table 6.2**. Additional first trimester findings in T21 fetuses are shown in images in various chapters of this book.

## Trisomy 18 and Trisomy 13

Thickened NT is not specific to T21 as it can be also found in other aneuploidies. In T18 and T13, NT median values were

shown to be 5.5 and 4.0 mm, respectively.[5,6] The PAPP-A value is also reduced in both trisomies with a median value of 0.2 MoM for T18 and 0.3 MoM for T13. Unlike in T21, free β-hCG values are decreased in T18 and T13 with median values of 0.2 MoM and 0.5 MoM, respectively (**Table 6.1**). For physicians and sonographers with expertise in the first trimester ultrasound examination, T18 or T13 is often first suspected by the presence of typical ultrasound features, rather than by biochemical screening. In a study involving 5,613

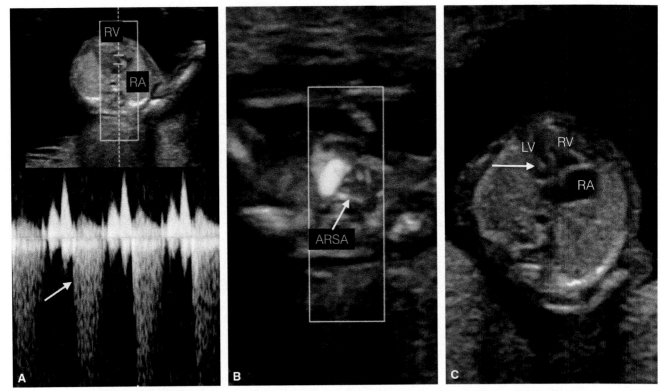

**Figure 6.4:** Additional sonographic findings in fetuses with trisomy 21 in the first trimester. Tricuspid regurgitation shown in **A** on color and pulsed (*arrow*) Doppler, an aberrant course of the right subclavian artery (ARSA) shown in **B** and an echogenic intracardiac focus shown in the left ventricle (LV) in **C** (*arrow*). RA, right atrium; RV, right ventricle.

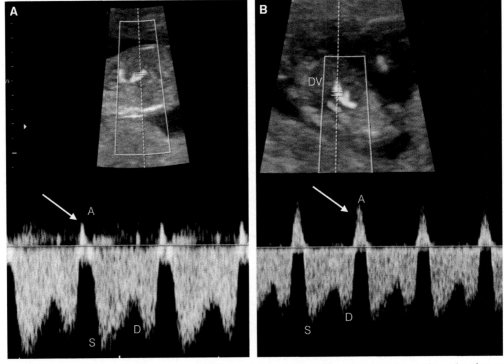

**Figure 6.5:** Ductus venosus (DV) Doppler flow assessment in two fetuses **(A and B)** with trisomy 21 at 13 weeks of gestation. Note the presence of reverse flow during the atrial contraction phase **(A)** of the cardiac cycle (*arrow*). Fetus **A** had no associated cardiac defect, whereas fetus **B** had a cardiac defect, which may explain the more severe reverse flow of the A-wave (*arrow* in **B**). Normal Doppler waveforms of the ductus venosus show antegrade flow throughout the cardiac cycle with low impedance. S, systolic flow; D, diastolic flow.

**Table 6.2** • First Trimester Features of Trisomy 21

Thickened nuchal translucency (NT)
High human chorionic gonadotropin (HCG, β-hCG)
Low pregnancy-associated plasma protein A (PAPP-A)
Absent or hypoplastic nasal bone
Reversal of flow in diastole or high impedance flow in ductus venosus
Tricuspid regurgitation
Increased fronto-maxillary-facial (FMF) angle, short maxilla reflecting midface hypoplasia
Aberrant right subclavian artery
Echogenic focus
Echogenic bowel
Renal tract dilation
Increased peak velocity in the hepatic artery
Ductus venosus directly draining into the inferior vena cava
Structural anomalies such as atrioventricular septal defect, tetralogy of Fallot, and others

normal fetuses and 37 fetuses with T18, the first trimester ultrasound examination was found to be a good screening test for T18.[7] The mean NT thickness was 5.4 mm in T18 fetuses as compared to 1.7 mm in euploid fetuses.[7] Congenital heart defects were observed in 70.3% of T18 fetuses and in 0.5% of euploid fetuses and extracardiac malformations were identified in 35.1% of T18 fetuses and in 0.8% of euploid fetuses.[7] Only one case of T18 demonstrated no sonographic markers of aneuploidy.[7]

Figures 6.6 to 6.17 show common sonographic features of T18 in the first trimester, including thickened NT (Figs. 6.6, 6.8, and 6.9), absent/hypoplastic nasal bone (Figs. 6.6 and 6.8), dilated fourth ventricle/abnormal posterior fossa (Figs. 6.6 to 6.8), megacystis (Fig. 6.7), spina bifida (Figs. 6.7 and 6.8), cardiac malformations (Figs. 6.10 to 6.12), small omphalocele (Figs. 6.6, 6.7, and 6.13), abnormal extremities (Figs. 6.14 and 6.15), cleft lip and palate (Figs. 6.6 and 6.15), short CRL (Figs. 6.6, 6.7, and 6.15), and single umbilical artery/cord abnormalities (Fig. 6.16 and 6.17).[1,8]

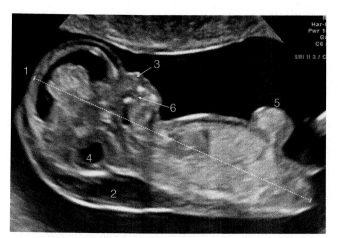

**Figure 6.6:** Midsagittal view of the body of a fetus with trisomy 18 at 12 weeks of gestation showing several typical abnormalities. Note the short crown-lump length (*1*), the thickened nuchal translucency (*2*), the absence of an ossified nasal bone (*3*), the dilated fourth ventricle (*4*), the small omphalocele with bowel content (*5*), and the maxillary gap as a sign of cleft lip and palate (*6*). See Figures 6.7 to 6.11 for associated fetal abnormalities with trisomy 18.

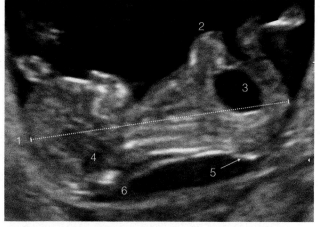

**Figure 6.7:** Midsagittal view of the body of a fetus with trisomy 18 at 13 weeks of gestation showing typical associated abnormalities. Note the presence of a short crown-rump length (*1*), an omphalocele (*2*), a megacystis (*3*), an abnormal posterior fossa (*4*), and thickened brainstem and no fluid in the fourth ventricle due to an open spina bifida (*5*). Note that the nuchal translucency (*6*) is not markedly thickened.

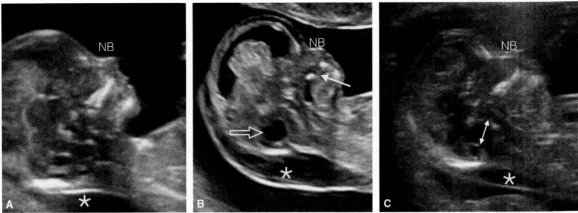

**Figure 6.8:** Midsagittal view of the fetal face in three fetuses **(A–C)** with trisomy 18 at 13, 12, and 14 weeks of gestation, respectively. Note the presence of a normal nuchal translucency (NT) in **A**, a mildly increased NT in **C**, and a markedly increased NT in **B**. All three fetuses have an absent or poorly ossified nasal bone (NB). The posterior fossa is an interesting marker in trisomy 18 and can be normal as in fetus **A**, but is often dilated as seen in fetus **B** (*open arrow*) and occasionally compressed as in fetus C (*double headed arrow*) in the presence of an open spina bifida. Fetus **A** was diagnosed with trisomy 18 due to the presence of radius aplasia (see Fig. 6.14) and cardiac abnormalities. Fetus **B** has a cleft in the maxilla (*arrow*) suggesting the presence of a facial cleft.

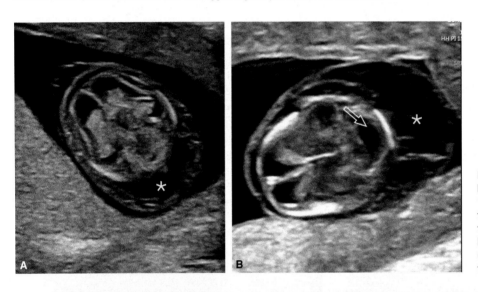

**Figure 6.9:** Axial views of the fetal head in two fetuses with trisomy 18 at 12 weeks of gestation. Note the presence of early hydrops and thickened nuchal translucency/cystic hygroma (*asterisk*) in both fetuses **(A and B)**. Fetus **B** also has a dilated fourth ventricle (*open arrow*).

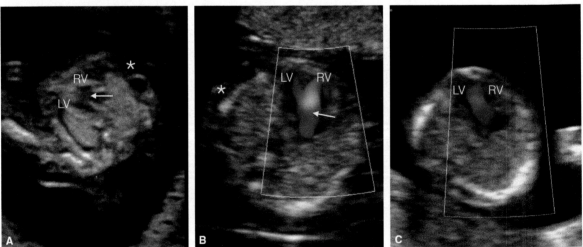

**Figure 6.10:** Axial views of the chest in three fetuses **(A–C)** with trisomy 18 and cardiac anomalies at 11, 13, and 13 weeks of gestation, respectively. In fetus **A** and **B**, an atrioventricular septal defect (AVSD) is shown in gray scale in **A** (*arrow*) and in color Doppler in **B** (*arrow*). Fetus C initially appeared to have a univentricular heart, but a follow-up ultrasound a week later confirmed the presence of an AVSD as well. Hydrops and skin edema (*asterisk*) are often found as shown in **A** and **B**. LV, left ventricle; RV, right ventricle.

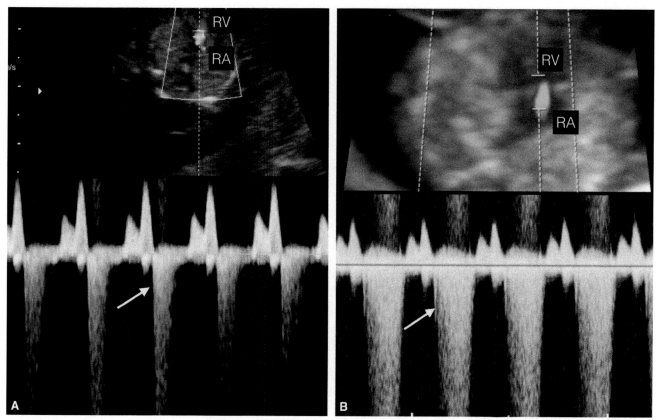

**Figure 6.11:** Cardiac valves are often insufficient in fetuses with trisomy 18 in the first trimester of pregnancy. **A:** Color and pulsed Doppler across the tricuspid valve in a fetus with trisomy 18 at 13 weeks of gestation showing the presence of mild tricuspid regurgitation (*arrow*). **B:** Color and pulsed Doppler across the tricuspid valve in a fetus with trisomy 21 at 13 weeks of gestation showing the presence of severe tricuspid regurgitation (*arrow*). RA, right atrium; RV, right ventricle.

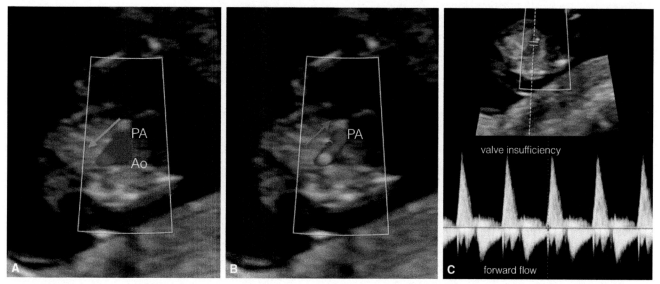

**Figure 6.12:** Three-vessel-trachea view in color and pulsed Doppler in a fetus at 12 weeks of gestation with dysplastic or polyvalvular pulmonary valve with stenosis and insufficiency, a finding that is typical for trisomy 18 and 13. **A:** Antegrade flow across the pulmonary artery (PA) in systole (*blue arrow*). **B:** Retrograde flow in PA in diastole (*red arrow*). **C:** The spectral Doppler across the PA demonstrating the bidirectional flow. This finding can also affect the aortic valve and is often accompanied by fetal hydrops and fetal demise. Ao, aorta.

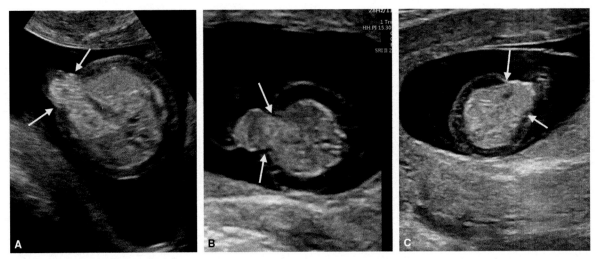

**Figure 6.13:** Axial views of the fetal abdomen at the level of the umbilical cord insertion in three fetuses **(A–C)** with trisomy 18 at 13, 12, and 12 weeks of gestation, respectively. Note the presence of an omphalocele (*arrows*) in each fetus, which is a typical finding in trisomy 18. In fetus **A** and **B**, the omphalocele is small with bowel content, which is commonly seen in trisomy 18. In fetus **C**, the liver is in the omphalocele sac. Note the presence of fetal hydrops in all fetuses.

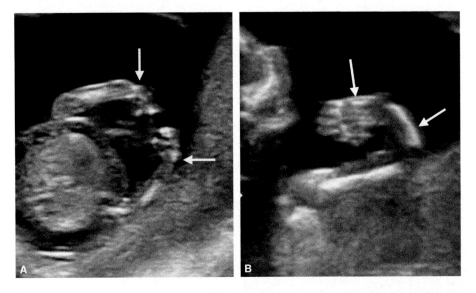

**Figure 6.14:** Abnormal hands in two fetuses **(A and B)** with trisomy 18 at 12 and 13 weeks of gestation, respectively. Note the presence of bilateral clubbed hands in fetus **A** (*yellow arrows*) and radial aplasia in fetus **B** (*white arrows*).

**Figure 6.15:** Midsagittal view **(A)** and 3D surface mode view **(B)** of a fetus at 12 weeks of gestation with trisomy 18. Note the presence of the following features: short crown-rump length (*1*), normal nuchal translucency thickness (*2*), facial cleft with protrusion and maxillary gap (yellow arrow) (*3*), and an omphalocele (*4*). **B:** The facial cleft (*yellow arrow*) and bilateral radial aplasia (*white arrows*), which are not demonstrated in **A**.

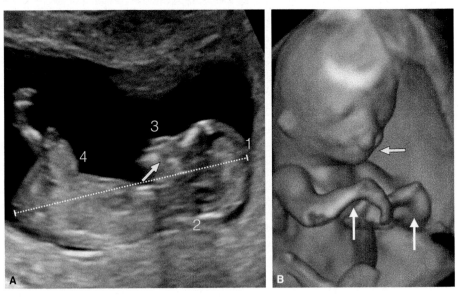

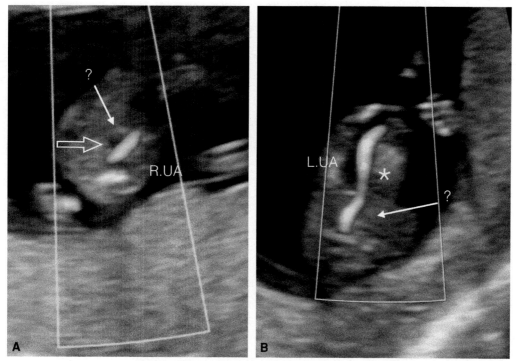

**Figure 6.16:** Axial planes of the lower abdomen in two fetuses **(A and B)** with trisomy 18 at 12 weeks of gestation. Note in fetus **A** the presence of a single right umbilical artery (R.UA) next to the bladder (*open arrow*), with the absence of the left UA (*solid arrow* with "?"). Fetus **B** has a single left umbilical artery (L.UA) in addition to an omphalocele (*asterisk*). The solid arrow with "?" in **B** denotes the absence of the R.UA.

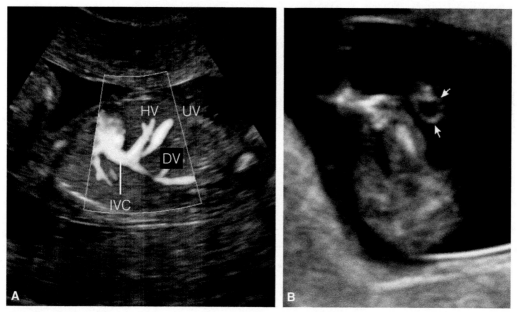

**Figure 6.17: A:** A parasagittal plane of the fetal abdomen and chest in color Doppler in a fetus with trisomy 18 at 12 weeks of gestation. Note the direct connection of the ductus venosus (DV) with the inferior vena cava (IVC) in **A**. **B:** A cross section of the umbilical cord in the amniotic cavity of another fetus with trisomy 18 at 12 weeks of gestation. Note the presence of a cord cyst in **B** (*arrows*). These cord and umbilical vessel abnormalities represent subtle findings in trisomy 18 and also in trisomy 13 (see Fig. 6.24). Additional malformations were found in both fetuses. HV, hepatic vein; UV, umbilical vein.

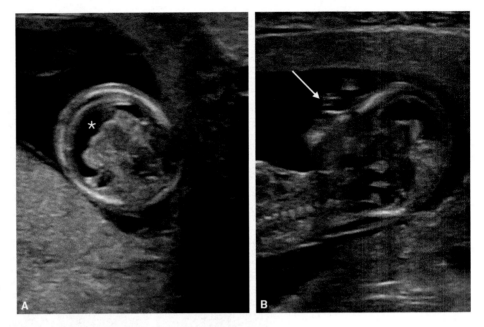

**Figure 6.18:** Axial plane of the fetal head **(A)** and midsagittal plane of the face **(B)** in a fetus with trisomy 13 at 12 weeks of gestation. Note the presence of typical craniofacial abnormalities with holoprosencephaly, demonstrated in **A** (*asterisk*) and severe facial cleft in **B** (*arrow*).

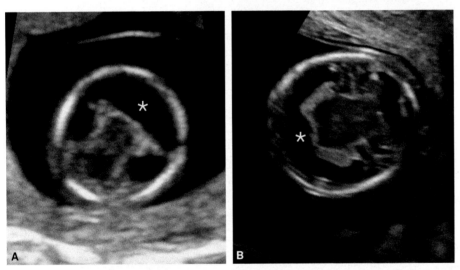

**Figure 6.19:** Axial planes of the fetal head in two fetuses **(A and B)** with trisomy 13 at 12 and 13 weeks of gestation respectively with alobar holoprosencephaly (*asterisk*). **A** is obtained by the transabdominal approach and **B** is obtained by the transvaginal approach.

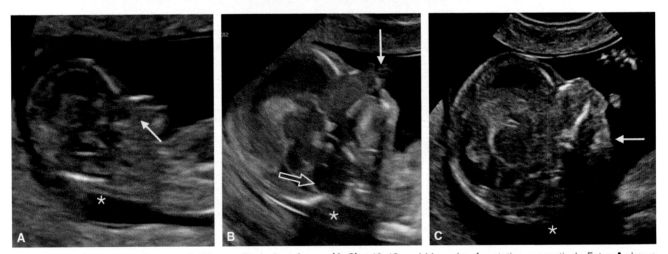

**Figure 6.20:** Trisomy 13 with severe facial anomalies in three fetuses **(A–C)** at 13, 13, and 14 weeks of gestation, respectively. Fetus **A** shows a median cleft in association with holoprosencephaly, no maxilla is seen (*arrow*), and the nuchal translucency (NT) (*asterisk*) is not thickened. Fetus **B** is examined transvaginally and shows a thickened NT (*asterisk*), a bilateral cleft with protrusion (*solid arrow*), and a dilated fourth ventricle (*open arrow*). Fetus **C** had no thickened NT (*asterisk*), a normal fourth ventricle, and retrognathia (*arrow*). All three fetuses had severe additional anomalies.

Features of T13 on first trimester ultrasound include craniofacial abnormalities (Figs. 6.18 to 6.20), cleft lip/palate (Figs. 6.18 and 6.20), thickened NT (Fig. 6.20), abnormal extremities with polydactyly (Fig. 6.21), cardiac abnormalities (Fig. 6.22), renal abnormalities (Fig. 6.23), and umbilical cord/abdominal venous abnormalities (Figs. 6.23 and 6.24).[1,8]

First trimester features of fetuses with T18 and T13 are listed in Table 6.3. Additional first trimester findings in T18 and T13 fetuses are shown in images in various chapters of this book.

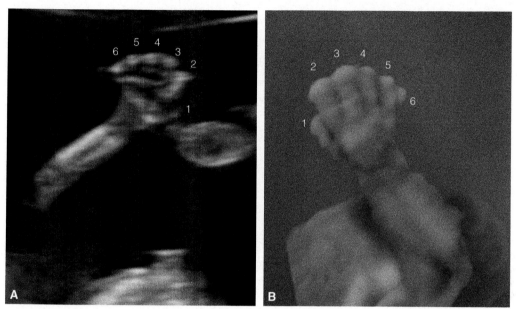

**Figure 6.21:** Polydactyly in two fetuses with trisomy 13 at 14 weeks and in gray scale in fetus **A** and at 12 weeks and in 3D surface mode in fetus **B**.

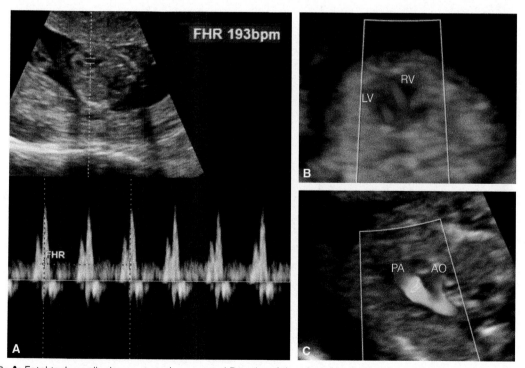

**Figure 6.22: A:** Fetal tachycardia demonstrated on spectral Doppler of the tricuspid valve in a fetus with trisomy 13 at 12 weeks of gestation, with fetal heart rate (FHR) at 193 beats per minute (bpm). **B:** Color Doppler at the four-chamber view in a fetus with trisomy 13 at 14 weeks of gestation. Note the presence in **B** of discrepant ventricular filling with a narrow left ventricle (LV). **C:** The three-vessel-trachea view of the fetus shown in **B**. Note in **C** the narrow aortic arch (AO) in comparison with the pulmonary artery (PA). Cardiac findings in fetuses with trisomy 13 are common and include tachycardia (>175 per minute), intraventricular echogenic foci, an aberrant right subclavian artery, and cardiac defects, predominantly left ventricular outflow tract obstruction. RV, right ventricle.

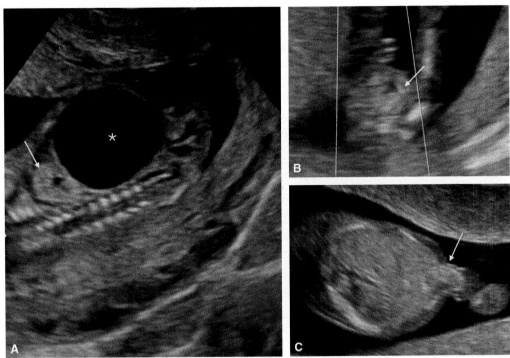

**Figure 6.23: A:** A parasagittal view of the abdomen in a fetus at 12 weeks of gestation with trisomy 13 and renal abnormalities. Note the presence in **A** of hyperechogenic kidneys (*arrow*) and megacystis (*asterisk*). Fetus in **B** also has trisomy 13 at 14 weeks of gestation. Note in **B** the presence of a single umbilical artery, a finding similar to trisomy 18. Fetus in **C** has trisomy 13 at 12 weeks of gestation and shows a small omphalocele, another finding commonly seen in trisomy 18 fetuses in early gestation.

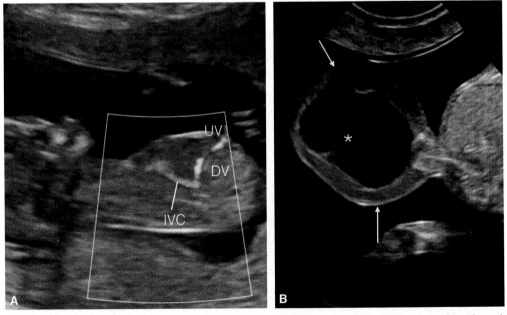

**Figure 6.24: A:** A parasagittal plane of the fetal abdomen and chest in color Doppler in a fetus with trisomy 13 at 13 weeks of gestation. Note the direct connection of the ductus venosus (DV) with the inferior vena cava (IVC) in **A**. **B:** A cross section of the umbilical cord in the amniotic cavity of another fetus with trisomy 13 at 14 weeks of gestation. Note the presence of a large cord cyst (*asterisk/arrows*) in **B**. These cord and umbilical vessel abnormalities represent subtle findings in trisomy 13 and in trisomy 18 as shown in Figure 6.17. Additional malformations were found in both fetuses. UV, umbilical vein.

**Table 6.3** • First Trimester Features of Trisomy 18 and 13

|  | Trisomy 18 | Trisomy 13 |
|---|---|---|
| Nuchal translucency (median) | 5.5 mm | 4.0 mm |
| Free β-hCG (median) | 0.2 MoM | 0.5 MoM |
| PAPP-A (median) | 0.2 MoM | 0.3 MoM |
| Fetal growth | Growth restriction | Growth restriction |
| Brain | Rarely holoprosencephaly | Typically holoprosencephaly |
|  | Occasionally choroid plexus cysts | Occasionally choroid plexus cysts |
| Posterior fossa | Cystic dilation of posterior fossa. Signs of brainstem thickening and IT compression as marker for open spina bifida | Cystic dilation of posterior fossa |
| Face | Absent nasal bone, flat profile, retrognathia, occasionally median clefts | Severe midline facial anomalies: hypotelorism, pseudocyclopia, proboscis, arrhinia, median clefts, retrognathia, absent nasal bone |
| Neck and skin | Thickened NT and severe hydrops | Thickened NT and severe hydrops |
| Heart | Tricuspid regurgitation, aberrant right subclavian artery, echogenic focus, structural cardiac anomalies especially septal defects (AVSD; VSD), conotruncal anomalies such as tetralogy of Fallot and double outlet right ventricle, polyvalvular dysplastic semilunar valves | Tachycardia, tricuspid regurgitation, echogenic focus, aberrant right subclavian artery, structural cardiac anomalies, especially left ventricular outflow tract obstruction (HLHS, CoA, etc.), and polyvalvular dysplastic semilunar valves |
| Abdomen | Omphalocele (often with bowel only), Diaphragmatic hernia | Rarely omphalocele or other bowel anomalies, abnormal ductus venosus course with connection with inferior vena cava |
|  | Abnormal ductus venosus course with connection with inferior vena cava |  |
| Urogenital anomalies | Horseshoe kidneys | Megacystis, hyperechogenic kidneys |
| Skeletal anomalies | Radius aplasia, club hands, clenched fingers, spina bifida | Polydactyly |
| Umbilical cord | Single umbilical artery, cord cyst | Single umbilical artery, cord cyst |

Free β-hCG, free β human chorionic gonadotropin; PAPP-A, pregnancy-associated plasma protein A; NT, nuchal translucency; AVSD, atrioventricular septal defect; VSD, ventricular septal defect; HLHS, hypoplastic left heart syndrome; CoA, coarctation of aorta.

## Monosomy X

The NT is often enlarged in fetuses with monosomy X (Turner syndrome). This enlarged NT has a median value of 7.8 mm[5] and has often been described as a cystic hygroma (Figs. 6.25 and 6.26). The occurrence of monosomy X is not related to maternal age. Typically, lymphatic disturbances in monosomy X are not limited to the neck region but involve the whole body including the presence of hydrothorax, ascites, and skin edema (Fig. 6.27). Nasal bone is generally present in fetuses with monosomy X.[8] Maternal serum-free β-hCG is normal (1.1 MoM) and PAPP-A is low (0.49 MoM).[9] Typical first trimester features in monosomy X are listed in Table 6.4 and include fetal tachycardia and left ventricular outflow tract obstruction (Fig. 6.28), renal anomalies such as the presence of horseshoe kidneys as well as feet edema. Some of these anomalies are often difficult to diagnose in the first trimester. In a first trimester study involving 31 cases of monosomy X and 5,613 euploid controls, NT measurement (8.8 mm) and fetal heart rate (171 beats per minute) in monosomy X were significantly greater than in euploid controls (NT = 1.7 mm and fetal heart rate 160 beats per minute).[10] In monosomy X fetuses, congenital heart defects and hydrops were noted in 54.8% and 43.8%, respectively.[10] None of the monosomy X cases demonstrated absent sonographic markers of aneuploidy.[10] Additional first trimester findings in monosomy X fetuses are shown in images in various chapters of this book.

## Triploidy

In triploidy, there is a complete additional haploid set of chromosomes resulting in 69 chromosomes in each cell instead of 46 chromosomes. The additional haploid set can be of maternal or paternal origin. The "paternal" type is called diandric triploidy and the "maternal" type is called digynic

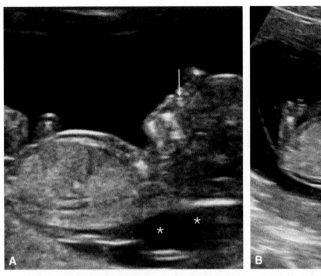

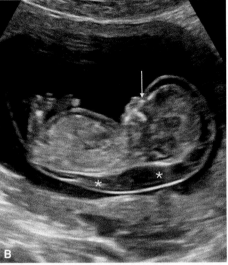

**Figure 6.25:** Midsagittal planes of the fetal body in two fetuses **(A and B)** with monosomy X (Turner syndrome) at 11 and 13 weeks of gestation, respectively. Note the presence of a marked thickened nuchal translucency (*asterisks*) in **A** and fetal hydrops and cystic hygroma in **B**. Maternal age is often not increased and the nasal bone is typically ossified (*arrows*).

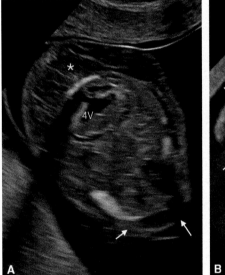

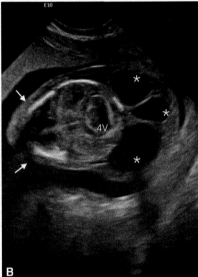

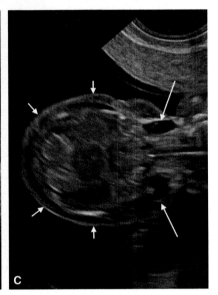

**Figure 6.26:** Three fetuses **(A–C)** with Turner syndrome and neck abnormalities, all at 13 weeks of gestation. Fetus **A** and **B** has cystic hygromas (*asterisks*), whereas fetus **C** has lateral neck cysts (*long arrows*). Fetal scalp edema is seen in all fetuses (*short arrows*). Intracerebral structures are normal in all fetuses. 4V, fourth ventricle.

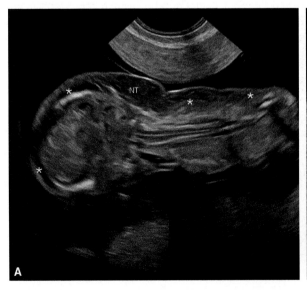

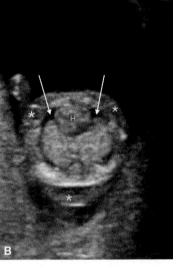

**Figure 6.27: A:** A midsagittal plane of the body in a fetus with monosomy X at 13 weeks of gestation. Note the presence in **A** of marked thickened nuchal translucency (NT)/cystic hygroma with body edema (*asterisks*). **B:** An axial plane of the chest in another fetus with monosomy X at 11 weeks of gestation. Note the presence in **B** of bilateral pleural effusion (*arrows*). H, heart.

**Table 6.4** • First Trimester Features of Monosomy X

Marked thickened nuchal translucency (NT), cystic hygroma, early hydrops

High human chorionic gonadotropin (HCG, β-hCG)

Low pregnancy-associated plasma protein A (PAPP-A)

Normal nasal bone

Cardiac abnormalities: tachycardia, left ventricular outflow obstruction, hypoplastic left heart syndrome, coarctation of the aorta, aberrant right subclavian artery, tricuspid regurgitation

Renal anomalies: horseshoe kidney, renal pelvis dilation

Ductus venosus abnormalities: directly draining into inferior vena cava, reversal flow of A-wave or high impedance

Female gender

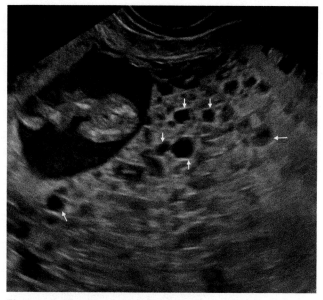

**Figure 6.29:** Ultrasound of the placenta in a pregnancy at 11 weeks of gestation with diandric triploidy. Note the presence of molar placental changes (*arrows*). See text for details.

triploidy. These two types of triploidy have different features, which can be often differentiated on ultrasound.

NT can be thickened in both diandric and digynic triploidy, but is often within the normal range. The typical pattern of diandric triploidy includes the presence of a molar placenta (Fig. 6.29), with a normally grown fetus, whereas in digynic triploidy, severe growth restriction is noted with a small but not molar placenta. These placental differences are reflected

in the profile of biochemistry with diandric triploidy associated with increased maternal serum-free β-hCG and mildly decreased PAPP-A and digynic triploidy associated with markedly decreased maternal serum free β-hCG and PAPP-A.[11,12] Another important first trimester feature of digynic triploidy

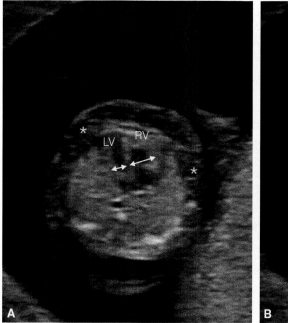

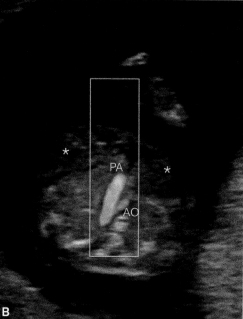

**Figure 6.28:** Axial plane at the level of the four-chamber view in gray scale **(A)** and the three-vessel-trachea view in color Doppler **(B)** in a fetus with monosomy X at 13 weeks of gestation. Note the presence in **A** of ventricular disproportions with a narrow left ventricle (LV). In **B**, a narrow aortic arch (AO) is noted in comparison with the pulmonary artery (PA), suggesting the presence of aortic coarctation. Also note the presence of skin edema (*asterisks*) in **A** and **B**. The presence of left ventricular outflow tract anomaly including aortic coarctation or hypoplastic left heart syndrome is a typical finding in fetuses with monosomy X. RV, right ventricle.

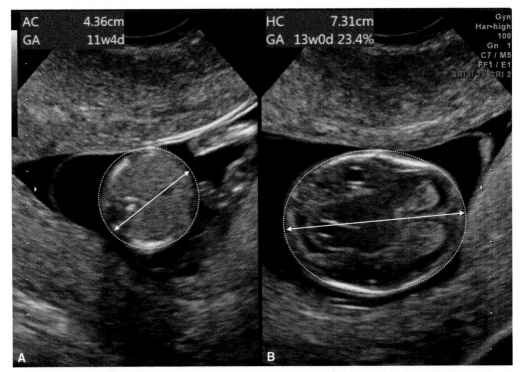

**Figure 6.30:** Axial planes of the fetal abdomen **(A)** and head **(B)** in a fetus with digynic triploidy at 12 weeks of gestation. Note the marked difference in size between the abdominal **(A)** and head **(B)** circumference, of more than "2 weeks" of gestational age. See text for details.

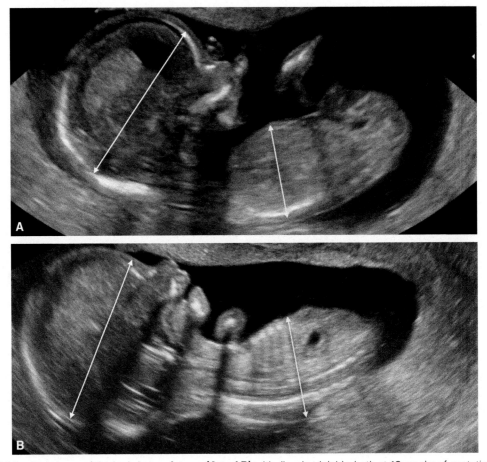

**Figure 6.31:** Midsagittal planes of the body in two fetuses **(A and B)** with digynic triploidy, both at 13 weeks of gestation. Note in both fetuses the marked difference in size between the abdominal (*yellow arrows*) and head (*white arrows*) dimensions. This discrepancy in dimensions between the head and abdomen is an almost pathognomonic sign of digynic triploidy. In addition, the crown-rump length is significantly short, reflecting the presence of early growth restriction. See 6.32 for the 3D surface mode views.

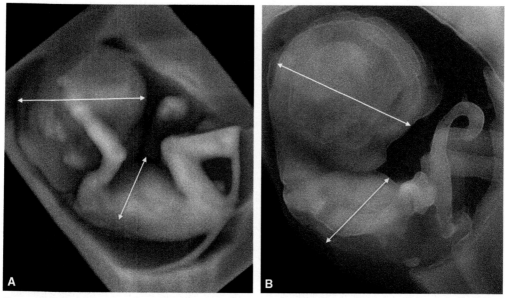

**Figure 6.32:** Three-dimensional ultrasound in surface mode in two fetuses **(A and B)** with digynic triploidy; same fetuses as in Figure 6.31. Note the marked difference in dimensions between the abdomen (*yellow arrows*) and the head (*white arrows*) in both fetuses. See text for details.

is the presence of significantly short CRL and a marked difference in size between the abdominal and head circumference, typically of more than "2 weeks" of gestational age[13] (Figs. 6.30 to 6.32). This discrepancy in dimensions between the head and abdomen is an almost pathognomonic sign of digynic triploidy.

A high detection rate for triploidy is also achieved with first trimester screening for T21. In a study involving 198,427 women with singleton pregnancies who underwent first trimester screening between 11+2 and 14+0 weeks of gestation, the overall detection rate of triploidy was 25/30 (83.3%), primarily resulting from an abnormal first trimester screening in 23/30 and structural abnormalities in 2/30.[12] A smaller CRL than

expected was found in 95% of the fetuses with data available for evaluation and eight of 30 fetuses had a larger biparietal diameter than expected for gestational age.[12] Typical features of triploidy are presented in **Table 6.5** and additional first trimester findings in triploidy fetuses are shown in images in various chapters of this book.

# NONINVASIVE PRENATAL TESTING

Noninvasive prenatal testing (NIPT) is a relatively new genetic testing that is offered as a screening test in the first

## Table 6.5 • First Trimester Features of Triploidy

|  | Digynic (Maternal) Triploidy | Diandric (Paternal) Triploidy |
|---|---|---|
| Nuchal translucency | Normal | Increased |
| Free β-hCG (median) | 0.18 MoM | 8 MoM |
| PAPP-A (median) | 0.06 MoM | 0.75 MoM |
| Growth | Short crown-rump length, severe growth restriction with discrepant head/abdominal circumference >2 wk | Normal growth or short crown-rump length |
| Head | Proportional large head, dilated fourth ventricle, compressed posterior fossa as a clue for spina bifida, holoprosencephaly | |
| Heart | Cardiac anomalies, aberrant right subclavian artery, echogenic focus, tricuspid regurgitation | |
| Abdomen | Echogenic bowel, single umbilical artery, absent gall bladder, echogenic kidneys | |
| Limbs, skeletal | Clenched hands, syndactyly, club feet, spina bifida | |

Free β-hCG, free β human chorionic gonadotropin; PAPP-A, pregnancy-associated plasma protein A.

(and second trimester of pregnancy) for trisomies 21, 13, 18, monosomy X, and sex chromosome abnormalities. The test is based upon the presence of fetal cell-free DNA (cfDNA) in the maternal circulation primarily from placental cells apoptosis. Placental cell apoptosis releases into the maternal circulation small DNA fragments that can be detected from about 4 to 7 weeks of gestation.[14] It is estimated that about 2-20% of circulating cfDNA in the maternal circulation is fetal in origin.[14] The half-life of cfDNA is short and is typically undetectable within hours after delivery.[15] Details of the technical aspect of NIPT are beyond the scope of this book but the various tests that are clinically available are based upon the isolation and counting of cfDNA using sequencing methods.

NIPT has very good performance with regard to screening for T21. In published studies, the detection rate for T21 is at 99% for a false-positive rate of 0.16%.[16,17] Detection rate for T18 is at 97% for a false-positive rate of 0.15%.[16] The use of NIPT is rapidly expanding and is now being offered as the primary screening test in pregnancy. Even if the NIPT test has an excellent detection rate for T21, T18, and T13, other aneuploidies remain missed.[18–20]

It should be emphasized that NIPT is a screening and not a diagnostic test and thus caution should be used when NIPT is incorporated in the genetic evaluation of fetal malformations. Given a relatively high association of anomalies with chromosomal imbalance, the significance of a normal NIPT result in the setting of fetal anomalies should be explained with the patient and further invasive diagnostic testing should be recommended. Undoubtedly NIPT technology will expand over the next few years to allow for screening of chromosomal deletions and duplications and is already available for very few monogenic conditions.

## FIRST TRIMESTER DIAGNOSIS OF GENETIC DISEASES AND SYNDROMIC CONDITIONS

Screening for chromosomal aneuploidy in the first trimester with NT and other markers has expanded the use of ultrasound in early gestation. This expansion in first trimester ultrasound led to the detection of single or multiple fetal malformations, which in some cases suggested the possible presence of a genetic syndrome. We presented in Chapter 5 four possible pathways that result in the detection of fetal anomaly in the first trimester. These four pathways include: (1) the presence of an obvious structural anomaly on ultrasound, (2) the detection of a thickened NT with resultant workup leading to the fetal anomaly, (3) the presence of a positive family history leading to the detection of a recurrent case and (4) the detection of the anomaly by a detailed ultrasound examination. In the absence of a prior family history of a genetic syndrome with fetal anomalies, the de novo diagnosis of a genetic syndrome

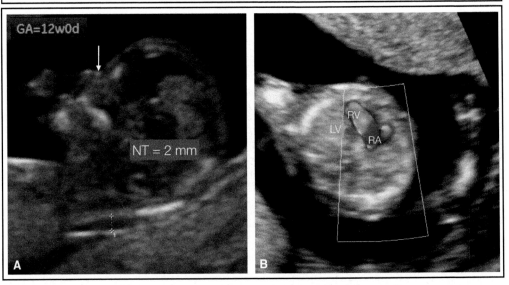

**Figure 6.33:** This figure shows the fetal profile **(A)** and the four-chamber view in color Doppler, obtained transvaginally **(B)** in a pregnant patient referred at 30 years of age for nuchal translucency (NT) screening at 12 weeks of gestation. **A:** An NT of 2 mm, within the normal range and an absent nasal bone (*arrow*). **B:** A hypoplastic left ventricle (LV), suspicious for a hypoplastic left heart syndrome with blood flow only demonstrated across the right atrium (RA) and ventricle (RV) on color Doppler. Chorionic villous sampling revealed a partial monosomy 9q and partial trisomy 2p as unbalanced translocation. Karyotyping of parents' chromosomes revealed a previously unknown balanced translocation in the father.

in the first trimester is quite challenging. When presented with a constellation of sonographic abnormalities in the second or third trimester of pregnancy, an expert sonologist is commonly able to suggest the presence of a specific syndrome. This is a more challenging task in the first trimester however as the full display of all of the sonographic features of a genetic syndrome is rare in early gestation. Nevertheless, there are four ways that syndromic conditions are diagnosed in the first trimester:

1. The presence of an abnormal karyotype following an invasive diagnostic procedure such as trisomies, triploidy, monosomy X and large unbalanced translocations, deletions, and duplications.
2. The presence of microdeletions and microduplications, detected either with fluorescent in situ hybridization (FISH) or with comparative genomic hybridization (CGH or microarray).
3. Monogenic diseases detected by selective molecular genetic examination of a special condition or with the use of next generation sequencing.
4. Genetic syndromes with "association" or "sequence" with no or not yet defined molecular genetic background.

## Abnormal Karyotype, Deletions, Duplications

If an anomaly is detected on ultrasound, the authors believe that it is not advisable to offer the NIPT test, as it is a screening test and will miss some significant chromosomal

abnormalities.[18] Invasive diagnostic testing, such as chorionic villous sampling (CVS), should be offered in that context. The traditional karyotypic analysis will detect the presence of large balanced or unbalanced translocations (Fig. 6.33), rare mosaic trisomies, marker chromosomes, and isochromosomes (Figs. 6.34 and 10.19) in addition to numerical chromosomal abnormalities. Large chromosomal deletions can also be identified on traditional karyotype analysis as in the majority of deletions 4p- (Wolf–Hirschhorn syndrome) (Fig. 6.35) or deletion 18p- (De Grouchy syndrome) (Fig. 6.36). Small deletions, termed microdeletions, such as 22q11 (DiGeorge syndrome), are typically too small to be identified by this method (Fig. 11.6). Microdeletions can be detected by the use of FISH, when such a condition is suspected (e.g., FISH for deletion 22q11 in conotruncal anomalies) or by examining the complete chromosome using CGH or microarray. This CGH technique has become popular recently despite its cost and limitations. Some centers offer CGH as a first-line genetic testing after CVS or amniocentesis, whereas others restrict its use to suspected DNA imbalance or as a second-line test following normal karyotype analysis. Recent studies suggest that CGH detects an additional 6% of chromosomal abnormalities over the aneuploidies in pregnancies with fetal malformations.[21,22]

## Monogenic Diseases and Other Syndromic Conditions

Many fetal anomalies identified in the first trimester can also be caused by a monogenic inherent disease (e.g., skeletal

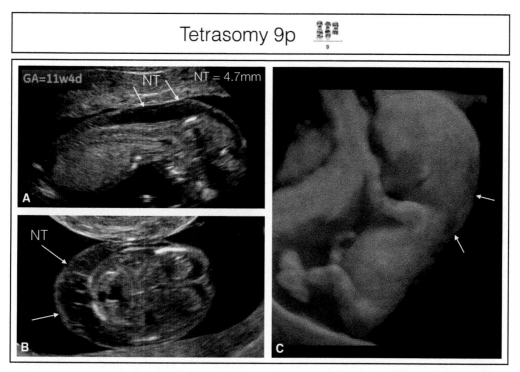

**Figure 6.34: A:** A thickened nuchal translucency (4.7 mm) in a fetus at 11 weeks of gestation. **B:** The corresponding axial plane of the head and **C** is the 3D ultrasound in surface mode. Note the thickened nuchal translucency (NT) in **B** and in **C** shown as transparent thickening in the dorsal aspect of the fetus (*arrows*). At this stage no other anomalies were seen. Chorionic villous sampling with prolonged cell culture revealed tetrasomy 9p.

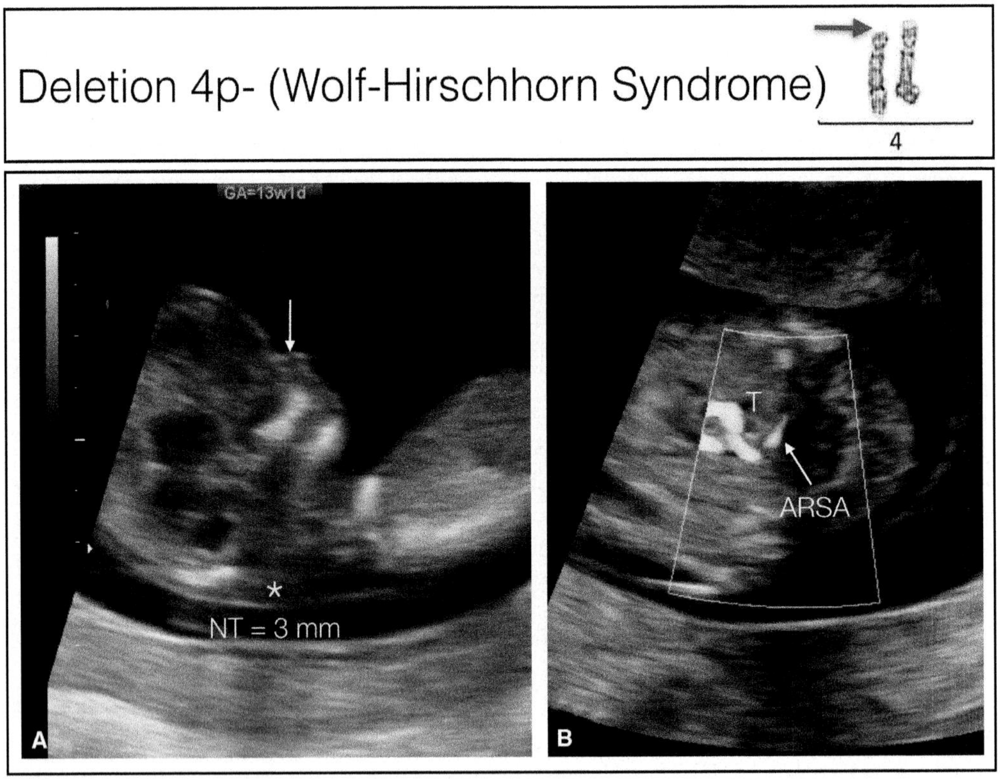

**Figure 6.35:** This 40-year-old pregnant woman was referred for first trimester screening. A nuchal translucency (NT) of 3 mm was measured (*asterisk*) along with absent nasal bone (*arrow*) as shown in **A**. An aberrant right subclavian artery (ARSA) was also found in **B** with a course behind the trachea (T). We had high suspicion for trisomy 21. Prolonged culture of cells from chorionic villous sampling revealed deletion 4p- (*red arrow*). The distal part of the short arm of chromosome 4 is absent. Keep in mind that noninvasive prenatal testing in such a condition would have missed the diagnosis.

anomalies, central nervous system anomalies associated with ciliopathies, polycystic renal diseases, and others) and may escape detection with CGH. In these cases, knowledge of typical sonographic features is needed in order to test for the specific gene(s) involved. Recently, there has been an increased use of selective panels for genetic diseases and in the future the use of next generation exon or genome sequencing will be more widely used. Until then, expert sonographers and sonologists should become familiar with fetal anomalies in the first trimester that are commonly associated with monogenic inheritance patterns.

The ability to suggest the presence of a possible association of a fetal anomaly with a monogenic type of inheritance vary based upon the expertise of the examiner and the types of fetal anomalies. It is relatively easy, for instance, to suggest the diagnosis of Meckel–Gruber syndrome (Figs. 8.21, 13.30, and 13.31), in the presence of an occipital encephalocele and polydactyly in the first trimester. Noonan syndrome is suggested when a markedly thickened NT is associated with normal karyotype and persists into the second trimester (Fig. 9.45). The diagnosis of monogenic syndromes is difficult when anomalies are subtle and expressivity of sonographic markers is incomplete in the first trimester. In this setting, follow-up ultrasound examinations in the early second trimester

are required. In two cases, the authors have observed the presence of short femur and polydactyly at 12 to 13 weeks of gestation and CVS revealed normal karyotype. Follow-up ultrasound at 15 weeks revealed short ribs, which led us to suggest the presence of short-rib-polydactyly or Ellis–Van Creveld syndrome, and molecular genetic testing confirmed the diagnoses in both cases (Figs. 14.18 and 14.22). Often, genetic diseases are diagnosed in early gestation due to routine screening or in diagnostic testing in the presence of maternal or paternal carrier status, and before any sonographic markers are present. Examples of such conditions include cystic fibrosis, tuberous sclerosis, fragile X, thalassemia, sickle cell, storage diseases, and others. There are also associations as VATER association, or autosomal recessive inherited conditions such as Fryns syndrome (Fig. 10.20) with no specific genetic identification to date. Table 6.6 lists several genetic syndromes and conditions that the authors diagnosed in the first trimester of pregnancy along with their corresponding ultrasound figures, presented in various chapters of this book.

Detailed discussion of ultrasound features and genetic testing of all genetic syndromes is beyond the scope of this book. Interested readers are referred to reference books[23] and Internet sites such as Online Mendelian Inheritance in Man (www.OMIM.org) and Orphanet (www.orphanet.net).

# Deletion 18p- (De Grouchy Syndrome)

18

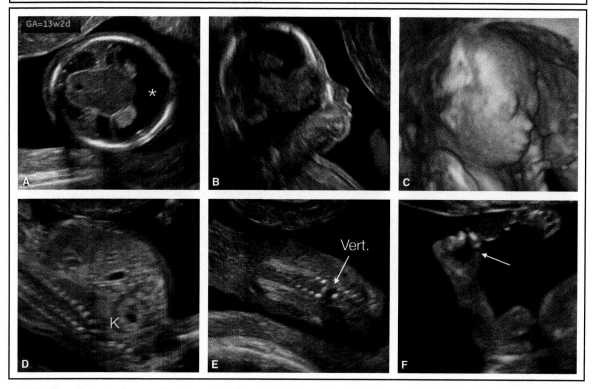

**Figure 6.36:** First trimester ultrasound at 13 weeks of gestation showing the presence of alobar holoprosencephaly (*asterisk*) in **A**, abnormal face in **B** and **C**, dysplastic kidneys (K) in **D**, vertebral anomalies (Vert.) in **E**, and clenched fingers (*arrow*) in **F**. Chorionic villous sampling revealed a deletion of the small arm of chromosome 18 (*red arrow*). 18p- deletions are typically associated with holoprosencephaly as the TGIF gene is present on the short arm of chromosome 18 as well as spinal and others anomalies. Keep in mind that noninvasive prenatal testing in such a condition would have missed the diagnosis.

**Table 6.6 •** Genetic and Syndromic Conditions Presented in This Book along with the Corresponding Figures

| | |
|---|---|
| Beckwith–Wiedemann syndrome | Figure 12.18 |
| Campomelic dysplasia | Figure 14.23 |
| CHARGE syndrome | Figure 9.32 |
| Diastrophic dysplasia | Figure 14.20 |
| Ellis–Van Creveld syndrome | Figure 14.22 |
| Femur-fibula-ulna (FFU) complex | Figures 14.25 and 14.32 |
| Fryns syndrome | Figure 10.20 |
| Grebe dysplasia | Figure 14.33 |
| Holoprosencephaly, autosomal-dominant nonsyndromic | Figure 8.30 |
| Joubert syndrome Type 14 | Figure 8.22 |
| Meckel–Gruber syndrome | Figures 8.21, 13.30, and 13.31 |
| Noonan syndrome | Figure 9.45 |
| Osteogenesis imperfecta Type II | Figures 14.18 and 14.19 |
| Short-rib-polydactyly syndrome | Figure 14.18 |
| Thanatophoric dysplasia | Figure 14.21 |
| VACTERL–VATER association | Figure 12.36 |
| Walker–Warburg syndrome | Figure 8.35 |

## REFERENCES

1. Syngelaki A, Guerra L, Ceccacci I, et al. Impact of holoprosencephaly, exomphalos, megacystis and high NT in first trimester screening for chromosomal abnormalities. *Ultrasound Obstet Gynecol.* 2016. doi:10.1002/uog.17286.

2. Szabó J, Gellén J. Nuchal fluid accumulation in trisomy-21 detected by vaginosonography in first trimester. *Lancet.* 1990;336:1133.

3. Schulte-Vallentin M, Schindler H. Non-echogenic nuchal oedema as a marker in trisomy 21 screening. *Lancet.* 1992;339:1053.

4. Nicolaides KH, Azar G, Byrne D, et al. Fetal nuchal translucency: ultrasound screening for chromosomal defects in first trimester of pregnancy. *BMJ (Clin Res ed).* 1992;304:867–869.

5. Nicolaides KH. Screening for fetal aneuploidies at 11 to 13 weeks. *Prenat Diagn.* 2011;31:7–15.

6. Santorum M, Wright D, Syngelaki A, et al. Accuracy of first trimester combined test in screening for trisomies 21, 18 and 13. *Ultrasound Obstet Gynecol.* 2016. doi:10.1002/uog.17283.

7. Wiechec M, Knafel A, Nocun A, et al. How effective is ultrasound-based screening for trisomy 18 without the addition of biochemistry at the time of late first trimester? *J Perinat Med.* 2016;44:149–159.

8. Wagner P, Sonek J, Hoopmann M, et al. First-trimester screening for trisomies 18 and 13, triploidy and Turner syndrome by detailed early anomaly scan. *Ultrasound Obstet Gynecol.* 2016;48:446–451.

9. Spencer K, Tul N, Nicolaides KH. Maternal serum free beta-hCG and PAPP-A in fetal sex chromosome defects in the first trimester. *Prenat Diagn.* 2000;20:390–394.

10. Wiechec M, Knafel A, Nocun A, et al. What are the most common first-trimester ultrasound findings in cases of Turner syndrome? *J Matern Fetal Neonatal Med.* 2016. doi:10.1080/14767058.2016.1220525.

11. Spencer K, Liao AW, Skentou H, et al. Screening for triploidy by fetal nuchal translucency and maternal serum free beta-hCG and PAPP-A at 10-14 weeks of gestation. *Prenat Diagn.* 2000;20:495–499.

12. Engelbrechtsen L, Brøndum-Nielsen K, Ekelund C, et al. Detection of triploidy at 11–14 weeks' gestation: a cohort study of 198 000 pregnant women. *Ultrasound Obstet Gynecol.* 2013;42:530–535.

13. Zalel Y, Shapiro I, Weissmann-Brenner A, et al. Prenatal sonographic features of triploidy at 12–16 weeks. *Prenat Diagn.* 2016;36:650–655.

14. Illanes S, Denbow M, Kailasam C, et al. Early detection of cell-free fetal DNA in maternal plasma. *Early Hum Dev.* 2007;83:563–566.

15. Lo YM, Zhang J, Leung TN, et al. Rapid clearance of fetal DNA from maternal plasma. *Am J Hum Genet.* 1999;64:218–224.

16. Lo JO, Cori DF, Norton ME, et al. Noninvasive prenatal testing. *Obstet Gynecol Surv.* 2014;69:89–99.

17. Norton ME, Jacobsson B, Swamy GK, et al. Cell-free DNA analysis for noninvasive examination of trisomy. *N Engl J Med.* 2015;372:1589–1597.

18. Syngelaki A, Pergament E, Homfray T, et al. Replacing the combined test by cell-free DNA testing in screening for trisomies 21, 18 and 13: impact on the diagnosis of other chromosomal abnormalities. *Fetal Diagn Ther.* 2014;35:174–184.

19. Norton ME, Baer RJ, Wapner RJ, et al. Cell-free DNA vs sequential screening for the detection of fetal chromosomal abnormalities. *Am J Obstet Gynecol.* 2016;214:727.e1–.e6.

20. Wellesley D, Dolk H, Boyd PA, et al. Rare chromosome abnormalities, prevalence and prenatal diagnosis rates from population-based congenital anomaly registers in Europe. *Eur J Hum Genet.* 2012;20:521–526.

21. Wapner RJ, Martin CL, Levy B, et al. Chromosomal microarray versus karyotyping for prenatal diagnosis. *N Engl J Med.* 2012;367:2175–2184.

22. Srebniak MI, Diderich KE, Joosten M, et al. Prenatal SNP array testing in 1000 fetuses with ultrasound anomalies: causative, unexpected and susceptibility CNVs. *Eur J Hum Genet.* 2016;24:645–651.

23. Jones KL, Jones MC, del Campo M. *Smith's Recognizable Patterns of Human Malformation.* 7 ed. Philadelphia, PA: Saunders; 2013.

# CHAPTER 7

# Multiple Pregnancies in the First Trimester

## INTRODUCTION

The widespread use of assisted reproductive technologies along with increasing maternal age has resulted in a steady rise in the frequency of multiple pregnancies over the past two decades.[1] Pregnancies with twins and higher order multiples are at an increased risk for many maternal and fetal/child complications to include miscarriage, gestational diabetes, hypertensive disorders, preterm birth, fetal genetic and congenital malformation, fetal growth restriction, perinatal death, and cerebral palsy.[2,3]

Ultrasound is an integral part of the clinical care of multiple pregnancies, from the initial diagnosis to guiding the delivery of the neonates. In this chapter, we review the utility of ultrasound in the diagnosis and management of multiple pregnancies in the first trimester with a focus on twin pregnancies. Detailed evaluation of fetal congenital abnormalities is covered in subsequent chapters of this book. Table 7.1 lists the benefits of first trimester ultrasound in multiple pregnancies.

## PREGNANCY DATING IN TWINS

There are no significant differences in the first trimester fetal biometric measurements between fetuses of multiple pregnancies and singleton fetuses and thus singleton-derived reference

---

**Table 7.1 • Benefits of First Trimester Ultrasound in Multiple Pregnancies**

- Diagnosis of multiple pregnancies
- Pregnancy dating
- Determining chorionicity
- Evaluation of fetal anatomy
- Assessment for the presence of multiple pregnancy complications
- Guiding chorionic villous sampling and other interventions

---

measurements of crown-rump length (CRL), biparietal diameter (BPD), head circumference (HC), abdominal circumference (AC), and femur length can be used in multiple pregnancies.[4] Criteria for first trimester assignment of gestational age on ultrasound are also similar in twins and singletons and are discussed in detail in Chapter 4 of this book. Twin pregnancies are best dated when the CRL measurement is performed between 11+0 and 13+6 weeks of gestation.[5] In twin pregnancies conceived by in vitro fertilization, the oocyte retrieval date or the embryonic age should date the pregnancy.[5] In early gestation, the growth rate of twins is no different than that of singletons. On occasions, differential growth in twin fetuses can be detected by differences in biometric measurements such as CRL, BPD, and HC. When this situation is noted, it is recommended to date the twin pregnancy based on the biometric measurements (CRL) of the larger twin.[5] For twin pregnancies presenting after 14 weeks of gestation, the larger HC should be used for pregnancy dating when biometric discrepancy is noted.[6]

## ETIOLOGY AND PLACENTATION IN TWINS

Twin pregnancies are classified into two main categories—dizygotic and monozygotic—based upon the number of eggs fertilized at conception.

### Dizygotic Twins

Dizygotic twins, also called fraternal, occur when two eggs are fertilized with two separate sperms resulting in two fetuses that are distinct genetically but share the same uterus. Dizygotic twins are always dichorionic/diamniotic, as each fetus has its own set of placenta and membranes. Several factors affect the rate of dizygotic twinning including maternal age, race, increasing parity, geographic area and presence of assisted reproduction.[7] The rate of dizygotic twinning varies significantly around the world with high rates reported in parts of Nigeria and low rates reported in Southeast Asia and Latin America.[7,8]

## Monozygotic Twins

Monozygotic twins (also referred to as identical) occur when one egg is fertilized by one sperm followed by division of the embryo into two. These twins are therefore typically identical genetically. Unlike dizygotic twins, the rate of monozygotic twins is fairly constant throughout the world at 1/250 pregnancies[9] excluding pregnancies of assisted reproduction. Monozygotic twins are associated with higher pregnancy complications and perinatal morbidity and mortality than dizygotic twins. Monozygotic twins can have various types of placentation based upon the timing of the division of the fertilized egg. Table 7.2 shows types of placentation in monozygotic twins in relation to the timing of embryo cleavage. Although conceptually monozygotic twins are identical, post-fertilization genetic events result in genetic heterogeneity between the twin pairs.[10,11] Furthermore, discordance in fetal malformations, which poses significant challenges in clinical management, is not uncommon in monozygotic twins.

## Zygosity and Chorionicity in Twins

Zygosity refers to whether the twins are genetically identical or not, whereas chorionicity refers to the type of placentation in twins. As shown in Table 7.2, monozygotic twins (identical) can have different types of placentation based upon the time of division of the fertilized egg, whereas dizygotic twins always have two separate placentas that on occasions can appear fused on ultrasound. Parents commonly ask at the time of the ultrasound examination whether their unborn twins are identical or not. It is important to note that the sonographic diagnosis of identical twins can only be made when the criteria for a monochorionic pregnancy (discussed later in this chapter) are met. When a dichorionic spontaneous twin pregnancy is diagnosed by ultrasound, the chance of identical twins in this setting is about 10%. From the point of view of pregnancy care chorionicity is therefore more important than zygosity.

## DETERMINING CHORIONICITY/ AMNIONICITY IN TWINS

First trimester ultrasound can determine the type of placentation in twins with high accuracy. The diagnosis of dichorionic/diamniotic twin pregnancy can be made accurately when two separate and distinct chorionic sacs are seen in the endometrial cavity as early as the fifth week of gestation (Fig. 7.1). Indeed, until about 8 weeks of gestation, the presence of two distinct gestational sacs on ultrasound with embryos/cardiac activities confirms a dichorionic/diamniotic twin gestation (Fig. 7.2). Later on in early gestation, when two adjoining gestational sacs or fetuses are seen within the endometrial cavity, the characteristic of the dividing membrane(s), when present, is the most accurate way for determining chorionicity. Indeed, chorionicity should be ideally determined between 11 + 0 and 13 + 6 weeks of gestation if feasible.[6] If the placenta

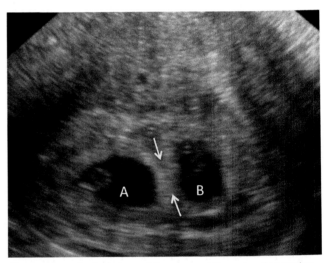

**Figure 7.1:** Sagittal plane of the uterus at 5 weeks of gestation with two distinct chorionic sacs *A* and *B*. The thick separation of the chorionic sacs (*arrows*) suggests a dichorionic twin gestation.

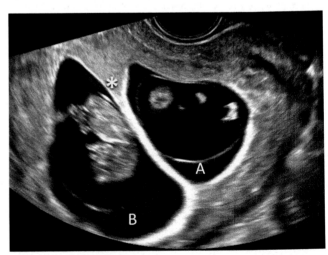

**Figure 7.2:** Dichorionic-diamniotic twins (*A* and *B*) at 9 week of gestation. Note the thick dividing membrane with a twin-peak sign (*asterisk*) at the placental insertion of the membranes.

| Table 7.2 • Types of Placentation in Monozygotic Twins in Relation to Timing of Embryo Cleavage | | |
| --- | --- | --- |
| **Embryo Cleavage (d)** | **Placentation Type** | **Frequency** |
| 0–3 | Dichorionic/diamniotic | ~25% |
| 4–8 | Monochorionic/diamniotic | ~75% |
| 9–12 | Monochorionic/monoamniotic | ~1% |
| 13–15 | Conjoined | Rare |

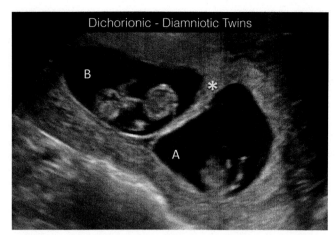

Figure 7.3: Dichorionic-diamniotic twins (*A* and *B*) at 11 weeks of gestation. Note the thick dividing membrane with a twin-peak sign (*asterisk*) at the placental insertion of the membranes.

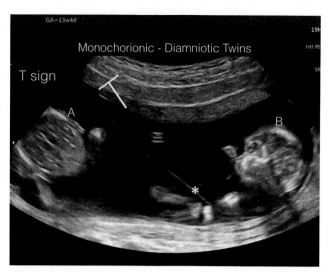

Figure 7.5: Monochorionic-diamniotic twins (*A* and *B*) at 13 weeks of gestation. The dividing membrane (*asterisk*) is thin with a T-shape configuration at placental insertion (*T*). See Figure 7.6.

appears to fill the junction of the dividing membrane(s) at its insertion into the placenta, resulting in a thick wedge-shaped configuration (lambda or twin-peak sign), this is diagnostic of dichorionic/diamniotic placentation (**Figs. 7.2 to 7.4**).

In monochorionic pregnancies, the dividing membrane attach to the uterine wall in a thin T-shaped configuration without any placental tissue at its insertion site (**Figs. 7.5 and 7.6**). The shape of the placental attachment of the dividing membranes (T-shaped) has a very high sensitivity and specificity for the diagnosis of monochorionicity between 11 and 14 weeks of gestation. Commonly, the presence of communicating fetal vessels on the surface of the twin placenta can be documented by ultrasound in color Doppler and this finding confirms the presence of monochorionic pregnancy (**Fig. 7.6**). The demonstration of such vessels however has no clinical relevance to twin pregnancy management. Although in general the number of yolk sacs correlates with the number of amnions (**Fig. 7.7**),

this rule has many exceptions, as monoamniotic twins can be associated with a single yolk sac, a partially divided yolk sac, or two yolk sacs. For pregnancies beyond 8 weeks of gestation, the number of placental masses can be assessed as the presence of two distinct placental masses signifies a dichorionic gestation. The reliability of the number of placental masses is questionable, however, as in about 3% of monochorionic twin pregnancies two placental masses can be seen on ultrasound.[12] The thickness of the twin separating membrane can also be used for determining chorionicity, and similar to findings

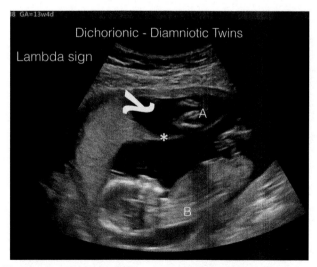

Figure 7.4: Dichorionic-diamniotic twins (*A* and *B*) at 13 weeks of gestation. The separating membrane (*asterisk*) is thick with a twin-peak or lambda sign (*λ*) at the placental insertion of the membranes.

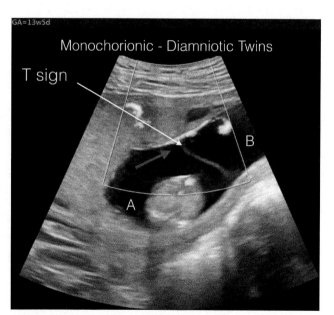

Figure 7.6: Monochorionic-diamniotic twin pregnancy at 13 weeks of gestation. A thin separating membrane is visible with a T-shape configuration at placental insertion separating twin *A* from twin *B*. The use of color Doppler shows in this case an artery with a course from twin *A* to *B* (*red arrow*). Such connections are present in almost all monochorionic placentas and can occasionally be demonstrated on ultrasound by color Doppler as shown here.

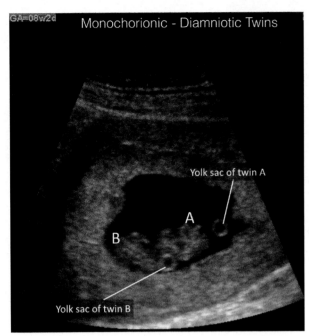

Figure 7.7: Monochorionic-diamniotic twins (*A* and *B*) at 8 weeks of gestation. Note the presence of two yolk sacs. A thin separating membrane is not visible in this image. The presence of two yolk sacs at this gestation suggests monochorionic-diamniotic pregnancy but does not confirm it. The presence of a dividing membrane on follow-up ultrasound examinations with high-resolution transducers, confirmed this diagnosis.

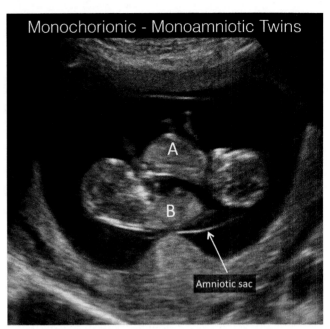

Figure 7.9: Monochorionic-monoamniotic twins (*A* and *B*) at 10 weeks of gestation. Note the presence of a single amniotic sac (labeled) with no dividing membrane.

in the second trimester, this technique is not reliable to be solely used for chorionicity diagnosis. Occasionally the use of three-dimensional ultrasound can help in assessing membrane thickness in the first trimester of pregnancy (Fig. 7.8). Discordance in fetal gender at 13 weeks of gestation and beyond implies the presence of dichorionic gestation.

When no dividing membrane is noted on ultrasound, especially with high-frequency transvaginal or transabdominal transducer, the diagnosis of monoamniotic twins can be performed (Fig. 7.9). Color and pulsed Doppler confirms the diagnosis of monoamniotic twins by demonstrating the presence of cord entanglement (Fig. 7.10), which is almost universally seen in these pregnancies (discussed later in this chapter). Conjoined twins are diagnosed by ultrasound in the first trimester when shared tissue is noted between twins and

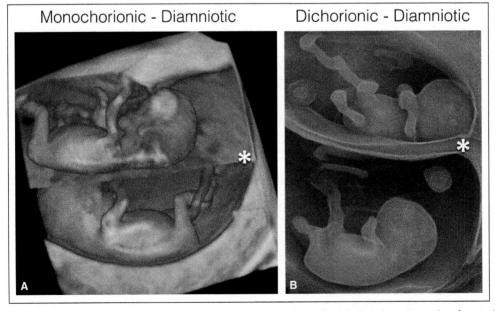

Figure 7.8: Three-dimensional (3D) ultrasound in surface mode in a monochorionic-diamniotic twin at 11 weeks of gestation with a thin membrane (*asterisk*) **(A)** and in a dichorionic-diamniotic twin at 10 weeks of gestation with a thick separating membrane (*asterisk*) **(B)**. 3D can support but not replace 2D gray scale ultrasound in the diagnosis of chorionicity.

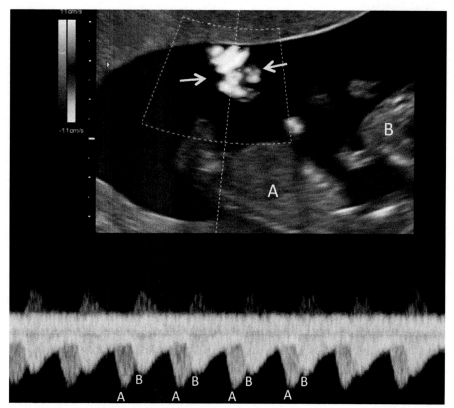

**Figure 7.10:** Monochorionic-monoamniotic twins (*A* and *B*) at 13 weeks of gestation with cord entanglement seen on color and pulsed Doppler modes. Note the presence of a mass of cord (*arrows*) on color Doppler. Pulsed Doppler with a wide sample gate confirms cord entanglement by demonstrating two distinct Doppler waveforms (*A* and *B*) within the same Doppler spectrum.

confirmed on color Doppler evaluation demonstrating shared vasculature (discussed later in this chapter).

The first trimester ultrasound is thus very accurate in determining chorionicity in twin pregnancies with rates approaching 100% when correlated with delivery. Chorionicity should be determined before 14 weeks of gestation if feasible as the accuracy of ultrasound in determining chorionicity decreases with advancing gestation. It is therefore imperative that an early gestation ultrasound, preferably in the first trimester, be part of the management of twin gestation and that chorionicity is determined and reported at that time when feasible. As pregnancy advances, the accuracy of determining chorionicity and amnionicity decreases. The accuracy of determining chorionicity and amnionicity is estimated around 90% in the second and third trimester of pregnancy with the twin-peak or lambda sign being the most accurate and reliable method.[13,14]

## ULTRASOUND LABELING OF TWIN FETUSES

Accurate labeling of twin pregnancy by ultrasound is important and should be clearly reflected in the report. Traditionally, twins have been labeled as twin A and twin B based upon fetal presentations in relationship to the cervix. This is confusing as fetal presentations may change during pregnancy and it is not uncommon for twin B to be born first at cesarean section,

which presents confusion for parents. It is recommended to follow a descriptive process for twin labeling that takes into account the location of each gestational sac in relationship to maternal right or left side and the position of the sac in the uterus as upper or lower.[5] For instance, twin A can be referred to as "on maternal left with posterior placenta and lower gestational sac." This can be performed in the first trimester by the 13th week of gestation.

## MONITORING OF TWIN PREGNANCY

One of the most important benefits of first trimester ultrasound is the diagnosis of twins and the designation of chorionicity. When dichorionic twins are diagnosed in the first trimester, follow-up ultrasound is recommended at 18 to 20 weeks of gestation and if uncomplicated every 4 weeks thereafter.[5] When monochorionic twins are diagnosed in the first trimester, follow-up ultrasound is recommended at 16 weeks and every 2 weeks thereafter in order to detect monochorionic complications such as twin-twin transfusion syndrome (TTTS) and twin anemia polycythemia syndrome (TAPS; both discussed later in this chapter).[5] With each ultrasound examination in the second trimester and beyond, fetal biometry, amniotic fluid volume, and umbilical artery Doppler should be obtained to screen for twin discordance and in monochorionic pregnancies, middle cerebral artery Doppler is also recommended to screen for fetal anemia.[5] In the presence of twin complications, more rigorous follow-up is recommended.

In one study, a combined risk assessment approach in the first and second trimester (16 weeks) ultrasound identified a subgroup of monochorionic twin pregnancies with a risk of complicated fetal outcome, reported as greater than 70% with a survival rate of only 69%.[15] The presence of intertwin CRL difference or discordant amniotic fluid volumes in the first trimester along with 16 weeks of gestation differences in AC, discordance in amniotic fluid volumes, or site of cord insertions predicted poor outcome.[15]

## SCREENING AND TESTING FOR CHROMOSOMAL ABNORMALITIES IN TWINS

First trimester screening for chromosomal abnormalities in twins can be performed with maternal age, nuchal translucency (NT), and biochemical markers such as free beta-human chorionic gonadotropin ($\beta$-HCG) and pregnancy-associated plasma protein A (PAPP-A), with maternal age and NT alone or with cell-free DNA (cfDNA). In monochorionic twins, Down syndrome risk is calculated as the average risk of both fetuses, whereas in dichorionic twins, the risk is calculated per fetus A and B. It is unclear whether the detection rate of Down syndrome is lower in twins than in singletons, as studies have shown conflicting results.[6,16] In the presence of a vanishing twin with a visible fetal pole, screening for chromosomal abnormalities is best performed with maternal age and NT alone, as the demised twin will alter biochemical markers. cfDNA is a Down syndrome screening modality associated with very high sensitivity and low false-positive rate. More data are accumulating on the role of cfDNA as a robust screening test in twin gestation with Down syndrome–reported detection rates of 94.4% with a near 0% false-positive rate.[17]

Invasive testing with chorionic villous sampling and amniocentesis for diagnostic purposes appears to carry a higher loss rate in twins than in singletons irrespective of the modality and approach used.[18] It is important therefore to council pregnant women with twins appropriately and discusses the complexity inherent in genetic screening and diagnostic testing and the clinical implication of an abnormal diagnostic test. The option for selective feticide should also be discussed with the patient during genetic counseling.

## CONGENITAL ANOMALIES IN TWINS

The risk of fetal anomalies is greater in twins when compared with singletons and this risk is especially increased for monochorionic and monoamniotic twin pregnancies.[15,19,20] In a retrospective analysis of prospectively collected data on 1,064 twin pregnancies, detection of structural abnormalities in the

first trimester occurred in 27.3% of cases.[21] This is compared to approximately half of fetal malformations detected in the first trimester in singleton pregnancies.[22] Similar to the pattern seen in singleton pregnancies, the likelihood for first trimester detection of structural abnormalities in twin pregnancies was best for cranial vault (Fig. 7.11), midline brain, and abdominal wall defects.[21,22] Monochorionicity and discordance on CRL and NT were associated with an increased risk of fetal anomalies with a moderate predictive accuracy.[21]

It is important to note that a smaller than expected CRL in a twin member is not only associated with an increased risk for fetal malformations, but also with an increased risk for chromosomal abnormalities, fetal loss, preterm delivery, and birth weight discordance.[4,5,23] The critical threshold for CRL-twin discordance in the first trimester has not been clearly defined. In general, studies addressing this issue defined twin discordance as a CRL difference of at least 10% or 7 days.[5,23–25] Pregnancy counseling, consideration for genetic testing, and detailed first trimester ultrasound examination is therefore appropriate when early gestation biometric discordance is noted in multiple pregnancies.

The presence of twin discordance in fetal anomalies presents a challenging clinical scenario. In such cases, management at a center with expertise in fetal medicine is recommended. When one fetus of a dichorionic twin pregnancy presents with a lethal anomaly that carries a high risk for in utero demise, conservative management is generally recommended (Fig. 7.11),[5] whereas in monochorionic twin pregnancy, this situation may warrant an intervention with cord occlusion, laser, or radiofrequency cord ablation of the anomalous twin in order to protect the health of the normal twin should a demise occur.[5]

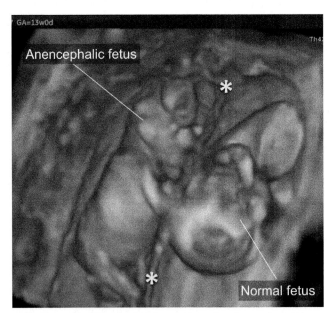

**Figure 7.11:** Dichorionic twins at 13 weeks of gestation with a thick dividing membrane (*asterisks*). These twins are discordant for anomaly as seen on three-dimensional ultrasound in surface mode. Note the presence of anencephaly in one twin and a normal head in the other twin.

# COMPLICATIONS OF TWIN GESTATION

## Vanishing Twin and Twin Demise

Vanishing twin describes the clinical situation where following documentation of a twin gestation by ultrasound, subsequent follow-up ultrasounds demonstrate the disappearance of one of the gestational sacs or the demise of one of the twins (Fig. 7.12). Vanishing twin is not an uncommon phenomenon. When ultrasound examinations are performed in the first trimester, about a third of twin pregnancies will ultimately result in singletons.[26] This is even more common in higher order multiples, occurring in about 50% of triplets.[27] In general, patients with vanishing twins are asymptomatic and the pregnancy outcome does not appear to be affected. As stated previously, biochemical markers for genetic screening are typically affected, especially when the vanishing twin occurs later in the first trimester. In case of a vanishing twin with a still measurable fetal pole, NT alone or in combination with maternal age and other sonographic markers should be used for aneuploidy risk assessment.[28]

The presence of a single demise in a twin pregnancy complicates the clinical management, especially in the presence of monochorionic placentation. In this setting, careful attention should be given to ultrasound imaging with the application of color Doppler to rule out the presence of an acardiac twin with twin-reversed arterial perfusion (discussed later in this chapter). Follow-up ultrasound examinations in the second trimester are also important to rule out the presence of malformations in the surviving twin, especially involving the central nervous system. Of note, the earlier in gestation that the demise of a co-twin occurs in a monochorionic twin pregnancy, the lower is the risk of neurologic complication in the surviving twin member. In general, demise of a co-twin embryo/fetus in the first trimester in a dichorionic pregnancy typically results in a favorable outcome for the surviving twin member.

## Twin-Twin Transfusion Syndrome

TTTS, which complicates 10% to 20% of monochorionic twins,[29] is an abnormality that is seen predominantly in the second and third trimesters of pregnancy. TTTS is believed to occur when vascular anastomoses exist in a monochorionic placenta with net blood flow going to one fetus at the expense of the other. The recipient twin fetus is typically plethoric, larger in size, and has polyhydramnios due to excess urination. The donor twin fetus is anemic, smaller in size, and has a "stuck" appearance due to oligohydramnios with restricted movements. TTTS can progress quickly and lead to preterm labor and delivery if untreated. Risk factors for TTTS in monochorionic-diamniotic pregnancies include the presence of velamentous cord insertion and/or placental arteriovenous (AV) anastomosis without compensating arterioarterial anastomosis.[30] Given that placental vascular anastomoses cannot be accurately diagnosed prenatally on ultrasound, close ultrasound follow-up (every other week) of monochorionic-diamniotic twins is recommended starting at 16 weeks of gestation.[5]

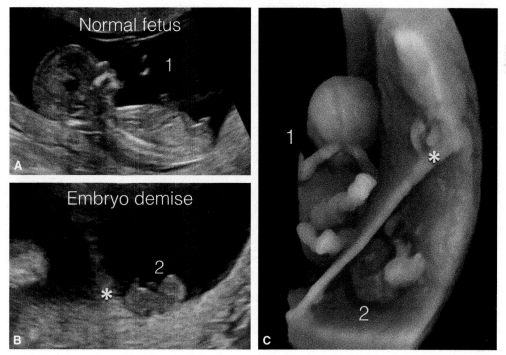

**Figure 7.12:** Dichorionic twins at 13 weeks of gestation with a normal fetus (*1*), shown in **A** on midsagittal plane and a small demised embryo (*2*), shown on gray scale ultrasound in **B**. In three-dimensional ultrasound in surface mode **(C)**, fetuses (*1*) and (*2*) are seen, separated by a thick membrane (*asterisk*).

Second and third trimester ultrasound is essential for the diagnosis and management of TTTS. Criteria for establishing the diagnosis of TTTS by ultrasound include a monochorionic placenta, polyhydramnios in one sac with a maximum vertical pocket of equal to or greater than 8 cm and oligohydramnios in the other sac with a maximum vertical pocket of less than 2 cm, in the absence of congenital abnormalities that may explain fluid and growth discrepancies. In Europe, the diagnosis of polyhydramnios is made when the maximum vertical pocket is greater to or equal to 8 cm by 20 weeks of gestation and 10 cm after 20 weeks.[5] Concurrent confirmatory features include a small or non-visible bladder in the donor twin and an enlarged bladder in the recipient twin.

On rare occasions, TTTS can be suspected in the first trimester by the presence of CRL and NT discordance in the setting of a monochorionic-diamniotic twin pregnancy.[31,32] Other first trimester warning signs include twin discordance on Doppler findings, especially of the ductus venosus (DV).[33] It is important to note however that the predictive value of CRL, NT, and DV for TTTS in the first trimester is relatively poor with significant false positives and negatives.[5] Close monitoring of the monochorionic pregnancy by ultrasound is still the optimal approach to the early diagnosis of TTTS.

## Twin Reversed Arterial Perfusion

Twin reversed arterial perfusion (TRAP), known as acardiac twinning, is a very rare condition characterized by monochorionic placentation and absence of a functioning heart in one fetus of a twin pregnancy (Figs 7.13 to 7.15). Color Doppler and three-dimensional ultrasound in the first trimester is helpful in confirming the presence of TRAP and in assessing the size of the acardiac twin in relationship to the normal twin (Figs. 7.13 to 7.15). TRAP can be considered as a severe form of TTTS. The normal fetus perfuses the acardiac mass by an arterial-to-arterial anastomosis on the placental surface. Typically in normal conditions, the umbilical arteries carry blood from the fetus to the placenta. In TRAP, the anastomosis allows for reverse perfusion to the acardiac mass (Fig. 7.15), thus the acronym TRAP. The acardiac fetus commonly has multiple anatomic and growth abnormalities. Given that the normal fetus has to perfuse his/her body and that of the acardiac mass, there is a significant increase in cardiac workload and a risk for cardiac failure and hydrops. The overall perinatal mortality of the normal fetus in TRAP syndrome is in the range of 30% to 50%.[34,35] Beyond the first trimester, frequent echocardiographic evaluation of the normal twin in TRAP syndrome may help recognize cardiovascular stress and help guide management. The ratio of the estimated weight of

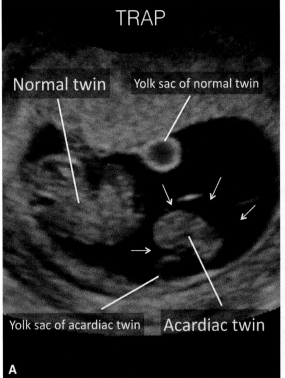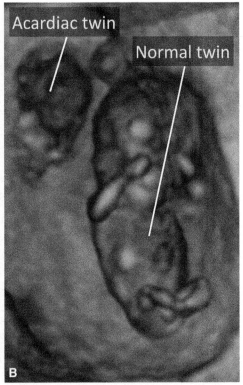

**Figure 7.13: A:** Gray scale ultrasound of an acardiac twin reversed arterial perfusion (TRAP) in a monochorionic twin pregnancy at 9 weeks of gestation. Note the presence of an amorphous mass of tissue with an amniotic membrane covering (*small arrows*) and a yolk sac, representing the acardiac twin. The normal twin is seen with its own yolk sac. **B:** Three-dimensional ultrasound in surface mode 2 weeks later showing the amorphous acardiac twin with the TRAP and the adjoining normal fetus.

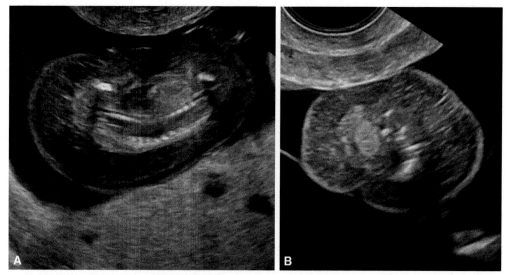

**Figure 7.14:** Two acardiac twin fetuses **(A** and **B)** in monochorionic-diamniotic pregnancies at 14 and 13 weeks of gestation, respectively, complicated by twin reversal arterial perfusion (TRAP) sequence. Acardiac twins may have various appearances but typically body edema is present. Often, a part of a spine **(A)** and some bones **(A** and **B)** are found and occasionally some parts of the lower body may be present along with lower extremities. In general, the mass appears amorphous without any typical anatomic features. See Figure 7.15.

the acardiac twin to that of the normal twin has been used to assess mortality risk.[34] Treatment options include expectant management with close observation, or cord coagulation of the acardiac twin. Bipolar cord coagulation of the acardiac twin appears to be the most feasible option for cord occlusion and is best performed before 24 weeks of gestation. Treatment intervention before 16 weeks of gestation is preferable when technically feasible.[36]

## Twin Anemia Polycythemia Syndrome

TAPS is another form of TTTS characterized by significant discrepancy in fetal hemoglobin in monochorionic twins with normal fluids in both sacs. Suggested pathophysiology includes small AV placental anastomosis with slow blood transfusion from one twin member to the other. Incomplete

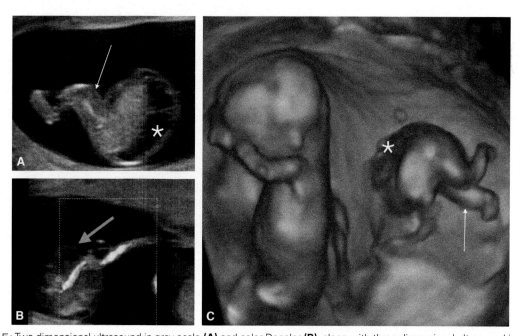

**Figure 7.15:** Two-dimensional ultrasound in gray scale **(A)** and color Doppler **(B)**, along with three-dimensional ultrasound in surface mode **(C)** of a monochorionic twin pregnancy at 12 weeks of gestation with twin reversal arterial perfusion (TRAP) sequence. Note in **A** the presence of edema (*asterisk*) and a lower extremity with a femur bone (*arrow*). Color Doppler of the umbilical artery in **B** shows opposite flow (*blue color*), with flow directed from the placenta to the acardiac fetus (*blue arrow*), typical of the TRAP sequence. Three-dimensional ultrasound shows the acardiac twin with both legs (*arrow*) and lower body formed with edema (*asterisk*).

laser treatment of TTTS may also lead to TAPS.[37] The diagnosis is typically performed in the late second or third trimester of pregnancy. Intertwin discordance in peak systolic velocities of the middle cerebral arteries (anemia in one twin member) suggests the diagnosis. Pregnancy outcome of TAPS is generally more favorable than the classic forms of TTTS and TRAP.[37]

## Cord Entanglement in Monoamniotic Twins

Monochorionic/monoamniotic twins (monoamniotic twins) account for about 1% of all monochorionic twins. The diagnosis is established when a monochorionic placenta is noted in a twin pregnancy in the absence of a dividing membrane. It is important to confirm this diagnosis after multiple sonographic evaluations. The transvaginal approach is recommended in the first trimester given the high resolution of the transducer and its proximity to the pregnancy. Monoamniotic twins tend to have placental cord insertions that are in close proximity and are at significant risk of cord entanglement. Cord entanglement can be suspected in the first trimester by gray scale and confirmed by color and pulsed Doppler evaluation. In our experience, cord entanglement is an almost universal finding in monoamniotic pregnancies and can often be diagnosed in the first trimester.

In the first trimester, cord entanglement appears as a mass of cord between the two fetuses. Color Doppler will confirm that this mass is indeed entanglement of umbilical cords (Fig 7.10) and pulsed Doppler can confirm the diagnosis by documenting two distinct Doppler waveforms, with different fetal heart rate patterns (twin A and twin B) on one Doppler spectrum (Fig. 7.10). In order to obtain these waveforms, a wide Doppler gate should be applied to the suspected cord entanglement region. The authors have correlated the presence of umbilical artery waveform notching on pulsed Doppler evaluation in monoamniotic twins with cord entanglement in the second and third trimesters of pregnancy.[38] In the absence of signs of fetal compromise, the presence of cord entanglement with or without umbilical artery waveform notching in monoamniotic twins does not appear to contribute significantly to perinatal morbidity and mortality however.[39,40]

## Conjoined Twins

Conjoined twins are very rare complications of monochorionic twinning, which results from incomplete division of the fertilized egg between days 13 and 15 from conception. The incidence varies and is reported between 1 in 50,000 and 1 in 250,000 births.[41] The anatomic site of conjunction describes conjoined twins. Complex types are described by a combination of forms. The five common types of conjoined twins and their frequencies are listed in Table 7.3.

**Table 7.3 •** Types and Frequency of Conjoined Twins

| Type | Frequency |
|---|---|
| Craniopagus (head) | 1%–2% |
| Thoracopagus (chest) | 75% |
| Omphalopagus (abdomen) | Rare |
| Pygopagus (rump) | 20% |
| Ischiopagus (pelvis) | 5% |

The diagnosis of conjoined twins can be easily made in the first trimester by gray scale and color Doppler ultrasound by demonstrating shared tissue on gray scale (Figs. 7.16 to 7.19) and vasculature on color Doppler between twins (Figs. 7.16B, 7.17C, and 7.18A). Three-dimensional ultrasound in surface mode in the first trimester can also confirm the presence of conjoined twins by demonstrating the anatomic site of shared tissue (Figs. 7.17 to 7.19). The prognosis is generally poor and is dependent on the degree and site of fusion and the extent of joined organs. Sharing of major organs complicates postnatal management and worsens the prognosis. Extensive multidisciplinary counseling should be part of the prenatal management of conjoined twins.

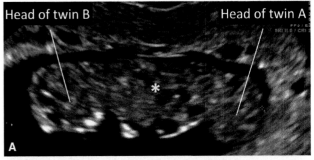

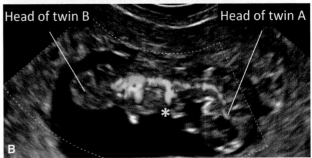

**Figure 7.16:** Conjoined twins noted on two-dimensional gray scale ultrasound at 9 weeks of gestation **(A)**. Note the fusion of twins in the pelvic area (*asterisk*). Cephalic regions of twins are labeled. **B:** The conjoined twins with color Doppler ultrasound confirming vascular connectivity between the two embryos (*asterisk*). Color Doppler can be used to confirm the diagnosis of conjoined twins, and differentiate it from monoamniotic non-fused embryos that are closely positioned in the amniotic cavity. Cephalic region of twins is labeled.

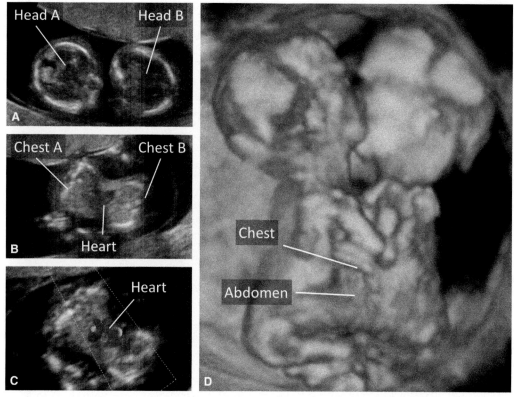

**Figure 7.17:** Thoracopagus conjoined twins have typically the heads close to each other **(A)**. At the level of the chest an abnormal heart is shared by both as shown in **B** and in color Doppler in **C**. In another fetus with thoracoomphalopagus at 12 weeks of gestation, three-dimensional ultrasound in surface mode **(D)** shows that the twins are joined at the chest and abdomen.

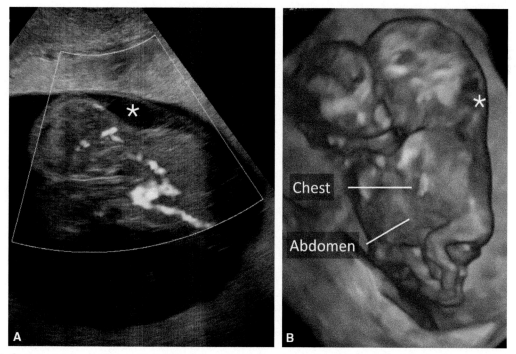

**Figure 7.18:** Conjoined twin gestation with thoracopagus at 10 weeks of gestation with joined hearts seen in color Doppler in a longitudinal view **(A)** and displayed in three-dimensional ultrasound in surface mode **(B)**. Thickened nuchal translucency (*asterisk*) is present in both fetuses.

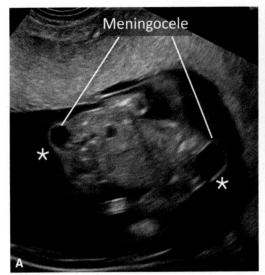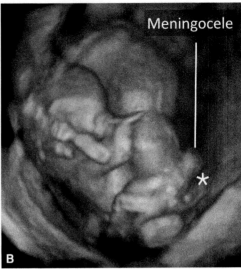

**Figure 7.19:** Conjoined twins at 13 weeks of gestation with thoracoomphalopagus. Note the presence of closed spina bifida, shown as cystic meningocele (*asterisks*), seen in an axial view at the level of the abdomen in **A** and in three-dimensional ultrasound in surface mode in **B** (*asterisk*).

## CONCLUSION

The first trimester ultrasound plays an important role in the management of multiple pregnancies. As discussed in this chapter, first trimester ultrasound allows for pregnancy dating and for determination of chorionicity with high accuracy. With recent improvements in transducer technology, ultrasound is currently able to diagnose a substantial number of major fetal malformations in the first trimester. This is of particular relevance to multiple pregnancies given an overall increased rate of fetal malformations as compared to singletons, especially for monochorionic pregnancies. Following chapters in this book present a systematic approach to the diagnosis of fetal malformations in the first trimester of pregnancy.

## REFERENCES

1. Martin JA, Hamilton BE, Ventura SJ, et al. Births: final data for 2011. *Natl Vital Stat Rep.* 2013;62(1):1–70.
2. Mathews TJ, MacDorman MF. Infant mortality statistics from the 2009 period linked birth/infant death data set. *Natl Vital Stat Rep.* 2013;61(8):1–28. http://www.cdc.gov/nchs/data/nvsr/nvsr61/nvsr61_08.pdf. Accessed March 17, 2017.
3. Topp M, Huusom LD, Langhoff-Roos J, et al. Multiple birth and cerebral palsy in Europe: a multicenter study. *Acta Obstet Gynecol Scand.* 2004;83(6):548–553.
4. Morin L, Lim K. Ultrasound in twin pregnancies. *J Obstet Gynaecol Can.* 2011;33(6):643–656.
5. Khalil A, Rodgers M, Baschat A, et al. ISUOG Practice Guidelines: role of ultrasound in twin pregnancy. *Ultrasound Obstet Gynecol.* 2016;47:247–263.
6. National Collaborating Center for Women's and Children's Health (UK). *Multiple Pregnancy. The Management of Twin and Triplet Pregnancies in the Antenatal Period.* Commissioned by the National Institute for Clinical Excellence. London: RCOG Press; 2011.
7. Nylander PP. The factors that influence twinning rates. *Acta Genet Med Gemellol.* 1981;30:189.
8. Smits J, Monden C. Twinning across the developing world, *PLoS One.* 2011;6(9):e25239.

9. MacGillivray I. Epidemiology of twin pregnancy. *Semin Perinatol.* 1986;10:4.
10. Silva S, Martins Y, Matias A, et al. Why are monozygotic twins different? *J Perinatal Med.* 2011;39(2):195–202.
11. Cheng PJ, Shaw SW, Shih JC, et al. Monozygotic twins discordant for Monosomy 21 detected by first trimester nuchal translucency screening. *Obstet Gynecol.* 2006;107(2, pt 2):538–541.
12. Lopriore E, Sueters M, Middeldorp JM, et al. Twin pregnancies with two separate placental masses can still be monochorionic and have vascular anastomoses. *Am J Obstet Gynecol.* 2006;194: 804–808.
13. Monteagudo A, Timor-Tritsch IE, Sharma S. Early and simple determination of chorionic and amniotic type in multifetal gestations in the first fourteen weeks by high-frequency transvaginal ultrasonography. *Am J Obstet Gynecol.* 1994;170(3):824–829.
14. Winn HN, Gabrielli S, Reece EA, et al. Ultrasonographic criteria for the prenatal diagnosis of placental chorionicity in twin gestations. *Am J Obstet Gynecol.* 1989;161(6, pt 1):1540–1542.
15. Lewi L, Jani J, Blickstein I, et al. The outcome of monochorionic diamniotic twin gestations in the era of invasive fetal therapy: a prospective cohort study. *Am J Obstet Gynecol.* 2008;199:493.e1–493.e7.
16. Prats P, Rodríguez I, Comas C, et al. Systematic review of screening for trisomy 21 in twin pregnancies in first trimester combining nuchal translucency and biochemical markers: a meta-analysis. *Prenat Diagn.* 2014;34:1077–1083.
17. Gil MM, Quezada MS, Revello R, et al. Analysis of cell-free DNA in maternal blood in screening for fetal aneuploidies: updated meta-analysis. *Ultrasound Obstet Gynecol.* 2015;45:249–266.
18. Agarwal K, Alfirevic Z. Pregnancy loss after chorionic villus sampling and genetic amniocentesis in twin pregnancies: a systematic review. *Ultrasound Obstet Gynecol.* 2012;40:128–134.
19. Vink, J, Wapner, R, D'Alton M. Prenatal diagnosis in twin gestations. *Semin Perinatol.* 2012;36:169–174.
20. Baxi LV, Walsh CA. Monoamniotic twins in contemporary practice: a single-center study of perinatal outcomes. *J Matern Fetal Neonatal Med.* 2010;23:506–510.
21. D'Antonio F, Familiari A, Thilaganathan B, et al. Sensitivity of first-trimester ultrasound in the detection of congenital anomalies in twin pregnancies: population study and systematic review. *Acta Obstet Gynecol Scand.* 2016;95:1359–1367.
22. Rossi AC, Prefumo F. Accuracy of ultrasonography at 11–14 weeks of gestation for detection of fetal structural anomalies: a systematic review. *Obstet Gynecol.* 2013;122:1160–1167.
23. Isada NB, Sorokin Y, Drugan A, et al. First trimester interfetal size variation in well-dated multifetal pregnancies. *Fetal Diagn Ther.* 1992;7(2):82–86.

24. Kalish RB, Gupta M, Perni SC, et al. Clinical significance of first trimester crown-rump length disparity in dichorionic twin gestations. *Am J Obstet Gynecol*. 2004;191(4):1437–1440.

25. D'Antonio F, Khalil A, Pagani G, et al. Crown-rump length discordance and adverse perinatal outcome in twin pregnancies: systematic review and meta-analysis. *Ultrasound Obstet Gynecol*. 2014;44(2):138–146.

26. Dickey RP, Taylor SN, Lu PY, et al. Spontaneous reduction of multiple pregnancy: incidence and effect on outcome. *Am J Obstet Gynecol*. 2002;186(1):77–83.

27. Goldman GA, Dicker D, Feldberg D, et al. The vanishing fetus. A report of 17 cases of triplets and quadruplets. *J Perinatal Med*. 1989;17(2):157–162.

28. Sankaran S, Rozette C, Dean J, et al. Screening in the presence of a vanished twin: nuchal translucency or combined screening test? *Prenat Diagn*. 2011;31:600–601.

29. Quintero RA. Twin-twin transfusion syndrome. *Clin Perinatol*. 2003;30(3):591–600.

30. Hack KE, Nikkels PG, Koopman-Esseboom C, et al. Placental characteristics of monochorionic diamniotic twin pregnancies in relation to perinatal outcome. *Placenta*. 2008;29(11):976–981.

31. El Kateb A, Nasr B, Nassar M, et al. First trimester ultrasound examination and the outcome of monochorionic twin pregnancies. *Prenatal Diagn*. 2007;27(10):922–925

32. Fratelli N, Prefumo F, Fichera A, et al. Nuchal translucency thickness and crown rump length discordance for the prediction of outcome in monochorionic diamniotic pregnancies. *Early Hum Dev*. 2011;87(1):27–30.

33. Maiz N, Nicolaides KH. Ductus venosus in the first trimester: contribution to screening of chromosomal, cardiac defects and monochorionic twin complications. *Fetal Diagn Ther*. 2010;28(2):65–71.

34. Moore TR, Gale S, Bernishke K. Perinatal outcome of forty nine pregnancies complicated by acardiac twinning. *Am J Obstet Gynecol*. 1990;163:907–912.

35. Healy MG. Acardia: predictive risk factors for the co-twin's survival. *Teratology*. 1994;50:205–213.

36. Pagani G, D'Antonio F, Khalil A, et al. Intrafetal laser treatment for twin reversed arterial perfusion sequence: cohort study and meta-analysis. *Ultrasound Obstet Gynecol*. 2013;42:6–14.

37. Slaghekke F, Kist WJ, Oepkes D, et al. Twin anemia-polycythemia sequence: diagnostic criteria, classification, perinatal management and outcome. *Fetal Diagn Ther*. 2010;27(4):181–190.

38. Abuhamad A, Mari G, Copel JC, et al. Umbilical artery flow velocity waveforms in monoamniotic twins with cord enlargement: can it be used in pregnancy management. *Obstet Gynecol*. 1995;86:674–677.

39. Rossi AC, Prefumo F. Impact of cord entanglement on perinatal outcome of monoamniotic twins: a systematic review of the literature. *Ultrasound Obstet Gynecol*. 2013;41(2):131–135.

40. Aurioles-Garibay A, Hernandez-Andrade E, Romero R, et al. Presence of an umbilical artery notch in monochorionic/monoamniotic twins. *Fetal Diagn Ther*. 2014;36:305–311.

41. Edmonds LD, Layde PM. Conjoined twins in the United States, 1970–1977. *Teratology*. 1982;25(3):301–308.

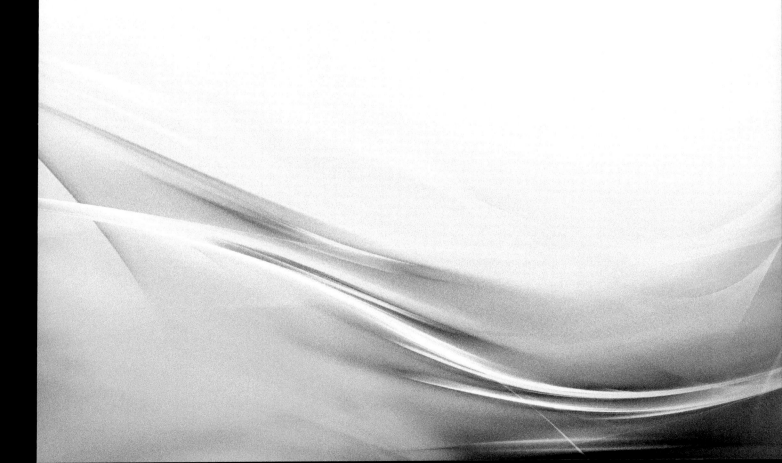

# SECTION two

# *First Trimester Ultrasound: Fetal Abnormalities*

# CHAPTER 8

# The Fetal Central Nervous System

## INTRODUCTION

The evaluation of the fetal central nervous system (CNS) is an important aspect of ultrasound in the first trimester given that several major malformations, such as anencephaly/exencephaly, holoprosencephaly (HPE), among others can be easily identified. However, detection of subtle malformations in the first trimester, such as small encephaloceles, neural tube defects, or posterior fossa abnormalities, requires a detailed ultrasound evaluation of the CNS. In this chapter we present a systematic detailed approach to the first trimester ultrasound examination of the normal CNS, followed by a comprehensive presentation of common CNS malformations that can be diagnosed in early gestation.

## EMBRYOLOGY

Formation of the fetal brain is seen as early as the fifth week of embryogenesis by outgrowth of the neural tube in its cephalic region to form three brain vesicles: the prosencephalon (forebrain), mesencephalon (midbrain), and rhombencephalon (hindbrain). By the sixth week of embryogenesis, the prosencephalon differentiates into the telencephalon and diencephalon, the mesencephalon remains unchanged, and the rhombencephalon divides into the metencephalon and myelencephalon. Ultrasound images of the fetal brain at 7 to 8 weeks of gestation (menstrual age) demonstrate these brain vesicles (**Figs. 8.1 and 8.2**). The falx cerebri, an echogenic structure that divides the brain

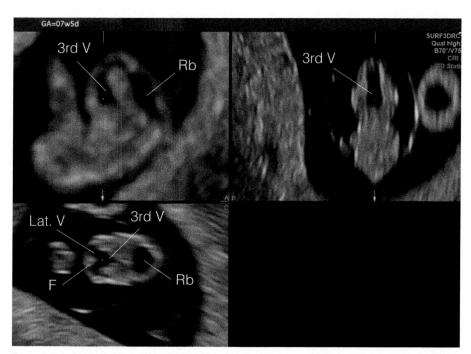

**Figure 8.1:** Three-dimensional ultrasound in multiplanar display of an embryo at 7 weeks 5 days gestation showing early development of the brain. Note the size of the rhombencephalic vesicle (Rb) in the posterior aspect of the brain as the largest brain vesicle at this stage of development. The lateral ventricles (Lat. V) and the third ventricle (3rd V) are also seen. F, falx cerebri.

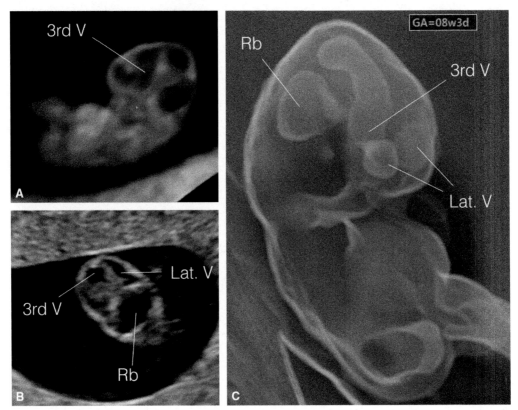

**Figure 8.2:** (**A**, **B** and **C**) Three-dimensional ultrasound volume of a fetus at 8 weeks of gestation showing early development of the brain. **A:** A sagittal view of the fetus in surface mode. **B:** A coronal plane of the fetal head retrieved from the multiplanar display. **C:** A rendered image of the fetus in Silhouette® mode. Note the anatomic relationships of the lateral (Lat. V), the third (3rd V), and the rhombencephalic (Rb) ventricles.

into two equal halves, and the choroid plexuses, which fill the lateral ventricles, are seen on ultrasound by the end of the eighth week and beginning of the ninth week of gestation (Fig. 8.3). The cerebellar hemispheres develop in the rhombencephalon and are completely formed by the 10th week of gestation, thus allowing for evaluation of the posterior fossa with optimal ultrasound imaging (Fig. 8.4). Prior to the 9th week of gestation, the cranium is not typically ossified (Fig. 8.5). Cranial ossification begins around the late 9th, early 10th week and is completed by the 12th week of gestation. Figure 8.5 shows progression in fetal cranial ossification from 9 to 13 weeks of gestation.

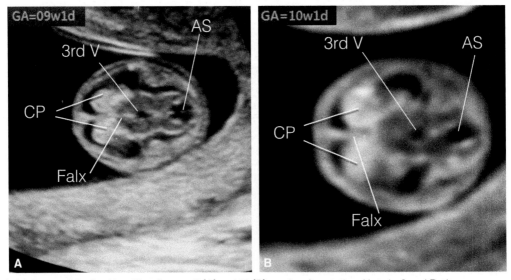

**Figure 8.3:** Axial planes of the fetal head in a fetus at 9 (**A**) and 10 (**B**) weeks of gestation. Note in **A** and **B**, the appearance of the choroid plexuses (CP) of the lateral ventricles and the falx cerebri (Falx), which are visible from 9 weeks onward. The third ventricle (3rd V) and the aqueduct of Sylvius (AS) are also recognized in these axial planes.

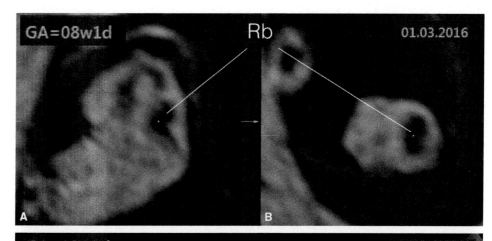

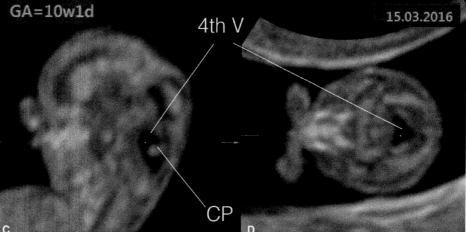

**Figure 8.4:** The posterior fossa, demonstrating the development of the rhombencephalic vesicle (Rb) into the fourth ventricle (4th V). The sagittal **(A)** and axial **(B)** planes of the fetal head at 8 weeks of gestation. Note the appearance of the Rb in the posterior aspect of the brain. The sagittal **(C)** and axial **(D)** planes of the fetal head at 10 weeks of gestation. Note the development of the 4th V at this gestational age. The choroid plexus (CP) of the 4th V is also visible in **C**.

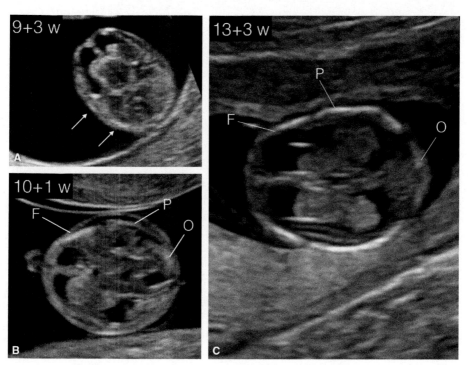

**Figure 8.5:** Axial planes of the fetal head at 9 **(A)**, 10 **(B)**, and 13 **(C)** weeks of gestation demonstrating the progression of skull ossification. Note at 9 weeks of gestation **(A)**, the presence of small islands of ossification (*arrows*). At 10 weeks of gestation **(B)**, partial ossification of the frontal (F), parietal (P) and occipital (O) bones is seen. At 13 weeks of gestation **(C)**, the frontal (F), parietal (P) and occipital (O) bones are clearly seen. The occipital bone (O) is better imaged in a more posterior plane at the level of basal ganglia (see Figs. 8.6 and 8.10).

# NORMAL SONOGRAPHIC ANATOMY

Ultrasound evaluation of the fetal intracranial anatomy is commonly performed in the axial (transverse) and midsagittal planes of the fetal head (**Figs. 8.6 to 8.12**). Axial (**Figs. 8.6 to 8.11**) and midsagittal (**Fig. 8.12**) planes of the fetal head are commonly obtained in the first trimester for the measurement of the biparietal diameter (BPD) and nuchal translucency (NT), respectively. Furthermore, the midsagittal plane is also obtained for the evaluation of the fetal facial profile and nasal bones. The axial and midsagittal planes of the fetal head are also part of the International Society of Ultrasound in Obstetrics and Gynecology (ISUOG) practice guidelines for the performance of the first trimester ultrasound examination.[1] The coronal planes of the fetal head are also occasionally helpful in the visualization of midline structures when certain malformations are suspected. The authors recommend routine evaluation of the axial and midsagittal planes of the fetal head when ultrasound examinations are performed beyond the 12 weeks of gestation. Please refer to Chapter 5 for the systematic approach

to the detailed ultrasound examination of the fetus in the first trimester, with comprehensive presentation of standardized planes for the evaluation of the CNS in early gestation.

## Axial Planes

The systematic detailed examination of the fetal brain in the first trimester includes the acquisition of three axial planes, similar to the approach performed in the second trimester ultrasound examination (see Figs. 5.7 and 5.8). In these planes, the fetal head shape is oval and the skull can be identified from 10 weeks onward (Fig. 8.5). At this early gestation, bone ossification primarily involves the frontal, parietal, and occipital parts of the cranial bones (**Figs. 8.5 and 8.6**). The use of high frequency linear or transvaginal transducers improves imaging of the fetal CNS in early gestation (**Fig. 8.7**). The intracranial anatomy is divided by the falx cerebri into a right and left side of equal size (**Figs. 8.6 to 8.8**). The choroid plexus on each side is hyperechoic, typically fills the lateral ventricles, and is surrounded by cerebral spinal fluid (**Figs. 8.7 to 8.9**). In the first trimester, the shape of

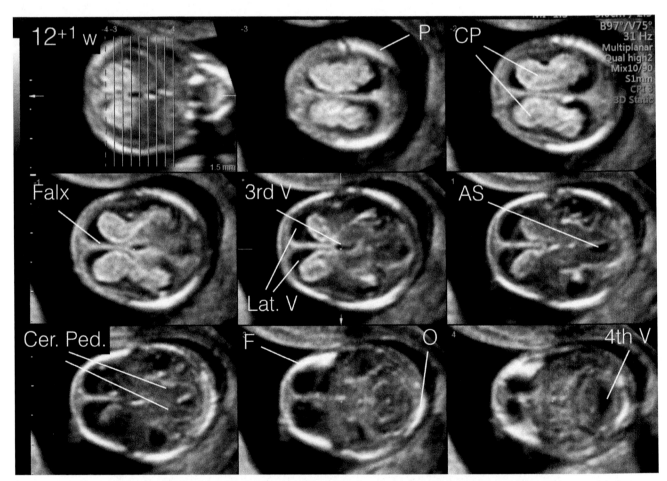

**Figure 8.6:** Three-dimensional (3D) volume of a fetal head at 12 weeks of gestation. The 3D volume was obtained from an axial plane and is displayed in tomographic view. From superiorly **(top)** to inferiorly **(bottom)** you can see the choroid plexuses (CP), the falx cerebri (Falx), the third ventricle (3rd V), the aqueduct of Sylvius (AS), the cerebral peduncles (Cer. Ped.), and the fourth ventricle (4th V). The lateral ventricles (Lat. V) are seen in the mid-axial plane. Note the appearance of the frontal (F), parietal (P), and occipital (O) bones.

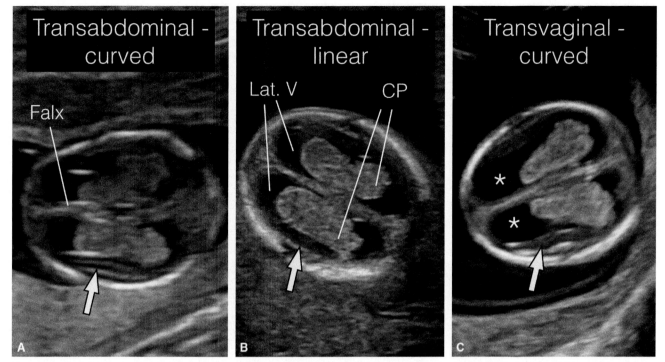

**Figure 8.7:** Axial view of the fetal head at 12 weeks of gestation from a lateral approach, obtained with three different high-resolution transducers: transabdominal curved array **(A)**, transabdominal linear **(B)**, and transvaginal **(C)**. Note the improved resolution in the transabdominal linear **(B)** and transvaginal **(C)** transducers. The falx cerebri (Falx) is seen along with the choroid plexuses (CP) and cerebrospinal fluid (*asterisks*) in the lateral ventricles (Lat. V). The rim of the developing cortex is also seen (*arrows*). Note that at this stage of development, the ventricular system occupies the majority of the brain.

the choroid plexus is described to be similar to a butterfly (Fig. 8.8).[2] The left and right choroid plexuses are rarely of similar size and shape, and this difference is considered part of the normal variation (Fig. 8.9).[3] A small rim of the developing cortex can be seen laterally surrounding the choroid plexuses

(Fig. 8.7). In an axial superior plane of the fetal head, a fluid rim can be seen surrounding the choroid plexus on each side, corresponding to the lateral ventricle (Fig. 8.10A). A more inferior axial plane toward the base of the skull shows the two thalami and the third ventricle, forming the diencephalon

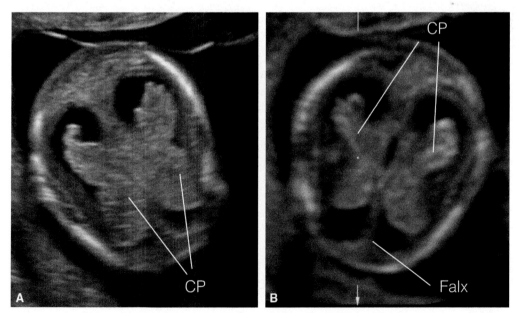

**Figure 8.8:** Axial view of the fetal head at the level of the choroid plexuses (CP) in a fetus at 11 weeks **(A)** and at 13 weeks **(B)** of gestation. Note that the right and left CP resemble the shape of a butterfly and are referred to as the "butterfly sign." The falx cerebri (Falx) is seen in the midline. Compare with Figures 8.24 and 8.25 obtained from fetuses with alobar holoprosencephaly.

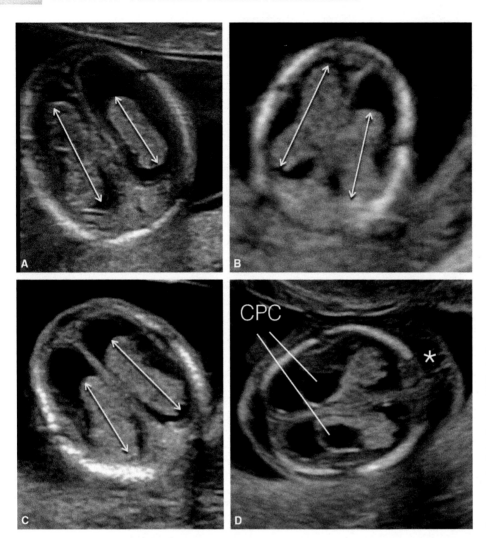

**Figure 8.9:** Axial views of the fetal head obtained in early gestation at the level of the choroid plexuses in three normal fetuses **(A–C)** and in a fetus with trisomy 13 **(D)**. Note in **A** to **C** the presence of choroid plexus asymmetry (*double arrows*), considered as a normal variant. Fetuses **A** to **C** had a normal subsequent second trimester ultrasound. Note the presence of choroid plexus cysts (CPC) and nuchal edema (*asterisk*) in the fetus with trisomy 13 **(D)**.

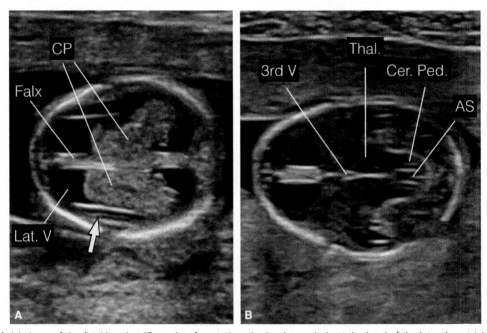

**Figure 8.10:** Axial views of the fetal head at 13 weeks of gestation obtained superiorly at the level of the lateral ventricles **(A)** and inferiorly at the level of the thalami **(B)**. In **A**, the two lateral ventricles (Lat. V), the choroid plexuses (CP), and the falx cerebri (Falx) are seen. In **B**, the thalami (Thal.) with the third ventricle (3rd V) are recognized and constitute the diencephalon. Posterior to the thalami, the cerebral peduncles (Cer. Ped.) with the aqueduct of Sylvius (AS) can be visualized and form the mesencephalon (see Fig. 8.11).

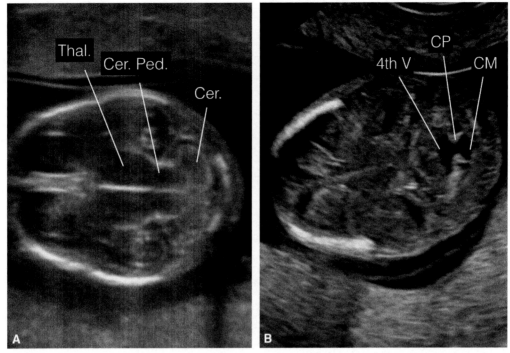

**Figure 8.11:** Axial view of the fetal head at 13 weeks of gestation obtained at the level of the posterior fossa (inferior to planes **A** and **B** in Fig. 8.10). **A:** At the level of the developing cerebellum (Cer.) and cerebral peduncles (Cer. Ped.). Note the thalami (Thal.) in a more anterior location. **B:** An oblique, slightly more inferior plane demonstrating the open fourth ventricle (4th V) connecting to the future cisterna magna (CM). The echogenic choroid plexus (CP) of the fourth ventricle can also be seen.

(Fig. 8.10B). Posterior to the thalami, the two small cerebral peduncles are identified surrounding the aqueduct of Sylvius and forming the mesencephalon (midbrain) (Fig. 8.10B). The developing cerebellum is identified in the posterior fossa primarily by transvaginal ultrasound and in an axial plane that is tilted toward the upper spine (Fig. 8.11A). A

slightly more inferior plane will show the fourth ventricle, the future cisterna magna, and the hyperechogenic choroid plexus of the fourth ventricle (Fig. 8.11B). Table 8.1 gives an overview of the anatomic landmarks and corresponding malformations that can be visualized in the axial planes of the fetal head in the first trimester.

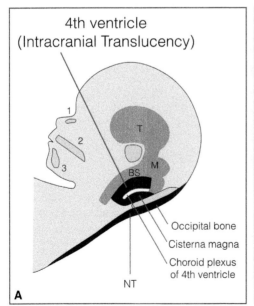
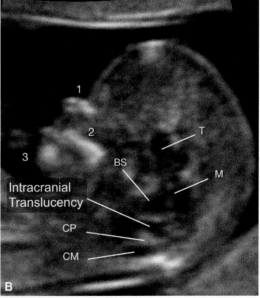

**Figure 8.12:** Schematic drawing **(A)** and corresponding ultrasound image **(B)** of the midsagittal plane of the fetal head in the first trimester (same as nuchal translucency [NT] plane). This plane enables a good assessment of the posterior fossa. The following structures can be seen: thalamus (T), midbrain (M), brainstem (BS), the fourth ventricle presenting as an intracranial translucency between the BS and the choroid plexus (CP), and the cisterna magna (CM). 1, 2, and 3 point to the nasal bone, maxilla, and mandible, respectively.

**Table 8.1** • Axial Planes of the Fetal Head and Associated Abnormalities in the First Trimester

| | Normal | Suspected Abnormalities |
|---|---|---|
| Head shape | Oval shape | • **Anencephaly/exencephaly:** Irregular shape, no skull identified<br>• **Holoprosencephaly**: circular head |
| Bony borders | Ossified bones<br>Clear head borders | • **Osteogenesis imperfecta:** no ossification (except for occipital bone). Additional findings such as short broken and bent femur and humerus<br>• **Thanatophoric dysplasia:** Increased ossification of head, additionally short or abnormally shaped long bones<br>• **Encephalocele:** Interrupted head contour, commonly in the occipital region |
| Falx cerebri | Hyperechogenic line from anterior to posterior dividing the brain in two halves | • **Holoprosencephaly:** absent falx cerebri<br>• **Encephalocele:** Often deviated falx cerebri |
| Choroid plexuses of lateral ventricles | Large hyperechogenic plexuses on both sides, could be slightly asymmetrical | • **Holoprosencephaly:** fused choroid plexuses<br>• **Choroid plexus cysts:** typically found in trisomy 13 or other aneuploidies (in general additional markers or abnormalities are present) |
| Biparietal diameter (BPD) | Within the reference range | • **Anencephaly:** No BPD measurable<br>• **Holoprosencephaly and spina bifida:** BPD often in the lower range |
| Thalami, cerebral peduncles, aqueduct of Sylvius | V-Shaped transition, visualized aqueduct. Some distance between occipital bone and cerebral peduncles | • **Spina bifida:** Parallel shaped transition between thalami and cerebral peduncles. Compressed aqueduct. Cerebral peduncles posteriorly shifted and touch or are close to the occipital bones |
| Fourth ventricle with its choroid plexus | Fourth ventricle well seen with hyperechogenic choroid plexus | • **Spina bifida:** Reduced fluid in fourth ventricle, choroid plexus not well identifiable<br>• **Dandy–Walker and Blake's pouch cyst:** Increased fluid in fourth ventricle, anteriorly shifted brainstem |

## Sagittal Plane

The midsagittal plane is commonly visualized in the first trimester, primarily due to NT measurement (Fig. 8.12). The midsagittal plane reveals more anatomic intracranial information when examined from the ventral approach (fetus back down) (Fig. 8.12). In this midsagittal plane (Fig. 5.6), the following anatomic landmarks can be evaluated: head shape, facial profile, nose with nasal bone, maxilla, mandible, thalamus, midbrain, brainstem (BS), fourth ventricle (called intracranial translucency [IT]) and its choroid plexus, the developing cisterna magna, the occipital bone, and the NT (Fig. 8.12).[4] Table 8.2 gives an overview of the anatomic landmarks and corresponding malformations that can be visualized in the midsagittal plane of the fetal head in the first trimester. In the context of spina bifida later in this chapter, the anatomy of the posterior fossa under normal and abnormal conditions is discussed.

## Coronal Planes

The coronal planes of the fetal head are obtained along the laterolateral axis of the fetus. In the second and third trimesters, coronal planes of the fetal head are primarily obtained to assess the frontal midline structures such as the interhemispheric fissure, the cavum septi pellucidi, frontal horns of the lateral ventricles, the Sylvian fissure, the corpus callosum, and the optic chiasm. Given that these midline anatomic structures are not fully developed in the first trimester, coronal planes of the fetal head are rarely obtained. Figure 8.13 shows coronal planes of the fetal head in a normal fetus at 12 weeks of gestation.

**Table 8.2 •** Midsagittal Plane of the Fetal Head and Associated Abnormalities in the First Trimester

| | Normal | Abnormalities Suspected |
|---|---|---|
| Head shape | Large head in comparison with body, physiologic slight frontal bossing | • **Anencephaly/exencephaly:** Irregular shape, no skull identified<br>• **Holoprosencephaly:** often abnormal shape |
| Nuchal translucency (NT) | NT within the normal range | Thickened NT in aneuploidies, complex cardiac malformations, and in many syndromic conditions |
| Posterior fossa: brainstem, fourth ventricle, cisterna magna | Brainstem diameter within the normal range, slightly s-shaped brainstem, fourth ventricle separated from cisterna magna with choroid plexus | • **Open spina bifida:** brainstem thickened and posteriorly shifted. Compressed or absent fourth ventricle. No cisterna magna seen<br>• **Dandy–Walker:** thin brainstem, large fourth ventricle<br>• **Aneuploidies**: often dilated fourth ventricle<br>• **Walker–Warburg syndrome**: Z-shaped brainstem (kinking) |
| Facial profile | Normal forehead, nasal bone, maxilla, and mandible | See Chapter 9 for details |

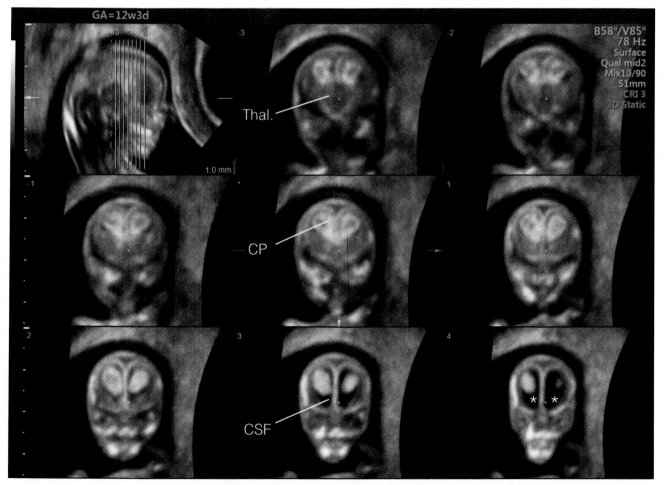

**Figure 8.13:** Coronal planes of the anterior fetal head obtained from a three-dimensional (3D) volume at 12 weeks of gestation and displayed in tomographic view. The posterior fossa is outside the range of the tomographic display and thus is not seen. Note the thalami (Thal.), the choroid plexuses (CP), and the presence of cerebrospinal fluid (CSF) in the anterior segments of the lateral ventricles (*asterisks*).

# CENTRAL NERVOUS SYSTEM ABNORMALITIES

## Acrania, Exencephaly, and Anencephaly

### Definition

Acrania, exencephaly, and anencephaly are neural tube defects that result from failure of closure of the rostral part of the neural tube in early embryogenesis (days 23 to 28 from fertilization). Acrania is defined by the absence of the cranial vault above the orbits. In exencephaly, the cranial vault is absent (acrania) and the abnormal brain tissue appears as bulging masses, covered by a membrane and exposed to the amniotic fluid. In anencephaly, the cranial vault, cerebral hemispheres, and midbrain are all absent. There is no overlying skin and a layer of angiomatous stroma covers the skull defect. Ample evidence suggests that anencephaly is at the end of the spectrum of acrania and exencephaly, and that it results from the destruction of brain tissue that is exposed to amniotic fluid in the first trimester. Except in rare cases of acrania, the exencephaly–anencephaly sequence is a lethal condition.

### Ultrasound Findings

The diagnosis of exencephaly/anencephaly in the first trimester is based upon the demonstration of an absent cranium along with the presence of "abnormal mass of tissue" arising from the base of the remaining skull (Figs. 8.14 and 8.15). On coronal views, the abnormal mass of tissue, representing the amorphous brain matter, has been described as the "Mickey Mouse" sign as it typically bulges to either side of the fetal head (Fig. 8.15A).[5] In anencephaly, the absence of the cranial vault is seen along with little to no brain tissue above the level of

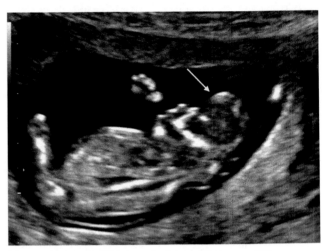

**Figure 8.14:** Sagittal view of a fetus with anencephaly–exencephaly at 12 weeks of gestation. Note the absence of normal brain tissue and the overlying calvarium. Amorphous brain tissue is seen protruding from the base of the head region (*arrow*).

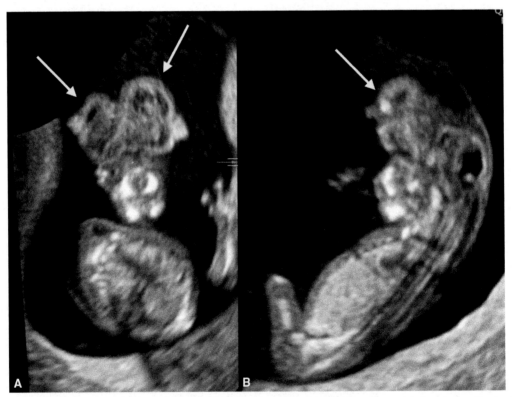

**Figure 8.15:** Coronal **(A)** and sagittal **(B)** views of a fetus with anencephaly–exencephaly at 11 weeks of gestation. The brain is replaced by amorphous tissue (*arrows*) with absence of the overlying calvarium. The shape of the amorphous brain tissue in the coronal view in **A** resembles the ears of Mickey Mouse and has been referred to as the "Mickey Mouse" sign. Note in **B** the absence of the forehead and the protruding brain tissue (*arrow*).

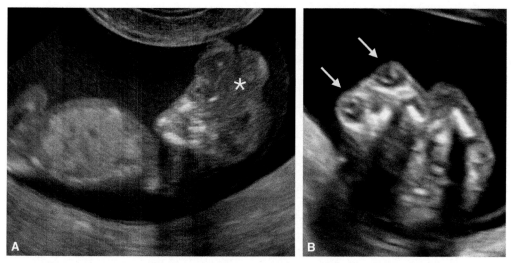

**Figure 8.16:** Coronal **(A)** and direct frontal **(B)** views of the face in a fetus with anencephaly–exencephaly at 12 weeks of gestation. **A:** The brain is replaced by amorphous tissue (*asterisk*) with absence of the overlying calvarium. The direct frontal view of the face in **B** is lacking the forehead and the eyes (*arrows*) appear prominent, a view called the "frog eyes."

the orbits (Fig. 8.16) and on coronal view of the fetal face, the characteristic "frog eyes" appearance is noted (Fig. 8.16B). By the 12th week of gestation, following complete ossification of the fetal skull, ultrasound diagnosis of exencephaly/anencephaly can be performed by the axial, sagittal, or coronal views of the

fetal head.[6] In these views, the absent calvarium, the abnormal fetal profile, and the disorganized brain tissue protruding from the fetal head can be demonstrated (Figs. 8.14 to 8.18). On transvaginal ultrasound, the amniotic fluid appears echogenic (Fig. 8.16A). The crown-rump length measurements are often

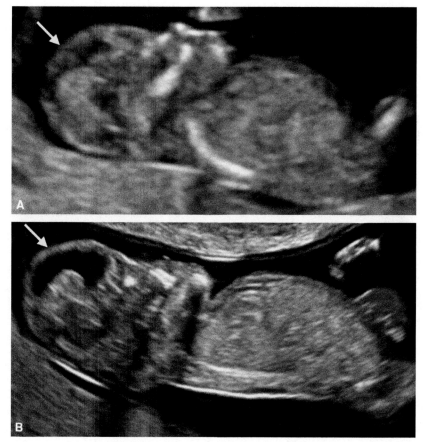

**Figure 8.17:** Sagittal views in two fetuses **(A and B)** with absence of the calvarium (acrania) in early gestation. Note in **A** and **B** the presence of a membrane (pia mater) covering the brain tissue (*arrows*). The shape of the brain and head is similar in both fetuses. In most cases of acrania, follow-up ultrasound examinations demonstrate amorphous brain tissue as shown in anencephaly–exencephaly cases.

smaller than expected due to loss of brain tissue. The diagnosis of exencephaly/anencephaly can be occasionally suspected at 9 weeks of gestation.[6] A follow-up ultrasound after 10 weeks is recommended in order to confirm the diagnosis, especially if pregnancy termination is being contemplated. On occasions, acrania can be diagnosed in the first trimester by the demonstration of absence of cranium and in the presence of membrane (pia mater) covering the brain tissue (Fig. 8.17). In most cases of acrania, follow-up ultrasound examination into the second trimester demonstrates amorphous brain tissue as shown in anencephaly–exencephaly cases. 3D ultrasound can help in providing a complete picture of face and head in anencephalic fetuses (Fig. 8.18).

The prenatal diagnosis of exencephaly/anencephaly in the first trimester requires a detailed transvaginal ultrasound looking for the presence of amniotic bands given the association of amniotic band sequence with exencephaly.

### Associated Malformations

Anencephaly is commonly associated with other fetal abnormalities to include neural tube malformations such as craniorachischisis, spina bifida, and iniencephaly.[6] Other fetal malformations such as cardiac, renal, gastrointestinal, and facial occur in association with anencephaly. Aneuploidy rates are also increased in anencephaly, especially when associated with other malformations. Amniotic band sequence, on the other hand, presents a sporadic association with no increased future risk for recurrence. The in utero mortality rate is high and the malformation is universally lethal.

## Cephalocele (Encephalocele)

### Definition

Cephalocele is a protrusion of intracranial content through a bony skull defect. If the herniated sac contains meninges and brain tissue, the term encephalocele is used. The term meningocele is used when the herniated sac contains meninges only. Given the difficulty involved in the first trimester in differentiating encephalocele from meningocele, the term encephalocele is used to describe both conditions. Most commonly an encephalocele is found posteriorly in the occipital region of the skull. Encephaloceles can also occur in other regions of the skull such as parietal, basal, and anterior. Encephaloceles are considered neural tube defects resulting from failure of closure of the rostral part of the neural tube.[7] In general, non-midline encephaloceles (lateral or parietal) have been associated with amniotic band sequence and considered to result from a disruptive process following normal embryogenesis.

### Ultrasound Findings

The detection of an encephalocele on ultrasound examination is often suspected in the axial view by the presence of a protrusion in the occipital or frontal region of the calvarium (Figs. 8.19, 8.20A, 8.21A, and 8.22A). A sagittal view can reveal the extent of the defect and the size of the encephalocele (Figs. 8.20B, 8.22B, and 9.23A). Transvaginal ultrasound along with image magnification can often reveal the bony defect in the skull (Figs. 8.19B and 8.22). Encephaloceles

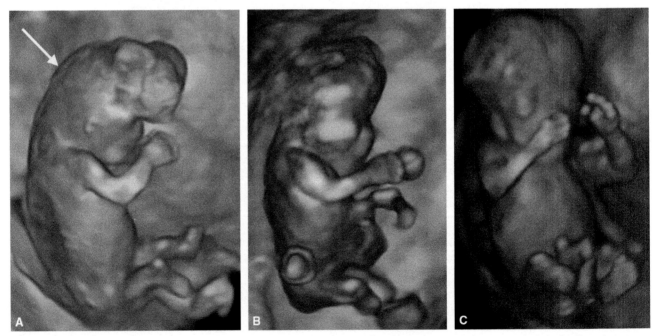

**Figure 8.18:** Three-dimensional ultrasound in surface mode in three fetuses **(A–C)** with anencephaly–exencephaly in the first trimester showing different appearances of the same malformation. Note the fetus in **A** has part of the calvarium formed (*arrow*), whereas fetuses in **B** and **C** do not.

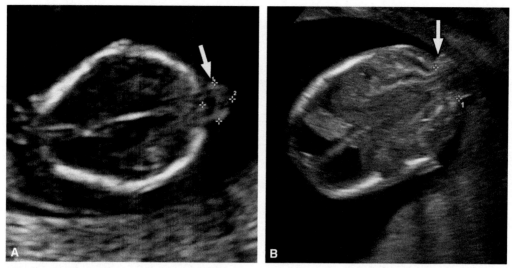

**Figure 8.19:** Axial plane of the head in two fetuses at 13 weeks of gestation with an occipital encephalocele (*arrows*) examined in A) with transabdominal and in B) with transvaginal transducer. Note the presence of brain tissue protruding out of the defect in the occipital region. The presence of an encephalocele is often associated with an abnormal shape of the head.

are often associated with abnormal brain anatomy that can be detected in the axial or sagittal views of the fetal head (**Figs. 8.19 to 8.22**). The larger the encephalocele, the more brain abnormality is seen on ultrasound. As encephaloceles are often part of genetic abnormalities and syndromes, detailed review of fetal anatomy is recommended.[7] Special attention should be given to the presence of polydactyly and polycystic kidneys given the association with Meckel–Gruber syndrome (**Figs. 8.21** and **13.31**).[7] Other autosomal recessive ciliopathies can present with posterior cephalocele, such as Walker–Warburg syndrome or the large group of Joubert syndrome–related disorders (**Fig. 8.22**). Three-dimensional

(3D) ultrasound in surface mode can be of help in showing the extent of the encephalocele. Not all cases of cephaloceles are detectable in the first trimester. Smaller defects and internal lesions are difficult to diagnose. The diagnosis of an encephalocele in the first trimester is commonly performed around 13 to 14 weeks unless a meningocele with a dilated posterior fossa is present, mimicking a Dandy–Walker malformation (DWM) enabling an earlier detection (**Figs. 8.22** and **13.31**). In isolated cases, an attempt should be made to differentiate between an encephalocele and a meningocele given a much improved prognosis of the latter. The absence of brain tissue in the herniated sac on transvaginal ultrasound along

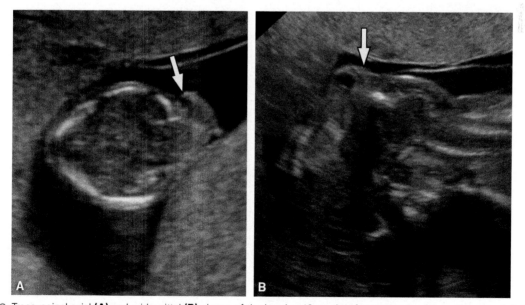

**Figure 8.20:** Transvaginal axial **(A)** and midsagittal **(B)** planes of the head at 12 weeks of gestation in a fetus with an occipital encephalocele (*arrows*). Note the presence of brain tissue protruding through the encephalocele. Additional findings, not shown here, include polydactyly and polycystic kidneys, typical signs for Meckel–Gruber syndrome.

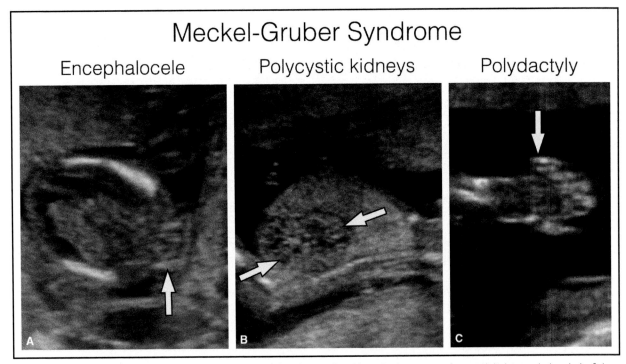

**Meckel-Gruber Syndrome**

Encephalocele    Polycystic kidneys    Polydactyly

**Figure 8.21:** Meckel–Gruber syndrome in a fetus at 12 weeks of gestation. Note the presence of an occipital encephalocele in **A** (*arrow*), large polycystic kidneys in **B** (*arrows*), and polydactyly in **C** (*arrow*). The presence of an occipital encephalocele in the first trimester should prompt a closer look at the fetal kidneys and extremities for associated abnormalities suggestive of Meckel–Gruber syndrome.

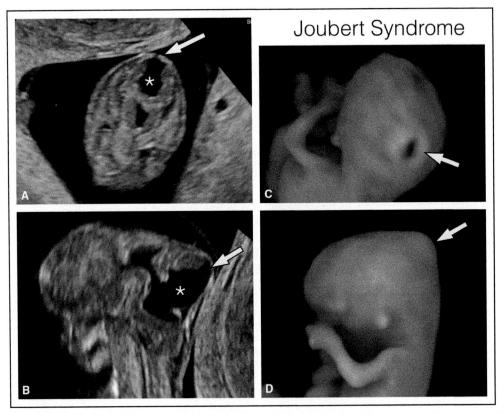

**Joubert Syndrome**

**Figure 8.22:** Axial **(A)** and midsagittal **(B)** planes of the head in a fetus with an occipital cystic encephalocele (*arrows*) at 11 weeks of gestation. Note the dilated fourth ventricle (*asterisk*). **C and D:** Three-dimensional ultrasound display in surface mode of the fetal head with the *arrows* pointing to the occipital encephalocele, posteriorly in **C** showing the defect and laterally in **D**, showing the encephalocele bulge. This case represented recurrence of Joubert syndrome type 14 (JBTS14). Note also that Joubert-related disorders may have no or only subtle findings in early gestation.

with normal intracranial anatomy make the diagnosis of a meningocele more likely.

## Associated Malformations

Encephaloceles or meningoceles can be isolated findings, or they can be associated with chromosomal abnormalities (trisomies 13 and 18) or genetic syndromes (ciliopathies). Encephaloceles are also often associated with other intracranial or extracranial abnormalities. Of note is the association of encephaloceles with one special ciliopathy, the Meckel–Gruber syndrome, an autosomal recessive disorder with 25% recurrence, but also with other ciliopathies such as Joubert syndromes and Joubert-related disorders (Fig. 8.22) as well as Walker–Warburg syndrome. The presence of lateral encephaloceles should raise the suspicion for the presence of amniotic bands. Differentiating occipital encephaloceles from cystic hygromas can occasionally be difficult in the first trimester. A cervical spina bifida (Fig. 8.23) can also be misdiagnosed as encephalocele but in this condition the defect is below the intact occipital bone (Figs. 8.23B and C), whereas in encephalocele the defect is cranial to or across the occipital bone. This is important as spina bifida is less commonly associated with a genetic syndrome than encephalocele.

## Holoprosencephaly

### Definition

HPE is a heterogeneous developmental abnormality of the fetal brain arising from failure of cleavage of the prosencephalon with varying degrees of fusion of the cerebral hemispheres.[2,6,8] It is the most common forebrain defect in humans. The incidence of HPE varies throughout pregnancy decreasing from 1:250 in embryos to 1:10,000 in live births.[9] In a recently published large study on 108,982 first trimester fetuses including 870 fetuses with abnormal karyotypes, HPE was found in 37 fetuses for a prevalence of 1:3,000 fetuses in first trimester screening.[10] HPE is subclassified into alobar, semilobar, lobar, and middle interhemispheric variants based upon the degrees of fusion of the cerebral hemispheres. The most common and severe form is the alobar form, which has a single ventricle of varying degree, fused thalami, and corpora striata with absent olfactory tracts and bulbs and corpus callosum. The single ventricle in alobar HPE may bulge dorsally to form a dorsal sac. In semilobar HPE, there is partial fusion of the posterior cerebral lobes with a posterior falx cerebri and a rudimentary corpus callosum. In lobar HPE, the falx cerebri is present and the cerebral lobes are distinct with the exception of the region of the ventricular frontal horns. In the interhemispheric variant of HPE, the posterior, parietal, and frontal lobes fail to separate. A feature common to all forms of HPE is an absent or dysplastic cavum septi pellucidi, which in normal conditions is first visible on ultrasound in the second trimester. Semilobar, lobar, and the interhemispheric variants of HPE are less severe and may escape detection until the second trimester of pregnancy. Anomalies of the face that range from severe, such as cyclopia and proboscis (Figs. 9.10 and 9.39), to mild, such as hypotelorism or single central maxillary incisor, are typically found in HPE and can be explained by the maldevelopment of the prosencephalon.

### Ultrasound Findings

The semilobar and lobar types of HPE are typically not detected in the first trimester and thus will not be discussed in this section. The transvaginal approach is preferred when

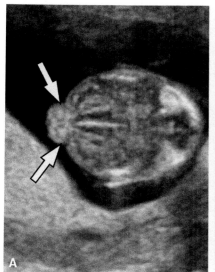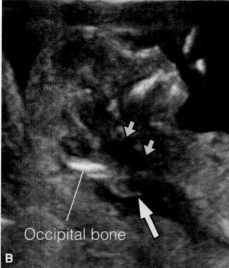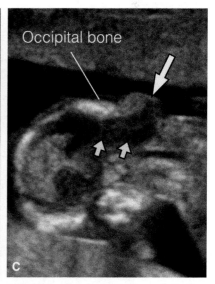

Figure 8.23: Axial (A), midsagittal anterior (B) and posterior (C) planes of the head in a fetus at 13 weeks of gestation with cervical spina bifida. In the axial (A) plane, the defect (*yellow arrows*) is suspicious for an encephalocele but in the midsagittal anterior (B) and posterior (C) views the lesion (*yellow arrows*) is below the occipital bone, at the level of the cervical spine. Note that the brainstem and posterior fossa (*short blue arrows*) are abnormal, typical findings for an open spina bifida in early gestation (see Figs. 8.40 and 8.43).

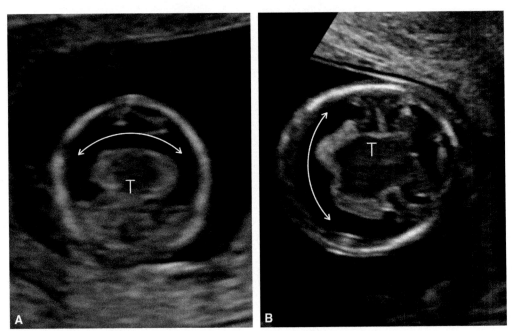

**Figure 8.24:** Coronal **(A)** and axial **(B)** planes of the head in two fetuses with alobar holoprosencephaly in early gestation. Note the presence of a crescent-shaped single ventricle (monoventricle) (*double headed arrows*). Fused thalami (T) are also noted. The falx cerebri is absent and no separated choroid plexuses can be visualized.

feasible given its higher resolution. A typical sonographic sign of HPE includes the absence of a falx cerebri, separating both hemispheres. This is easily detected in the axial or coronal planes of the fetal head (Figs. 8.24 to 8.27). The finding of two distinct choroid plexuses in each hemisphere (Fig. 8.8) rules out alobar HPE and the lack of the typical "butterfly" sign, seen in normal fetuses is an important clue to diagnosis in the first trimester (Figs. 8.24 to 8.27).[2] The coronal plane (Figs. 8.24A and 8.28) of the fetal head shows a single

ventricle anteriorly (monoventricle) with fused thalami. Biometric evaluation of the fetal head in HPE has shown small BPD measurements with or without associated aneuploidy.[11]

3D ultrasound is helpful in various modes (Figs. 8.27 to 8.29). The 3D tomographic display provides a better overview of the various planes of the fetal head (Figs. 8.27 and 8.28). 3D surface, Silhouette, or inversion modes are different tools that provide a spatial demonstration of the fused ventricles, thalami, and choroid plexus (Figs. 8.29 and 8.30).[12] Facial anomalies that are

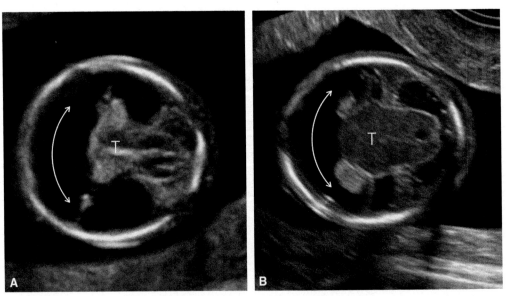

**Figure 8.25:** Axial plane of the head in two fetuses **(A and B)** with alobar holoprosencephaly at 12 and 13 weeks of gestation, respectively. Note the presence of a crescent-shaped single ventricle (monoventricle) (*double headed arrows*), fused thalami (T), and absence of the falx cerebri.

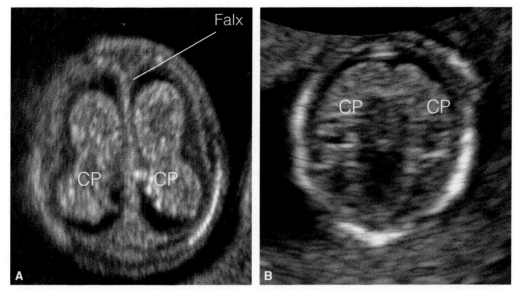

**Figure 8.26:** Axial planes at 13 weeks of gestation of the head comparing the choroid plexuses of the lateral ventricles in a normal fetus **(A)** and in a fetus with alobar holoprosencephaly **(B)**. The butterfly-like echogenic choroid plexuses (CP) are well recognized in the normal fetus **(A)**. In the fetus with holoprosencephaly **(B)**, the CP are fused and do no show the butterfly-like appearance. The falx cerebri (Falx) is noted in **A**, but absent in **B**. Note in **B** that the single ventricle (monoventricle) (as shown in Figs. 8.24 and 8.25) is not clearly displayed, but the fusion of CP and the absence of the falx cerebri suggest the diagnosis of holoprosencephaly.

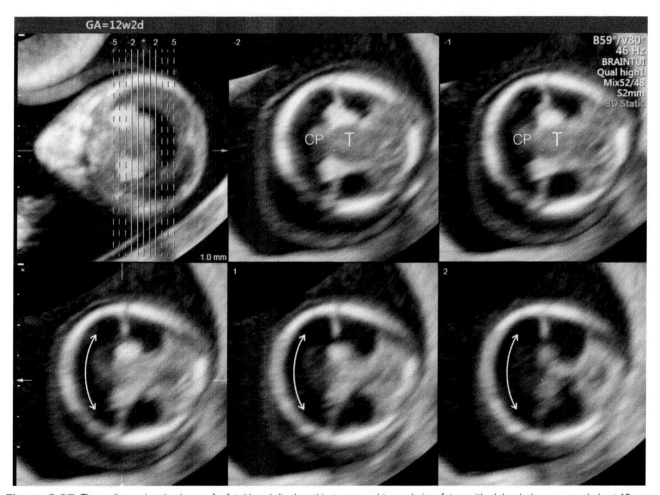

**Figure 8.27:** Three-dimensional volume of a fetal head displayed in tomographic mode in a fetus with alobar holoprosencephaly at 12 weeks of gestation. The parallel axial planes demonstrate the typical features of alobar holoprosencephaly such as the fused thalami (T) and choroid plexuses (CP) and the single anterior ventricle (*double headed arrow*) as shown in Figures 8.24 and 8.25.

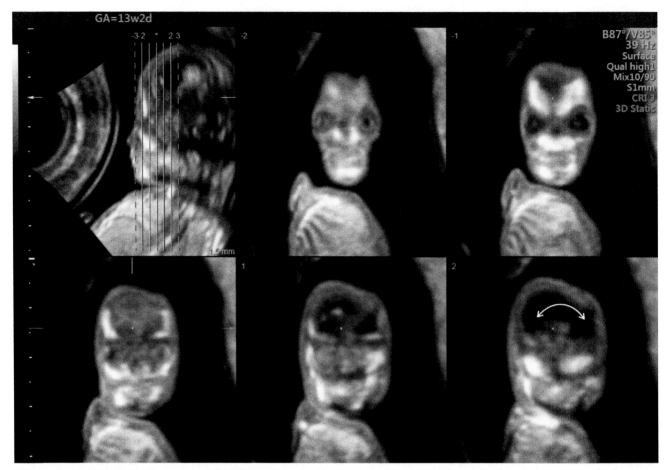

**Figure 8.28:** Three-dimensional volume of a fetal head displayed in tomographic mode in a fetus with alobar holoprosencephaly at 13 weeks of gestation. The parallel coronal planes demonstrate the single ventricle (*double headed arrow*) and the presence of an abnormal face, also shown in profile in the upper left plane.

found in HPE include a wide array and are mostly detected in the midsagittal and coronal facial planes[8] or with 3D ultrasound surface mode (Figs. 8.28, 8.30, 9.10, and 9.39). These facial abnormalities are discussed in more detail in Chapter 9. In expert

hands, alobar HPE can be detected from 9 weeks of gestation onward, with the demonstration of a lack of separation of both ventricles and choroid plexuses.[13] A follow-up evaluation at 12 to 13 weeks is prudent before a final diagnosis.

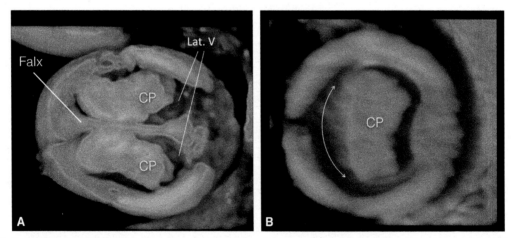

**Figure 8.29:** Three-dimensional ultrasound display in surface mode of an axial plane of the fetal head in a normal fetus **(A)** and in a fetus with alobar holoprosencephaly **(B)** at 13 weeks of gestation. Note the normal appearance of the choroid plexuses (CP) in **A**, separated by the falx cerebri (Falx). In the fetus with holoprosencephaly **(B)**, the CP are fused, the falx is absent and there is a single ventricle (*double headed arrow*). Lat. V, lateral ventricles.

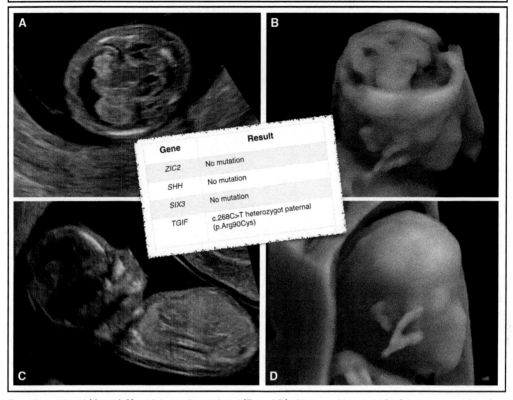

**Figure 8.30:** Two-dimensional **(A and C)** and three-dimensional **(B and D)** ultrasound images of a fetus at 13 weeks of gestation with holoprosencephaly (HPE), shown in **A** and **B** and abnormal face shown in **C** and **D**. A mutation in the TGIF was detected on genetic evaluation, which was also present in the otherwise healthy father, resulting in a recurrence risk of 50% with unpredictable penetrance. In cases of (isolated) HPE, in addition to chromosomal analysis and evaluation for syndromic conditions, workup for gene mutations of a specific group, called autosomal-dominant nonsyndromic HPE, including for instance the ZIC2, SHH, SIX3, TGIF genes, among others, maybe warranted if feasible.

## Associated Malformations

HPE is frequently associated with chromosomal abnormalities and genetic syndromes. Trisomy 13 accounts for the great majority of chromosomal aneuploidy along with triploidy and trisomy 18. In a recently published large study[10] on 108,982 first trimester fetuses including 37 fetuses with HPE, 78% (29/37) had an abnormal karyotype, including trisomy 13 (62%), trisomy 18 (17%), triploidy (17%), and others (4%) such as deletions and duplications (see also case of HPE with Del.18p in Fig. 6.36). Numerous genetic syndromes such as Smith–Lemli–Opitz, Meckel–Gruber, Otocephaly-HPE,[14] Rubinstein-Taybi syndrome among many others have been reported in association with the HPE spectrum.[9] Recently however, increased knowledge has been acquired on the molecular genetics of HPE and an important new group called autosomal-dominant nonsyndromic HPE was introduced.[9] To date, mutations in 14 genes are known to cause HPE, and the most common are SHH, ZIC2, SIX3, and TGIF1.[9] This is of importance as a parent can carry the mutation as well, having no or mild features, but a recurrence risk of HPE of 50%. The

case in Figure 8.30 shows an example of a nonsyndromic HPE with a mutation on the TGIF gene, with a carrier status of the same mutation in the apparently healthy father.

## Ventriculomegaly

### Definition

Ventriculomegaly is a nonspecific term and refers to the presence of excess cerebrospinal fluid within the ventricular system. Ventriculomegaly, the most frequent CNS malformation diagnosed prenatally refers to an enlargement of the lateral ventricle(s) and is defined as lateral ventricular width of 10 mm or greater at the level of the atria from the second trimester onward. There is currently no consensus definition on what constitutes ventriculomegaly before 20 weeks in general and in the first trimester in particular. Several definitions and reference curves were published, but their clinical value needs to be verified in prospective studies.[15–17] However, ventriculomegaly in the first trimester is rare in comparison with the second trimester.

## Ultrasound Findings

In the authors' centers, sonographic markers of ventriculomegaly in the first trimester include thinning and dangling of the choroid plexus, where the choroid plexus is seen to fill less than half of the ventricular space and its borders do not touch the medial and lateral ventricular walls (Figs. 8.31 to 8.37). Interestingly it was repeatedly observed that ventriculomegaly in the first trimester is commonly associated with thinning of the choroid plexus, rather than an increased width of the lateral ventricles (Figs. 8.31 to 8.37),

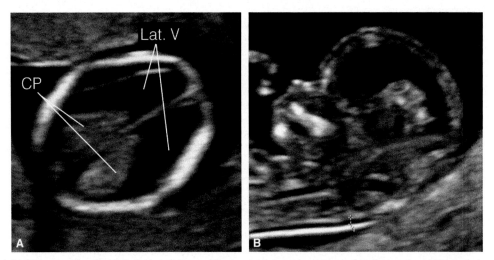

**Figure 8.31:** Axial **(A)** and midsagittal **(B)** views in a fetus with ventriculomegaly at 12 weeks of gestation. Note in **A** that the choroid plexuses (CP) are small and do not fill the lateral ventricles (Lat. V). The midsagittal plane **(B)** is not reliable for the diagnosis of ventriculomegaly in the first trimester. Follow-up ultrasound in the second trimester noted the presence of a small occipital meningocele.

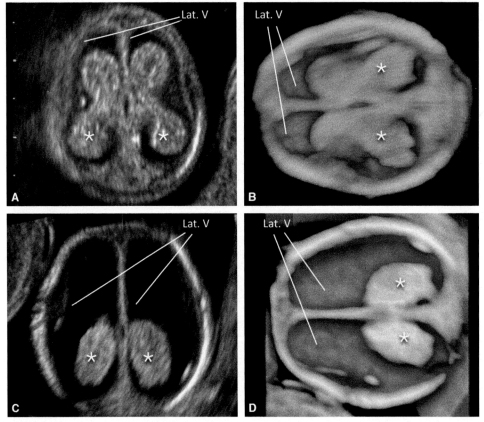

**Figure 8.32:** Axial view of the brain in two- and three-dimensional ultrasound of a normal fetus **(A and B)** and in a fetus with suspected ventriculomegaly **(C and D)**, both at 13 weeks of gestation. Note that the choroid plexuses (*asterisks*) fill the lateral ventricles (Lat. V) in the normal fetus **(A and B)** whereas the choroid plexuses occupy less than half of the lateral ventricles in the fetus with suspected ventriculomegaly **(C and D)**.

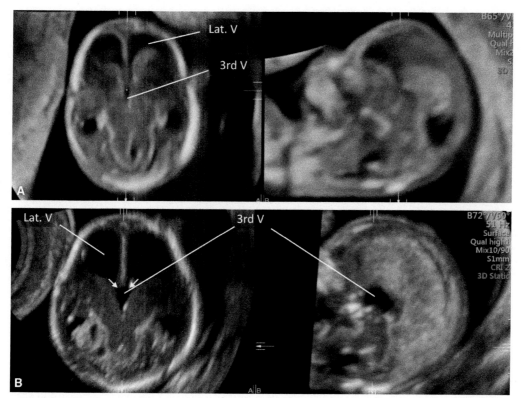

**Figure 8.33:** Orthogonal three-dimensional planes showing the axial **(left)** and sagittal **(right)** planes of the head in a normal fetus **(A)** and in a fetus with ventriculomegaly **(B)**. Note the dilated lateral (Lat. V) and third ventricle (3rd V) in **B**, as compared to the normal fetus in **A**. The foramen of Monroe communication (*arrows* in **B**) between the Lat. V and the 3rd V can be recognized.

which is also reflected by reference ranges of various studies on this subject.[15–17] One study reported on the ratio of the choroid plexus to the lateral ventricle in the assessment of ventriculomegaly in aneuploid fetuses at 11 to 14 weeks of gestation.[15] In another study, length, width, and area of the choroid plexus and the lateral ventricles were measured and the ratios calculated and compared with data from 17 fetuses with ventriculomegaly.[16] The authors found that the

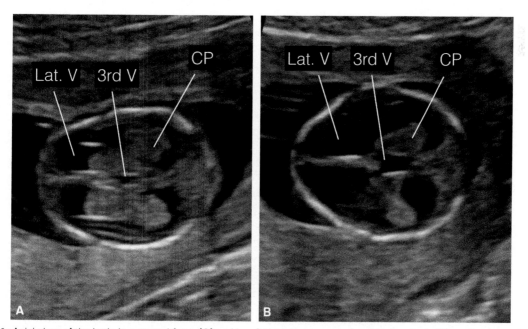

**Figure 8.34:** Axial view of the brain in a normal fetus **(A)** and in a fetus with suspected ventriculomegaly **(B)** at 12 weeks of gestation. When compared to the normal fetus **(A)**, the fetus with suspected ventriculomegaly **(B)** shows excess cerebrospinal fluid in the lateral ventricles (Lat. V), a dilated third ventricle (3rd V), and compressed, shortened choroid plexuses (CP).

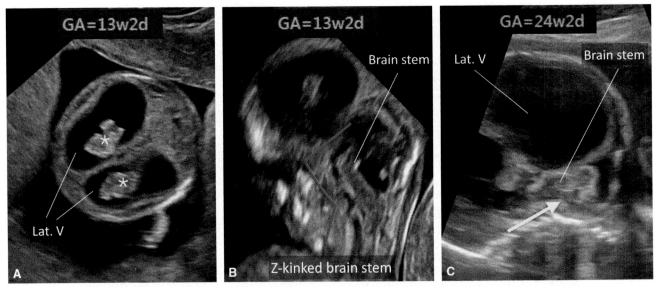

**Figure 8.35:** This pregnancy was referred at 13 weeks of gestation with a prior history of two fetal deaths with severe hydrocephaly and Walker–Warburg syndrome. **A:** An axial plane of the fetal head at 13 weeks of gestation, demonstrating the presence of dilated lateral ventricles (Lat. V) and small choroid plexuses (*asterisk*). A sagittal view of the posterior fossa **(B)** at 13 weeks of gestation shows the typical Z-kinked brainstem (*red line*), characteristic of Walker–Warburg syndrome. **C:** Midsagittal plane of the head at 24 weeks of gestation, demonstrating severely dilated lateral ventricles (Lat. V) and a kinked brainstem (*arrow*).

length and area ratio are the best parameters to be used.[16] In a recent study, ventriculomegaly was defined as bilateral separation of the choroid plexuses from superior borders of the lateral ventricles.[17] An enlarged third ventricle or an interruption of the falx can be found in ventriculomegaly in the first trimester, especially when associated with aqueductal stenosis (Figs. 8.33B and 8.34B) or semilobar HPE. Anomalies involving the posterior fossa can lead to

ventriculomegaly and therefore a careful examination of the posterior fossa is warranted (Figs. 8.35 and 8.36). As large data on outcome and associated findings in first trimester ventriculomegaly are still lacking, we recommend a detailed first trimester ultrasound examination, looking for associated malformations, when ventriculomegaly is encountered in early gestation. In addition, an invasive diagnostic procedure for genetic abnormalities should be offered, especially

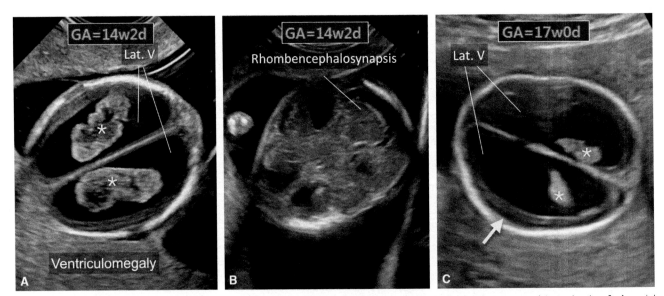

**Figure 8.36:** This pregnancy was referred at 14 weeks of gestation for evaluation of ventriculomegaly suspected 1 week prior. **A:** An axial plane of the fetal head demonstrating the presence of dilated lateral ventricles (Lat. V) and choroid plexuses (*asterisks*) that do not touch the ventricular walls. **B:** An axial view of the posterior fossa with abnormal cerebellar shape, typical for rhombencephalosynapsis, which is often associated with aqueductal stenosis, explaining the presence of ventriculomegaly. **C:** The follow-up ultrasound at 17 weeks of gestation showing the presence of ventriculomegaly with compression of choroid plexuses (*asterisks*) and effaced subarachnoid space (*arrow*).

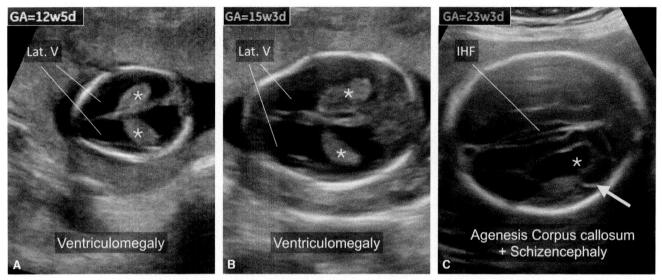

**Figure 8.37:** Axial planes of the fetal head at 12 **(A)**, 15 **(B)**, and 23 **(C)** weeks of gestation in the same fetus. Note in **A** the presence of dilated lateral ventricles (Lat. V) and dangling choroid plexuses (*asterisks*). **B**: Confirms the presence of ventriculomegaly without a known etiology. **C**: The presence of colpocephaly (*asterisk*) and widening of the interhemispheric fissure (IHF), suggesting agenesis of the corpus callosum. This fetus also had closed lip schizencephaly (*arrow* in **C**). Ventriculomegaly was not seen at 23 weeks of gestation (data not shown).

when ventriculomegaly is associated with other findings, which increases the risk for chromosomal aberrations.[15–17] A follow-up ultrasound examination between 15 to 17 weeks and at 20 to 22 weeks of gestation is recommended (Figs. 8.35 to 8.37). In our experience, many fetuses with ventriculomegaly in the second and third trimesters do not show ventricular dilation in the first trimester. This may be related to lack of clear diagnostic criteria in early gestation or a delayed onset into the second trimester of ventriculomegaly in many cases.

### Associated Malformations

Etiologic causes of ventriculomegaly are many and include various CNS malformations, genetic causes, and infections.[15,16] Extracranial-associated malformations are also common and include spina bifida, renal, cardiac, and skeletal abnormalities. In our experience, chromosomal anomalies including numerical aberrations and unbalanced translocations, deletions and duplications are commonly found in fetuses presenting with ventriculomegaly in the first trimester.[15–17] In addition, abnormalities of the posterior fossa such as DWM, Walker–Warburg syndrome (Fig. 8.35), Joubert syndrome, posterior fossa cysts, Chiari II malformation in spina bifida, and rhombencephalosynapsis may be associated with ventriculomegaly in early gestation.[16,17] Figure 8.36 describes a case of rhombencephalosynapsis diagnosed at 14 weeks of gestation. Ventriculomegaly in the first trimester can also be associated with anomalies of the prosencephalon and telencephalon, such as semilobar HPE or agenesis of the corpus callosum detected in the second trimester (Fig. 8.37).[16,17] Keep in mind that ventriculomegaly diagnosed in the first trimester can be an isolated finding or transient in nature, and as such is associated with good prognosis.

## Open Spina Bifida

### Definition

Spina bifida is defined as a midline defect in the spinal cord, primarily resulting from failure of closure of the distal neuropore during embryogenesis. Most commonly the defect is located dorsally. Ventral defects, which are very rare, result from splitting of the vertebral body, and are difficult to diagnose prenatally. Dorsal defects can be open or closed. Open defects occur in about 80% of cases and expose the neural tissue to the amniotic fluid given the absence of overlying muscle and skin. Closed defects are covered by skin and have a better prognosis than open defects, but are very difficult to diagnose in the first trimester and thus we will primarily discuss open spina bifida in this section. Most spina bifidas occur in the lumbosacral spinal region. Synonyms for open spina bifida include myelomeningocele and myelocele (or myeloschisis). Other spinal abnormalities are described in Chapter 14.

### Ultrasound Findings

The diagnosis of open spina bifida in the first trimester can be challenging, as the direct demonstration of the spinal lesion is difficult during ultrasound screening (Fig. 8.38) and the traditional CNS changes that are seen in the second trimester, such as lemon (frontal bone scalloping) and banana (obliteration of cisterna magna with abnormal shaped cerebellum) signs, are not typically visible before 12 to 14 weeks of gestation (Fig. 8.39).[4,18] The classic lemon and banana signs associated with an open spina bifida in the second trimester of pregnancy are thought to be the consequence of leakage of cerebrospinal fluid into the amniotic cavity and decreased pressure in the subarachnoid spaces leading to caudal displacement of the

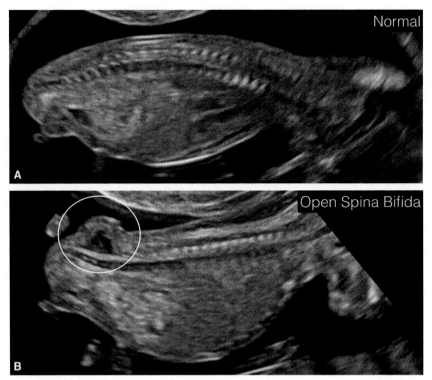

**Figure 8.38:** Dorsoanterior midsagittal view of a normal fetus **(A)** and a fetus with open spina bifida as myelomeningocele **(B)** at 12 weeks of gestation. Note in **B** the direct visualization of the spina bifida in the lower lumbosacral spine (*circle*).

brain and obstructive hydrocephalus (Chiari II malformation). The lemon and banana signs, when present, are best detected by transvaginal ultrasound in the first trimester, as they may not be visible on transabdominal scanning (Fig. 8.39).[6,19]

Chaoui et al. noted that in fetuses with open spina bifida, caudal displacement of the brain resulting in compression

of the fourth ventricle is evident in the first trimester, in the same midsagittal view of the fetal face, a plane commonly used for NT measurement and for assessment of the nasal bone[4,20] (cf. Figs. 8.12 and 8.40). This midsagittal plane in the normal fetus demonstrates the fourth ventricle as an IT parallel to the NT and delineated by two echogenic

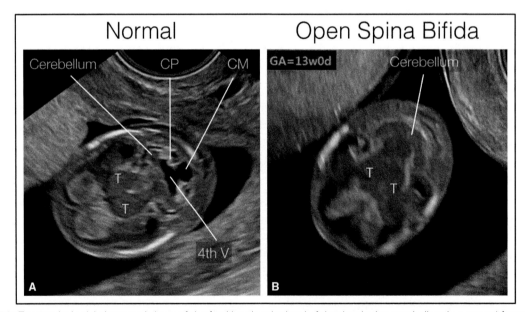

**Figure 8.39:** Transvaginal axial ultrasound views of the fetal head at the level of the developing cerebellum in a normal fetus **(A)** and a fetus with open spina bifida **(B)** at 13 weeks of gestation. In **A**, the structures of the posterior fossa including the fourth ventricle (4th V), the choroid plexus (CP) of the fourth ventricle, and the developing cisterna magna (CM) are well seen. In the fetus with spina bifida **(B)**, the posterior displacement of the posterior fossa structures leads to a change in the shape of the developing cerebellum, similar to the "banana sign" in the second trimester. T, thalamus.

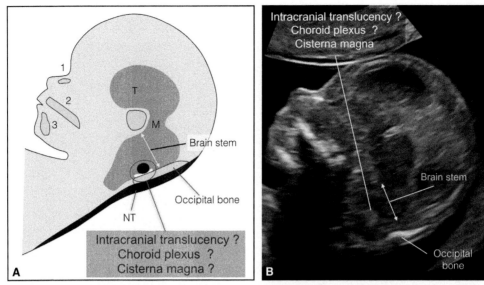

**Figure 8.40:** Schematic drawing **(A)** and corresponding ultrasound image **(B)** of the midsagittal plane of the fetal head in a fetus with open spina bifida (compare with normal anatomy in Fig. 8.12). In open spina bifida in the first trimester, there is a shifting of the posterior brain structures toward the occipital bone leading to brainstem thickening (*double headed arrow*), with partial or complete compression of the fourth ventricle (intracranial translucency), cisterna magna, and the choroid plexus of the fourth ventricle. All three structures are distorted and their normal anatomy cannot be visualized. The free floating choroid plexus in the cerebrospinal fluid of the fourth ventricle and cisterna magna is not seen anymore in open spina bifida and thus the typical normal lines in Figure 8.12 are not seen. See next Figures 8.41, 8.42 and 8.43. T, thalamus; M, midbrain; NT, nuchal translucency; 1, 2, and 3 point to the nasal bone, maxilla, and mandible, respectively.

borders—the dorsal part of the brain stem (BS) anteriorly and the choroid plexus of the fourth ventricle posteriorly (Figs. 8.12, 8.41A, 8.42A, 8.43A). In fetuses with open spina bifida, the IT space is small or not visible as the fourth ventricle and/or cisterna magna is obliterated and the posterior brain is displaced downward and backward (Figs. 8.23, 8.40, 8.41B, 8.42B, 8.43B, and 8.43C).[21,22] This leads to thickening of the brain stem (BS), and shortening of

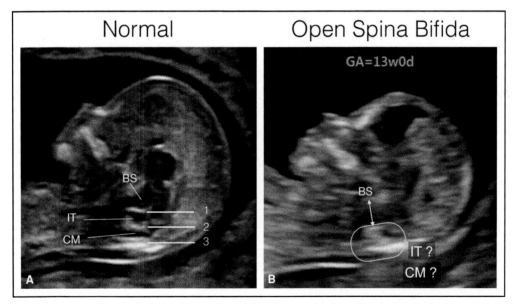

**Figure 8.41:** Midsagittal views of the head, obtained by transabdominal ultrasound at 13 weeks of gestation in a normal fetus **(A)** and in a fetus with open spina bifida **(B)**. In the normal fetus **(A)**, the brainstem (BS) is thin and posterior to it there is cerebrospinal fluid in the fourth ventricle called intracranial translucency (IT) and in the cisterna magna (CM). Typically three echogenic lines can be identified in the posterior fossa in the normal fetus: *line 1*—the posterior border of the brainstem; *line 2*—the choroid plexus of the fourth ventricle; and *line 3*—the occipital bone. In open spina bifida **(B)**, cerebrospinal fluid leaks out through the defect and leads to intracerebral changes, which can be seen in the midsagittal view. Changes in open spina bifida **(B)** include posteriorly shifted and thickened brainstem (BS) (*double headed arrow*) (see figures 8.42 and 8.43), decreased or absence of fluid in the intracranial translucency (IT ?), and cisterna magna (CM ?) (*circle*) and absence of the three anatomic lines that are seen in normal anatomy **(A)**. Also note the flat forehead in fetus **B**, leading to a small frontomaxillary facial angle (see Chapter 9 and Fig. 9.18).

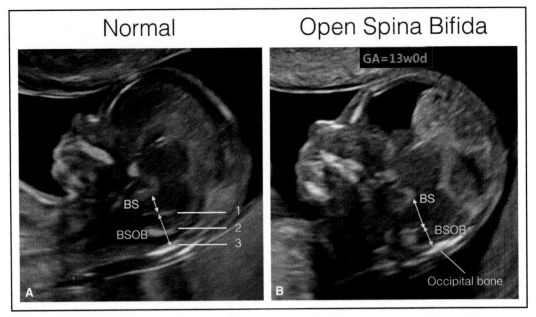

**Figure 8.42:** Transvaginal ultrasound of the midsagittal plane of the face and posterior brain in a normal fetus **(A)** and in a fetus with open spina bifida **(B)** at 13 weeks of gestation. See Figure 8.41 for more details on midsagittal brain anatomy in normal fetuses and in fetuses with open spina bifida. The three echogenic lines in **A** correspond to the posterior border of the brainstem (*1*), the choroid plexus of the fourth ventricle (*2*), and the occipital bone (*3*). Quantification of the posterior fossa can be achieved by measuring the brainstem diameter (BS) (*yellow double headed arrow*) and the distance from the BS to the occipital bone (BSOB) (*blue double headed arrow*). In normal fetuses **(A)** the BS is smaller than the BSOB and the ratio of both is smaller than 1. In open spina bifida **(B)** BS is larger and BSOB is shorter which leads to a ratio >1. See brainstem shape in Figure 8.43.

the distance between the brainstem and the occipital bone (BSOB), leading to an increase in the ratio of BS/BSOB of more than 1 in most cases (Fig. 8.42).[21,22] Another simple approach is to focus on the presence of three white lines in the normal fetus (Figs. 8.41A and 8.42A), which are not visible in open spina bifida (Figs. 8.41B, 8.42B and 8.42C). These changes in the IT and posterior fossa are not present in fetuses with closed spina bifida.[23] In a large prospective study in Berlin, performed by 20 specialists in fetal ultrasound, the detection of all 11 cases of open spina bifida during the first trimester scan was performed using the midsagittal plane.[24] Other intracranial signs reported with open spina bifida include posterior shifting of the cerebral peduncles and aqueduct of Sylvius[19,25] (Fig. 8.44) and an abnormal frontomaxillary facial angle (Figs. 8.41B and 9.18B).[26] The lateral and fourth ventricles are small due to loss of cerebrospinal fluid.[27] This results in a small BPD in the first trimester[28–30] and in comparison with normal fetuses, a ratio of BPD to abdominal transverse diameter of smaller than 1 has been reported.[31] It is important to note that despite the presence of numerous signs of open spina bifida in the first trimester, the diagnosis relies on the demonstration of the actual defect in the spine (Figs. 8.38B, 8.45B, 8.45C, 8.46B, and 8.47). When the diagnosis is suspected but not confirmed in the first trimester, follow-up ultrasound examination after the 15th week of gestation usually confirms the diagnosis.

## Associated Malformations

Spina bifida can occur as an isolated finding but is also found in association with aneuploidies such as trisomy 18, triploidy, or others. CNS abnormalities such as hydrocephaly appear later. Kyphoscoliosis may be present and could be a sign for the presence of Jarcho–Levin syndrome. Dislocation of the hips along with lower limb deformities such as bilateral clubbing and rocker bottom feet are typically seen in the second and third trimesters of gestation.

## Posterior Fossa Abnormalities

### Definition

Posterior fossa abnormalities include malformations of the cerebellar hemispheres, the cerebellar vermis, the cisterna magna, and the fourth ventricle. Given that the embryologic development of the posterior fossa is not completed until the second trimester of pregnancy with the formation and rotation of the vermis, many abnormalities of the posterior fossa cannot be detected in the first trimester. DWM is a posterior fossa abnormality characterized by the presence of a dilated cisterna magna, which communicates with the fourth ventricle, varying degrees of hypoplasia, or agenesis of the vermis and elevation of the tentorium.[32] The embryogenesis of DWM is thought to occur around the seventh week of gestation and thus its suspicion in the first trimester is possible. First

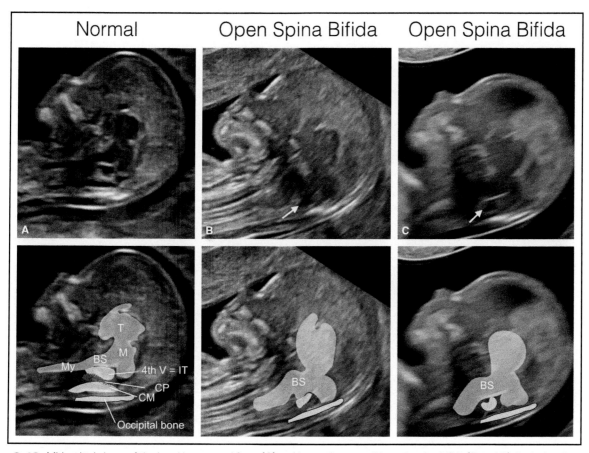

**Figure 8.43:** Midsagittal views of the head in a normal fetus **(A)** and in two fetuses with open spina bifida **(B and C)** displaying the anatomy of the midbrain and posterior fossa. The *upper panels* show the two-dimensional ultrasound images and the *lower panels* show an overlay to better highlight anatomy. *Green highlights* show brain structures to include the thalamus (T), midbrain (M), brainstem (BS), and myelencephalon (My). *Yellow highlights* show the cerebrospinal fluid in the posterior fossa, present in the fourth ventricle (4th V) or IT and in the future cisterna magna (CM). *Red highlights* show the choroid plexus (CP) of the fourth ventricle. In open spina bifida, in the first trimester there is a shifting of the posterior brain structures toward the occipital bone leading to thickening of BS (cf. *green highlights*; BS in **B** and **C** with **A**) and a partial or complete compression of the IT, the cisterna magna (*yellow highlights*), and the CP (*red highlights*). Some fetuses with spina bifida have no fluid in the fourth ventricle as shown in Figures 8.38B and 8.39B, whereas others may have some fluid as shown here in **B** and **C**.

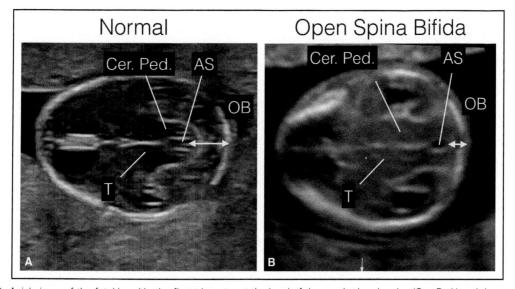

**Figure 8.44:** Axial views of the fetal head in the first trimester at the level of the cerebral peduncles (Cer. Ped.) and the aqueduct of Sylvius (AS) in a normal fetus **(A)** and in a fetus with open spina bifida **(B)**. Note in **B**, the posterior displacement of the Cer. Ped. and the AS toward the occipital bone (OB) (*double headed arrows*). This view is better evaluated in transvaginal sonography. T, thalamus.

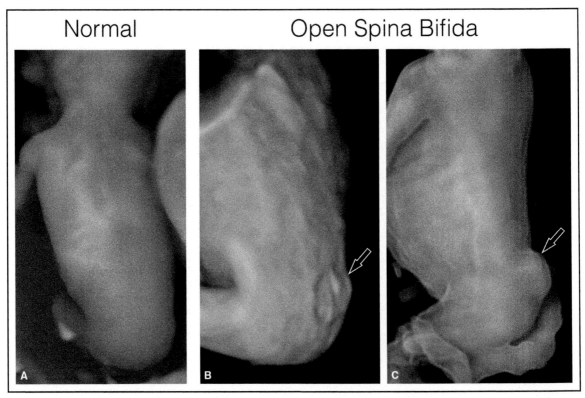

**Figure 8.45:** Three-dimensional ultrasound in surface mode of a normal fetus **(A)** and two fetuses with open spina bifida as myelomeningocele **(B and C)** at 13 weeks of gestation. Note in **B** and **C** the direct visualization of the spina bifida in the lower lumbosacral spine (*arrows*). The corresponding two-dimensional image of fetus **C** is displayed in Figure 8.33B.

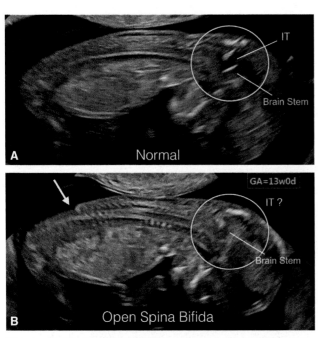

**Figure 8.46:** Dorsoanterior midsagittal view of a normal fetus **(A)** and a fetus with open spina bifida as myeloschisis **(B)** at 13 weeks of gestation. Note in **B** how difficult it is to directly visualize the spinal defect in the lower lumbosacral spine (*arrow*). Note however, changes in the posterior fossa (*circle*) in fetus **B** as compared to fetus **A**. The intracranial translucency (IT) and a slim brainstem (BS) is shown in **A** compared with no fluid (IT ?) and a compressed thickened BS in the fetus with spinal defect **(B)**. This fetus is also demonstrated in Fig.8.47.

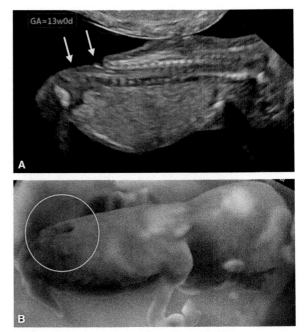

**Figure 8.47:** Dorsoanterior two-dimensional (2D) midsagittal view **(A)** of a fetus at 13 weeks of gestation with open spina bifida as myeloschisis (*arrows*) (see also Fig. 8.46) and corresponding three-dimensional ultrasound in surface mode **(B)**. Note that the open spina bifida is difficult to image in **A** on the 2D ultrasound image. **B:** The defect in the lower lumbosacral spine is shown (*circle*). Suspicion for the presence of an open spina bifida was achieved due to an abnormal posterior fossa, as shown in Figures 8.39, 8.40, and 8.46.

trimester ultrasound is not diagnostic of isolated mega cisterna magna, Blake's pouch cyst, cerebellar hypoplasia, cerebellar hemispheric asymmetry, and isolated vermian hypoplasia due to delayed embryogenesis of these structures.[33,34]

## Ultrasound Findings

The suspicious diagnosis of DWM in the first trimester is based upon the presence of an enlarged IT, a reduced thickness of the BS, and diminished visibility of the choroid plexus of the fourth ventricle in a midsagittal view of the fetal head (Figs. 8.48 and 8.49).[33] Axial and coronal views of the fetal head will show a large posterior fossa cyst separating the cerebellar hemispheres (Figs. 8.48 and 8.49). There is some evidence that midsagittal view measurements assessing the posterior brain such as the BS diameter, the BSOB diameter, and the ratio between both measurements (BS/BSOB ratio)

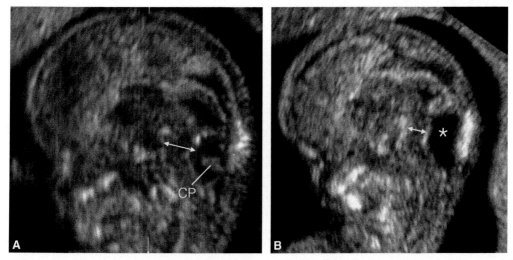

**Figure 8.48:** Midsagittal view of the head at 12 weeks of gestation demonstrating the posterior fossa in a normal fetus **(A)** and in a fetus with Dandy–Walker malformation **(B)**. Note in fetus **B** the presence of increased cerebrospinal fluid (*asterisk*) in the posterior fossa with absence of the choroid plexus (CP) as compared to fetus **A**. The brainstem (*double headed arrow*) is also thinned in the fetus with Dandy–Walker malformation.

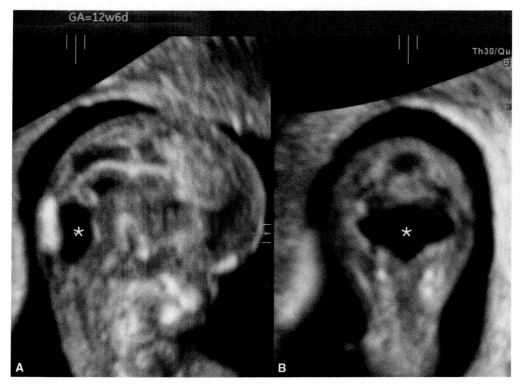

**Figure 8.49:** Sagittal **(A)** and coronal **(B)** views of the posterior fossa in a fetus with suspected Dandy–Walker malformation at 12 weeks of gestation. Note the dilated posterior fossa (*asterisk*) with absence of the choroid plexus.

might improve the screening for DWM in the first trimester (Figs. 8.48 and 8.49).[33] An increased BSOB (representing the fourth ventricle and cisterna magna complex) and a decreased BS/BSOB ratio should alert the sonographer to the possibility of DWM and encourage a detailed examination of the posterior fossa in the first trimester.[33] The examiner has to keep in mind that a true DWM is a fairly rare condition and a dilated fourth ventricle in the first trimester can also be a sign of aneuploidy (Figs. 8.50, 6.6, and 6.20B), syndromic conditions (Fig. 10.20), Blake's pouch cyst (Figs. 8.51A, 8.52 and 8.53A), encephalocele (Fig. 8.22B) but also a transient finding. Blake's pouch cyst also shows a dilation of the posterior fossa and may simulate the presence of a DWM (Figs. 8.52 and 8.53), especially when scanned in coronal views. In the presence of

Blake's pouch cyst, less fluid is present in the posterior fossa than DWM and follow-up ultrasound in the second trimester will demonstrate a normal cerebellum and vermis. When posterior fossa abnormalities are suspected in the first trimester, detailed ultrasound examination of the fetus and follow-up in the second trimester is recommended.

## Associated Malformations

Dilated posterior fossa and suspected DWM in the first trimester are associated with numerous malformations such as aneuploidies (trisomy 18, trisomy 13, triploidy, monosomy X, and trisomy 21),[35–37] genetic syndromes (Walker–Warburg syndrome), and other intracranial and extracranial abnormalities.

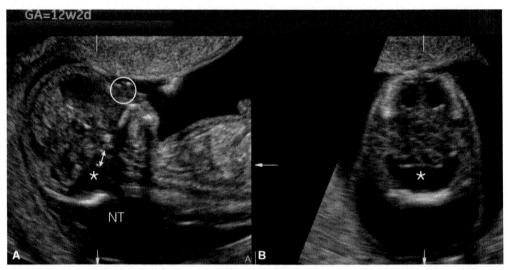

**Figure 8.50:** Midsagittal **(A)** and axial **(B)** views of the fetal head in a fetus with partial trisomy 11q, thickened nuchal translucency (NT), and absent nasal bone (*circle*) at 12 weeks of gestation. Note the cystic dilation of the posterior fossa (*asterisks*) with a thin brainstem (*double headed arrow*).

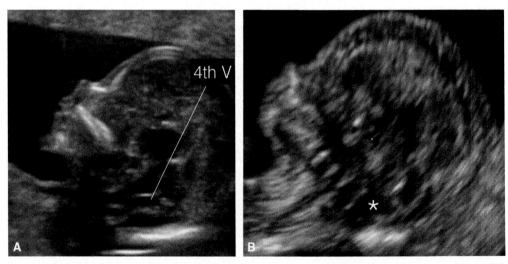

**Figure 8.51:** Sagittal view of a normal fetus **(A)** at 12 weeks and a fetus with suspected persistent Blake's pouch cyst **(B)** at 13 weeks of gestation. Note the normal appearing posterior fossa and fourth ventricle (4th V) in **A**. In the fetus with suspected persistent Blake's pouch cyst **(B)**, moderate dilation of the 4th V (*asterisk*) is seen.

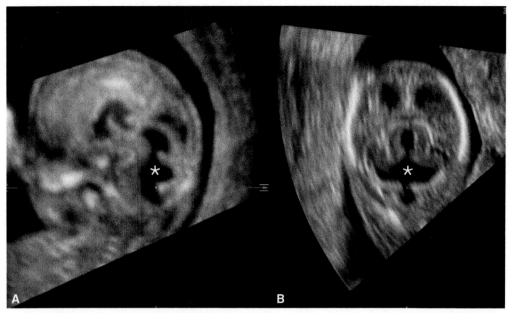

Figure 8.52: Midsagittal **(A)** and coronal **(B)** views of the fetal head at 12 weeks of gestation showing a moderately dilated posterior fossa (*asterisk*). The size of the posterior fossa is less than that showed in Dandy–Walker (Fig. 8.49). This fetus was suspected of having persistent Blake's pouch cyst, which was confirmed at 22 weeks of gestation.

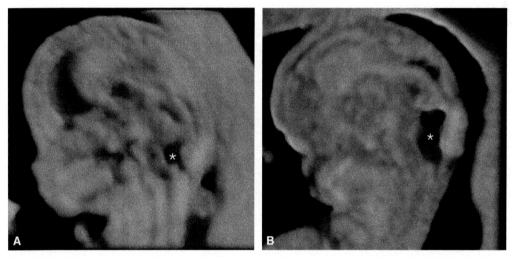

Figure 8.53: Three-dimensional volume in surface mode of the posterior fossa at 12 weeks of gestation in a fetus with persistent Blake's pouch cyst **(A)** and a fetus with Dandy–Walker malformation **(B)**. Note that the posterior fossa (*asterisks*) is moderately dilated in **A** as compared to markedly dilated in **B**.

## REFERENCES

1. Salomon LJ, Alfirevic Z, Bilardo CM, et al. ISUOG practice guidelines: performance of first-trimester fetal ultrasound scan. *Ultrasound Obstet Gynecol*. 2013;41:102–113.
2. Sepulveda W, Wong AE. First trimester screening for holoprosencephaly with choroid plexus morphology ("butterfly" sign) and biparietal diameter. *Prenat Diagn*. 2013;33:1233–1237.
3. Abu-Rustum RS, Ziade MF, Abu-Rustum SE. Reference Values for the right and left fetal choroid plexus at 11 to 13 weeks: an early sign of "developmental" laterality? *J Ultrasound Med*. 2013;32:1623–1629.
4. Chaoui R, Benoit B, Mitkowska-Wozniak H, et al. Assessment of intracranial translucency (IT) in the detection of spina bifida at the 11-13-week scan. *Ultrasound Obstet Gynecol*. 2009;34:249–252.
5. Chatzipapas IK, Whitlow BJ, Economides DL. The "Mickey Mouse" sign and the diagnosis of anencephaly in early pregnancy. *Ultrasound Obstet Gynecol*. 1999;13:196–199.
6. Blaas HG, Eik-Nes SH. Sonoembryology and early prenatal diagnosis of neural anomalies. *Prenat Diagn*. 2009;29:312–325.
7. Sepulveda W, Wong AE, Andreeva E, et al. Sonographic spectrum of first-trimester fetal cephalocele: review of 35 cases. *Ultrasound Obstet Gynecol*. 2015;46:29–33.
8. Blaas HGK, Eriksson AG, Salvesen KÅ, et al. Brains and faces in holoprosencephaly: pre- and postnatal description of 30 cases. *Ultrasound Obstet Gynecol*. 2002;19:24–38.
9. Solomon B, Gropman A, Muenke M. Holoprosencephaly overview—GeneReviews®. http:/www.genereviews.org. Accessed March 17, 2017.

10. Syngelaki A, Guerra L, Ceccacci I, et al. Impact of holoprosencephaly, exomphalos, megacystis and high NT in first trimester screening for chromosomal abnormalities. *Ultrasound Obstet Gynecol*. 2016. doi:10.1002/uog.17286.

11. Sepulveda W, Wong AE, Andreeva E, et al. Biparietal diameter-to-crown-rump length disproportion in first-trimester fetuses with holoprosencephaly. *J Ultrasound Med*. 2014;33:1165–1169.

12. Kim MS, Jeanty P, Turner C, et al. Three-dimensional sonographic evaluations of embryonic brain development. *J Ultrasound Med*. 2008;27:119–124.

13. Blaas HG, Eik-Nes SH, Vainio T, et al. Alobar holoprosencephaly at 9 weeks gestational age visualized by two- and three-dimensional ultrasound. *Ultrasound Obstet Gynecol*. 2000;15:62–65.

14. Chaoui R, Heling KS, Thiel G, et al. Agnathia-otocephaly with holoprosencephaly on prenatal three-dimensional ultrasound. *Ultrasound Obstet Gynecol*. 2011;37:745–748.

15. Loureiro T, Ushakov F, Maiz N, et al. Lateral ventricles in fetuses with aneuploidies at 11-13 weeks' gestation. *Ultrasound Obstet Gynecol*. 2012;40:282–287.

16. Manegold-Brauer G, Oseledchyk A, Floeck A, et al. Approach to the sonographic evaluation of fetal ventriculomegaly at 11 to 14 weeks gestation. *BMC Pregnancy Childbirth*. 2016;16:1–8.

17. Ushakov F, Chitty LS. Ventriculomegaly at 11–14 weeks: diagnostic criteria and outcome [Abstract]. *Ultrasound Obstet Gynecol*. 2016;48(suppl 1):267.

18. Blaas HG, Eik-Nes SH, Isaksen CV. The detection of spina bifida before 10 gestational weeks using two- and three-dimensional ultrasound. *Ultrasound Obstet Gynecol*. 2000;16:25–29.

19. Buisson O, De Keersmaecker B, Senat MV, et al. Sonographic diagnosis of spina bifida at 12 weeks: heading towards indirect signs. *Ultrasound Obstet Gynecol*. 2002;19:290–292.

20. Chaoui R, Nicolaides KH. From nuchal translucency to intracranial translucency: towards the early detection of spina bifida. *Ultrasound Obstet Gynecol*. 2010;35:133–138.

21. Lachmann R, Chaoui R, Moratalla J, et al. Posterior brain in fetuses with open spina bifida at 11 to 13 weeks. *Prenat Diagn*. 2011;31:103–106.

22. Chaoui R, Benoit B, Heling KS, et al. Prospective detection of open spina bifida at 11-13 weeks by assessing intracranial translucency and posterior brain. *Ultrasound Obstet Gynecol*. 2011;38:722–726.

23. Fuchs I, Henrich W, Becker R, et al. Normal intracranial translucency and posterior fossa at 11-13 weeks' gestation in a fetus with closed spina bifida. *Ultrasound Obstet Gynecol*. 2012;40:238–239.

24. Chen F, Gerhardt J, Entezami M, et al. Detection of spina bifida by first trimester screening—results of the prospective multicenter Berlin IT-study. *Ultraschall Med*. 2017;38:151–157.

25. Finn M, Sutton D, Atkinson S, et al. The aqueduct of Sylvius: a sonographic landmark for neural tube defects in the first trimester. *Ultrasound Obstet Gynecol*. 2011;38:640–645.

26. Lachmann R, Picciarelli G, Moratalla J, et al. Frontomaxillary facial angle in fetuses with spina bifida at 11-13 weeks' gestation. *Ultrasound Obstet Gynecol*. 2010;36:268–271.

27. Loureiro T, Ushakov F, Montenegro N, et al. Cerebral ventricular system in fetuses with open spina bifida at 11-13 weeks' gestation. *Ultrasound Obstet Gynecol*. 2012;39(6):620–624.

28. Karl K, Benoit B, Entezami M, et al. Small biparietal diameter in fetuses with spina bifida on 11-13-week and mid-gestation ultrasound. *Ultrasound Obstet Gynecol*. 2012;40:140–144.

29. Khalil A, Coates A, Papageorghiou A, et al. Biparietal diameter at 11-13 weeks' gestation in fetuses with open spina bifida. *Ultrasound Obstet Gynecol*. 2014;42(4):409–415.

30. Bernard JP, Cuckle HS, Stirnemann JJ, et al. Screening for fetal spina bifida by ultrasound examination in the first trimester of pregnancy using fetal biparietal diameter. *Am J Obstet Gynecol*. 2012;207:306.e1–306.e5.

31. Simon EG, Arthuis CJ, Haddad G, et al. Biparietal/transverse abdominal diameter ratio ≤ 1: potential marker for open spina bifida at 11-13-week scan. *Ultrasound Obstet Gynecol*. 2015;45:267–272.

32. Robinson AJ. Inferior vermian hypoplasia—preconception, misconception. *Ultrasound Obstet Gynecol*. 2014;43:123–136.

33. Lachmann R, Sinkovskaya E, Abuhamad A. Posterior brain in fetuses with Dandy-Walker malformation with complete agenesis of the cerebellar vermis at 11-13 weeks: a pilot study. *Prenat Diagn*. 2012;32:765–769.

34. Bornstein E, Goncalves Rodríguez JL, Álvarez Pavón EC, et al. First-trimester sonographic findings associated with a Dandy-Walker malformation and inferior vermian hypoplasia. *J Ultrasound Med*. 2013;32:1863–1868.

35. Loureiro T, Ferreira AFA, Ushakov F, et al. Dilated fourth ventricle in fetuses with trisomy 18, trisomy 13 and triploidy at 11-13 weeks' gestation. *Fetal Diagn Ther*. 2012;32:186–189.

36. Volpe P, Muto B, Passamonti U, et al. Abnormal sonographic appearance of posterior brain at 11-14 weeks and fetal outcome. *Prenat Diagn*. 2015;35:717–723.

37. Mace P, Quarello E. Analyse de la fosse posté rieure fœtale lors de l'é chographie du premier trimestre de la grossesse. *Gynecol Obstet Fertil*. 2016;44:43–55.

# CHAPTER 9

# The Fetal Face and Neck

## INTRODUCTION

Visualization of the fetal face and neck in early gestation is an important aspect of the ultrasound examination as it has been incorporated in the first-trimester fetal risk assessment for aneuploidy (Chapters 1 and 5). A midsagittal plane of the fetus is part of nuchal translucency (NT) measurement and is also used to assess for the presence or absence of nasal bones. A more detailed assessment of the fetal face and neck in the first trimester allows for the diagnosis of a number of abnormalities with high associations, including aneuploidy and genetic syndromes. In this chapter, we present a systematic approach to the evaluation of the fetal face and neck and discuss in detail major facial and neck abnormalities that can be diagnosed in the first trimester. The posterior fossa in the brain, which is also visualized in the midsagittal plane of the fetus, is separately discussed in Chapter 8 on central nervous system (CNS) anomalies.

## EMBRYOLOGY

Embryologic development of the fetal face and neck is a complex process, which involves coordination of multiple tissues including ectoderm, neural crest, mesoderm, and endoderm with involvement of six pairs of pharyngeal arches. The pharyngeal arches play a dominant role in building the face and neck, including its skeletal, muscular, vascular, and nerve structures.

The first evidence of facial development is seen during the third week of embryogenesis with the formation of the oropharyngeal (oral) membrane, which lies at the opening of the foregut and represents the future oral cavity. During the fourth to seventh week of embryogenesis, five facial swellings or processes merge and fuse to form the facial structures. These facial processes include one frontonasal process, arising from crest cells, and two maxillary and mandibular processes, arising from the first pharyngeal arch (Fig. 9.1). The frontonasal process gives rise to two medial and two lateral nasal

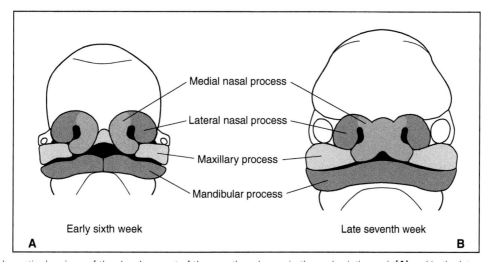

Figure 9.1: Schematic drawings of the development of the mouth and nose in the early sixth week (**A**) and in the late seventh week (**B**) of embryogenesis. The two medial and two lateral nasal processes fuse in the middle along with the lateral maxillary and mandibular processes to form the nose, as shown in **A**, and mouth, as shown in **B**. The primary palate is formed by the medial nasal and maxillary processes, whereas the secondary palate is formed by the fusion of the maxillary processes. The colors of nose, maxilla, and mandible in **A** and **B** show the process contributing to embryogenesis. See text for more details.

**Table 9.1** • Contributions of Embryologic Facial Prominences to Facial Structures

- Frontonasal: Forehead, dorsum of nose
- Lateral nasal: Lateral aspects of nose
- Medial nasal: Septum of nose
- Maxillary: Upper cheek, most of upper lip and secondary palate
- Mandibular: Lower cheek, chin, and lower lip

processes. **Table 9.1** and **Figures 9.1 and 9.2** list the various contributions of facial processes to the development of facial structures. Fusion and merging of the medial nasal and maxillary processes form the primary palate, and the secondary palate is formed by fusion of the maxillary processes, which completes facial development by the 12th week of embryogenesis. Facial growth continues during the fetal period with changes in proportions and features of facial structures. Detailed embryologic development of the face and neck is beyond the scope of this book. Failure of development or fusion of facial processes contributes to the majority of facial abnormalities, including clefting, which is discussed later in this chapter.

The pharyngeal arches contribute to the development of the neck. The third pharyngeal arch forms the skeletal structures of the hyoid bone. The parathyroid glands and the laryngeal cartilages are formed by fusion of the fourth and sixth pharyngeal arches. The thyroid gland originates around the 24th day of embryogenesis from the primitive pharynx and neural crest cells, forming the median and lateral thyroid, respectively. The median thyroid becomes the main thyroid gland. The thyroid descends in the neck until it reaches the front of the trachea in the seventh week of embryogenesis. The thyroid gland is the first endocrine organ to develop, and it starts producing thyroid hormones by the 12th week of menstrual age.

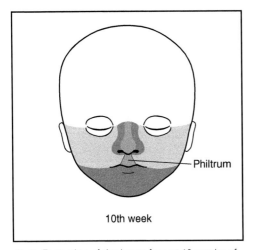

**Figure 9.2:** Formation of the lower face at 10 weeks of embryogenesis. Note that the face is completely formed, and note the contribution of various processes to the formation of the face. See Figure 9.1 for corresponding colors and text for details.

# NORMAL SONOGRAPHIC ANATOMY

The systematic visualization of the face and neck includes multiple approaches from the midsagittal, coronal, and axial planes. The midsagittal approach allows for the visualization of the facial profile and NT, and the coronal and axial planes allow for visualization of other facial and neck features. Several brain anatomic structures, such as the thalamus, brain stem, fourth ventricle, lateral ventricles, and choroid plexuses, can also be demonstrated in the midsagittal and parasagittal views of the head and face[1] and are discussed in detail in Chapters 5 and 8. We will hereby describe normal sonographic features of the face and neck in each anatomic plane.

## Sagittal Planes

The *midsagittal plane* of the fetal head (**Figs. 9.3 and 9.4**), demonstrating the fetal profile in the first trimester, enables the assessment of the forehead, nose with nasal bone, mouth with maxilla, mandible anteriorly, and NT posteriorly. In the first trimester, the fetal head appears slightly larger in proportion to the body than later on in gestation, and in this midsagittal view the forehead shows some normal-appearing "frontal bossing" (**Figs. 9.3 and 9.4**). At this stage of early gestation, the metopic suture is still wide and the frontal bones are not seen in the midsagittal view. The perpendicular insonation to the nasal structures in the midsagittal plane of the face enables clear visualization of facial structures. The midsagittal plane landmarks are important in order to correctly identify the nasal bone on midsagittal scanning, with the demonstration of the "equal sign" formed by the nasal bone inferiorly and the nasal skin superiorly (**Figs. 9.4, 9.5A, 9.6, and 1.1**). The maxilla is recognized in the midsagittal plane as a continuous ossified region in the face (**Figs. 9.4 to 9.6**). In the midsagittal plane, the anterior part of the mandible is seen as an echogenic dot under the anterior maxilla (**Fig. 9.6A**). In *parasagittal views*, a larger part of the mandible can be seen (**Fig. 9.6C**) as well as the maxillary process between the nasal bone and the maxilla (**Fig. 9.6B**). Several facial measurements in the midsagittal view have been proposed in the literature.[2–8] The significance of abnormal facial measurements and anatomic markers is discussed later in this chapter.

In the posterior aspect of the midsagittal view, the neck with NT is also demonstrated. A detailed discussion of NT measurement (**Figs. 9.3 and 9.4**) and its significance is presented in Chapters 1 and 6. Conditions associated with a thickened NT and cystic hygroma are discussed at the end of this chapter.

## Coronal Planes

A *frontal coronal view* of the bony face in the first trimester reveals both orbits and eyes and their relationships to the nasal bridge and maxilla (**Fig. 9.7**) (see Chapter 5). The position, size, and shape of the eyes and orbits are generally assessed in a subjective manner. A coronal view of the face demonstrates

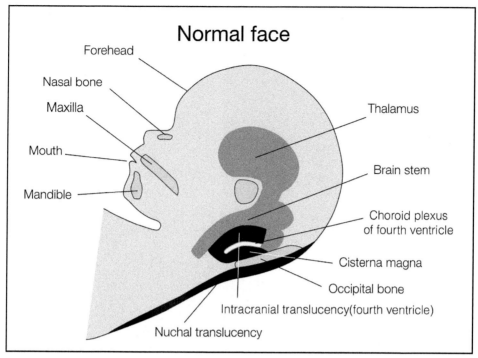

**Figure 9.3:** Schematic drawing of the midsagittal plane of the fetal head showing the fetal facial profile and displaying important anatomic structures evaluated by the first-trimester ultrasound, including forehead, nasal bone, maxilla, mouth, mandible, midline central nervous system structures, and nuchal translucency. See corresponding ultrasound in Figure 9.4 and text for details.

the anterior maxilla (alveolar ridge) (**Fig. 9.7**). The retronasal triangle is imaged in an oblique plane, between the coronal and axial planes of the face, in the region of the nose and maxilla (**Fig. 9.7B**)[9] (see Chapter 5 and Fig. 5.9). An oblique plane between the maxilla and the mandible normally reveals a mandibular gap (**Fig. 9.7B**).[10] Good visualization of facial structures is typically performed from a 3D surface rendering of the face, ideally obtained transvaginally.

## Axial Planes

In the experience of the authors, the systematic visualization of the *axial planes* of the face is of secondary importance to the midsagittal and coronal planes (Chapter 5). As performed in the second trimester, multiple axial planes obtained in the first trimester from cranial to caudal enable the demonstration of orbits, nasal bridge with nasal bones, the maxilla, and the mandible (**Fig. 9.8**) (Chapter 5). The fetal lips cannot be well identified on transabdominal scanning in the first trimester, and, when needed, imaging of these structures can be obtained transvaginally with high-resolution transducers.

## Three-Dimensional Ultrasound of the Fetal Face

Similar to the use of three-dimensional (3D) ultrasound in surface mode of the fetal face in the second and third trimesters of pregnancy, 3D ultrasound in the first trimester (**Fig. 9.9**) provides additional information to the 2D midsagittal (profile), frontal, and axial facial views.[11] When fetal abnormalities are suspected in the first trimester, 3D ultrasound of the fetal face in surface mode enables a detailed view of facial features, including the forehead, eyes, nose, mouth, chin, and ears (**Figs. 9.9 to 9.11**). Three-dimensional ultrasound of the

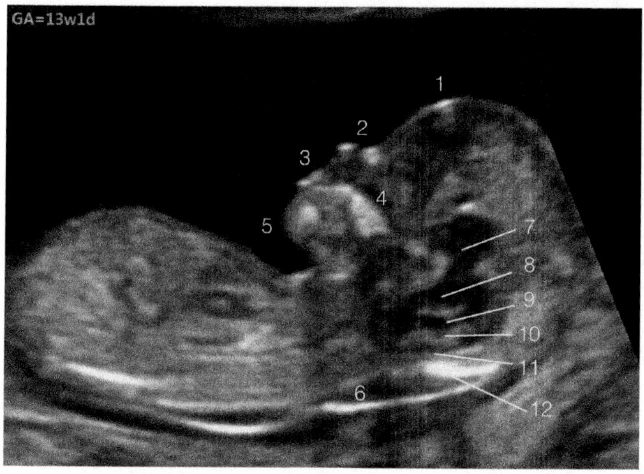

**Figure 9.4:** Midsagittal ultrasound plane of the fetal head at 13 weeks of gestation showing the profile with the forehead (*1*), nose with nasal bone (*2*), mouth (*3*), maxilla (*4*), and chin with mandible (*5*). The posterior aspect of the profile plane displays the nuchal translucency (*6*) and different anatomic structures of the midline brain to include the thalamus (*7*), brain stem (*8*), fourth ventricle as intracranial translucency (*9*), choroid plexus of the fourth ventricle (*10*), the developing cisterna magna (*11*), and the occipital bone (*12*). See Figure 9.3 for the corresponding schematic drawing.

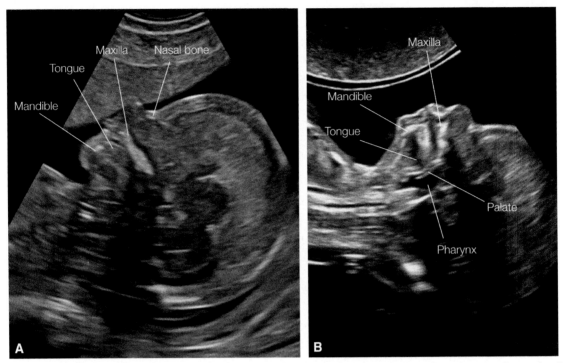

**Figure 9.5:** Transvaginal ultrasound of the midsagittal plane of the fetal face in two fetuses **(A and B)** at 13 weeks of gestation. In fetus **A**, the ultrasound beam is perpendicular to the long axis of the face and clearly displays the nose with nasal bone, the maxilla, and chin with mandible. Note in **A** the tongue between the maxilla and mandible. In fetus **B**, the ultrasound beam is inferior below the chin and shows the posterior aspect of the mouth region with the tongue, hard and soft palate, and the pharynx.

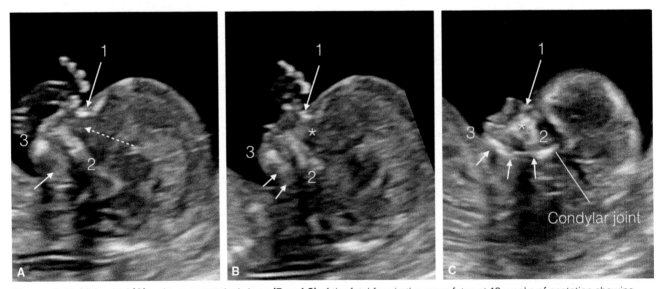

**Figure 9.6:** Midsagittal **(A)** and two parasagittal views **(B and C)** of the fetal face in the same fetus at 13 weeks of gestation showing the nasal bone (1), maxilla (2), and mandible (3). In **A**, obtained at the midsagittal view, the maxilla is seen (2), but the processus maxillaris (*broken arrow*) is not seen. In **A** also, the tip of the mandible is seen (3), but the mandibular body (*short arrow*) is not seen. **B** is a slight tilt to a parasagittal plane, where the processus maxillaris (*asterisk*) and the body of the mandible (*two arrows*) start to be seen. A more angulated parasagittal view is seen in **C,** showing the bony face with the processus maxillaris (*asterisk*) between nasal bone (1) and maxilla (2) and the lateral aspect of the mandible (3) with the body, the ramus, and the condylar joint (*short arrows*).

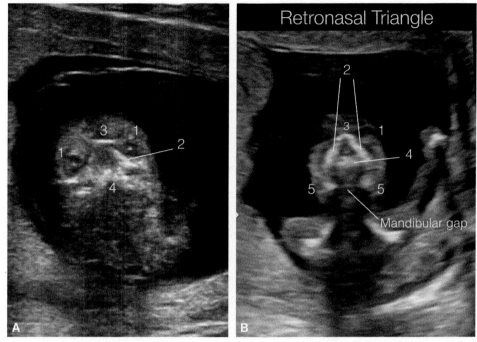

**Figure 9.7:** Coronal planes in two fetuses **(A and B)** at 12 weeks of gestation, obtained at the frontal aspects of the bony face. In fetus **A**, the coronal plane is at the level of the orbits and shows the two eyes (*1*) with orbits and lenses, between the maxillary processes (*2*), the nasal bones (*3*), and the anterior aspect of the maxilla (*4*) with the alveolar ridge. In fetus **B**, the plane is oblique and demonstrates the retronasal triangle (see text for details), which is formed by the nasal bones superiorly (*3*), the frontal processes of the maxilla laterally (*2*), and the alveolar ridge (primary palate) inferiorly (*4*). This coronal section **(B)** is posterior to the tip of the mandible, and therefore the two lateral bodies of the mandible are seen (*5*) with a normal gap between, called the mandibular gap. The presence of micrognathia results in disappearance of the mandibular gap in the retronasal triangle plane. See Figure 9.14 to help understand the anatomic facial location of the retronasal triangle plane.

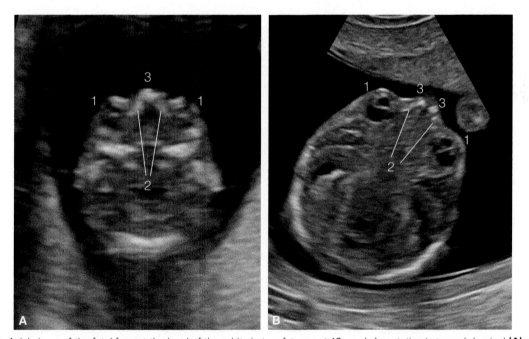

**Figure 9.8:** Axial views of the fetal face at the level of the orbits in two fetuses at 13 weeks' gestation in transabdominal **(A)** and transvaginal approach **(B)**. Note that the eyes (*1*), maxillary processes (*2*), and nasal bones (*3*) are seen in this plane. In the transvaginal approach **(B)**, the lenses in the eyes (*1*) and two separate nasal bones (*3*) are also seen.

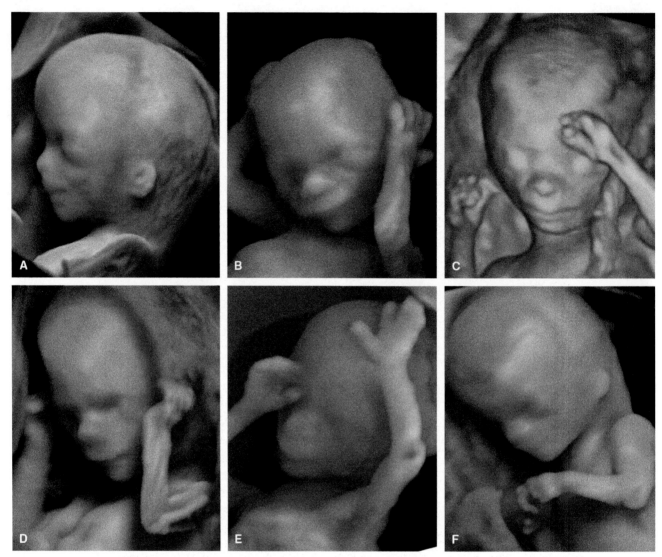

**Figure 9.9:** Three-dimensional ultrasound images in surface mode of the normal fetal face obtained in six fetuses **(A–F)** by the transvaginal approach. Note the physiologic frontal bossing and the clear anatomic regions of forehead, eyes, nose, mouth, chin, and ears. Compare with Figures 9.10 and 9.11 obtained in abnormal fetuses.

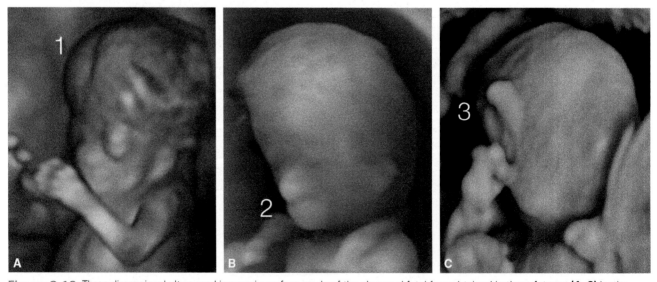

**Figure 9.10:** Three-dimensional ultrasound images in surface mode of the abnormal fetal face obtained in three fetuses **(A–C)** by the transvaginal approach. Fetus **A** has acrania/exencephaly (*1*); fetus **B** has trisomy 13 with holoprosencephaly, hypotelorism, and cebocephaly (*2*) (small nose with one nostril); and fetus **C** has trisomy 13 with proboscis (*3*).

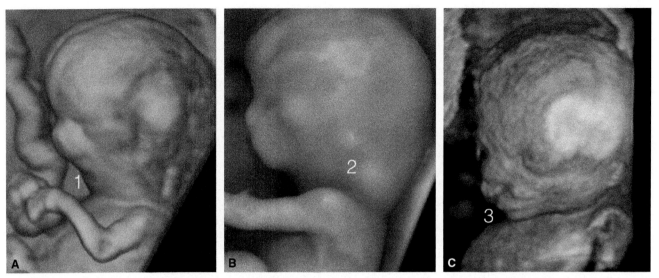

**Figure 9.11:** Three-dimensional ultrasound images in surface mode of the abnormal fetal face obtained in three fetuses **(A–C)** by the transvaginal approach. Fetus **A** has trisomy 13 with micrognathia (*1*), fetus **B** has trisomy 18 with abnormal profile and dysplastic ears (*2*), and fetus **C** has a syndromic condition with associated facial cleft (*3*).

fetal face can often be obtained by transabdominal acquisition, but when an abnormality is suspected the transvaginal approach provides for more details and higher resolution. Figures 9.9 to 9.11 show examples of normal and abnormal fetal faces on 3D ultrasound in the first trimester of pregnancy. Three-dimensional ultrasound can also be used in multiplanar display with reconstruction of planes for the specific evaluation of target anatomic regions (Figs. 9.12 to 9.14) such as the

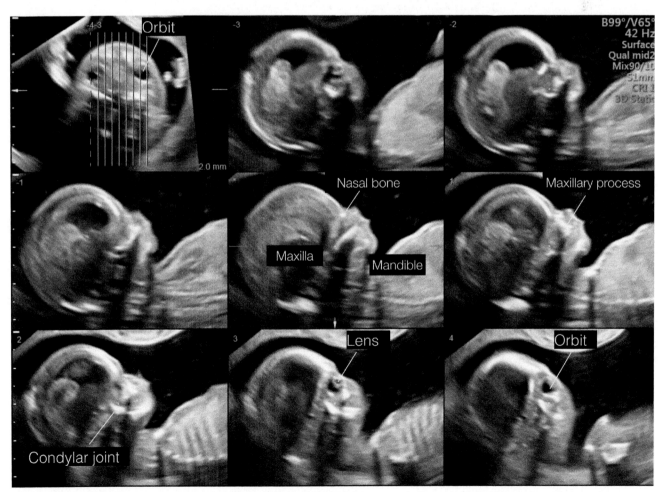

**Figure 9.12:** Three-dimensional ultrasound of a normal fetal face obtained transvaginally at 12 weeks of gestation and shown in tomographic display. Note the anatomic details assessed in the midsagittal and parasagittal views.

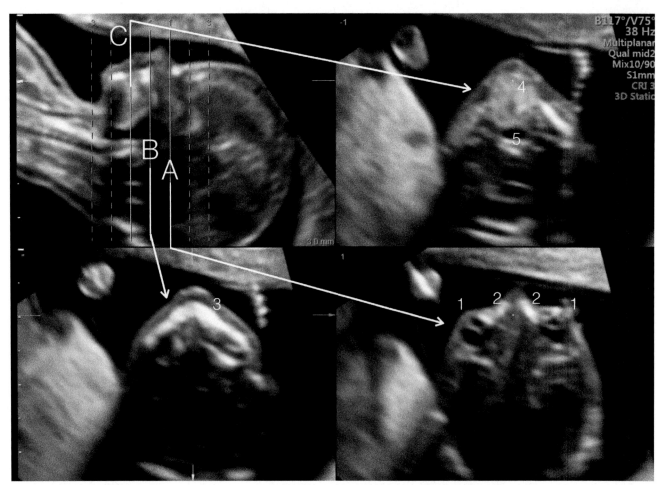

**Figure 9.13:** Three-dimensional ultrasound volume of the fetal face acquired transvaginally at 12 weeks of gestation and displayed in tomographic mode. In the reference image **(upper left)**, the midsagittal plane is shown and the corresponding tomographic coronal planes are displayed with *plane A* at the level of the eyes (*1*), *plane B* at the level of the maxilla (*3*), and *plane C* at the level of the tongue (*4*). The maxillary processes (*2*) and the pharynx (*5*) are also shown in *A* and *C*, respectively. Acquisition of a three-dimensional volume of the fetal head in early gestation allows for detailed assessment of facial anatomy.

bony face or the palate in the evaluation of facial anomalies (see later). For more details on the use of 3D ultrasound in the first trimester, refer to Chapter 3 in this book and a recent book on the clinical use of 3D in prenatal medicine.[11]

## BIOMETRIC MEASUREMENTS OF THE FACE

Several biometric measurements are currently published for the assessment of facial features in the second and third trimesters, and some of these are proposed for use in the first-trimester ultrasound screening. These measurements include diameters, ratios, and angles, primarily performed in the midsagittal plane of the fetal profile. They are used mainly in the first trimester in screening for aneuploidies or in the detection of facial clefts and micrognathia. Some of these measurements are discussed in the following sections.

### Nasal Bone Length

Reference ranges for nasal bone length in the fetus were reported in the second and third trimesters of pregnancy, and nasal bone has been described to be absent or short in fetuses with trisomy 21.[12] This observation was adapted to aneuploidy screening at 11 to 14 weeks of gestation, and Cicero et al.[2] demonstrated that nasal bones are hypoplastic or not ossified in the first trimester in the majority of fetuses with trisomy 21[2] (Figs. 9.15 and 6.1), and in other aneuploidies and syndromic conditions (Figs. 6.6, 6.8, 6.33, and 6.35).[13] Assessment of the nasal bone is also used to improve the efficiency of the combined first-trimester screening for Down syndrome.[13,14] Table 1.2 in Chapter 1 summarizes the essential criteria for an accurate nasal bone assessment in the first trimester.

### Prenasal Thickness

The observation that the skin of the forehead, called the "prenasal thickness," is increased in the second trimester in

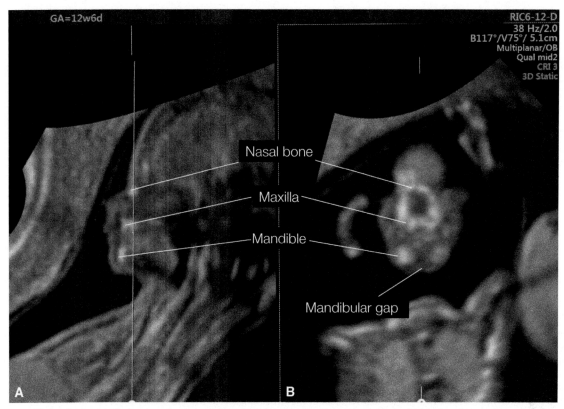

**Figure 9.14:** Three-dimensional ultrasound volume of the fetal face acquired transvaginally at 12 weeks of gestation and displayed in tomographic mode. In this figure, only two planes are displayed: *plane* **A**, showing a midsagittal plane of the head with facial profile, and *plane* **B**, obtained as the corresponding coronal plane at the level of the *yellow line*. Note that *plane* **B** shows the retronasal triangle view with the mandibular gap. See Figure 9.7 for details.

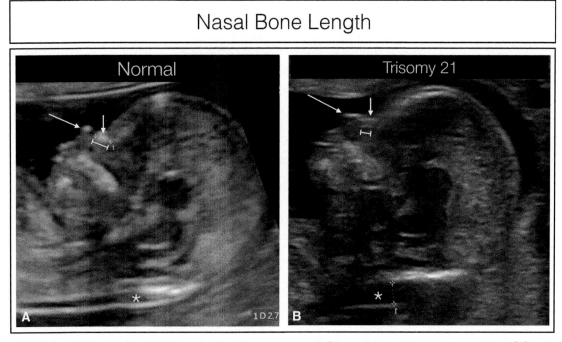

**Figure 9.15:** Midsagittal views of the fetal face showing the measurement of the nasal bone length in a normal fetus **(A)** and in a fetus with trisomy 21 **(B)**. In more than half of the fetuses with trisomy 21, the nasal bone is either completely nonossified or, as in this case, poorly ossified, resulting in a short and thin appearance. *Long arrows* point to the nose tip and *short arrows* to the nasal skin. Nuchal translucency measurement is also seen (*asterisk*). Compare with Figure 1.3 in Chapter 1 and with Fig. 9.16.

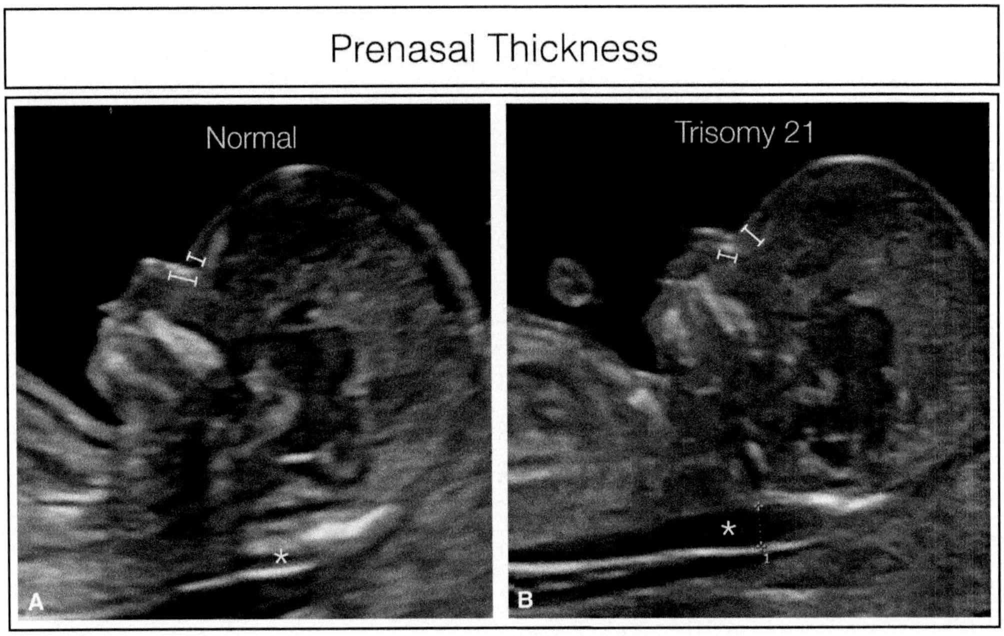

**Figure 9.16:** Midsagittal views of the fetal face showing the measurement of the prenasal thickness in a normal fetus **(A)** and in a fetus with trisomy 21 **(B)**. Prenasal thickness was adapted from the second trimester, where fetuses with trisomy 21 showed increased prenasal thickness. The prenasal thickness (*white line*) is measured as shown in **A** and **B**. Note the presence of increased prenasal thickness in fetus B with trisomy 21. In order to reduce the false-positive rate, the ratio of the prenasal thickness (*white line*) to nasal bone length (*yellow line*) was introduced. In normal fetuses, the ratio is smaller than 0.6 and is increased in trisomy 21. Note in **A** that the *white line* is shorter than the *yellow line*, whereas in **B** it is vice versa. Nuchal translucency measurement is also seen (*asterisk*).

fetuses with trisomy 21[15,16] has led to the use of this marker in the first trimester of pregnancy as well (Fig. 9.16).[5,8,17] To reduce the false-positive rate of prenasal thickness measurement, the ratio of the prenasal thickness to nasal bone length was proposed[5] (Fig. 9.16). In normal fetuses, the prenasal thickness is small and the nasal bone is relatively long, resulting in a ratio of approximately 0.6.[5] In trisomy 21 fetuses in the first trimester, the prenasal thickness increases, whereas the nasal bone length decreases, resulting in a ratio >0.8.[5]

## Maxillary Length

Fetuses with trisomy 21 have a flat profile due to midfacial hypoplasia, leading to the known feature of a protruding tongue. Measuring the maxillary length between 11 and 14 weeks of gestation is proposed as a method to quantify midfacial hypoplasia.[3] The measurement is performed in a slightly parasagittal view of the facial profile and includes the mandibular joint.[3] Maxillary length is short in fetuses with trisomy 21.[3] Midfacial hypoplasia can also be assessed by the use of the frontomaxillary facial angle, which indirectly includes the maxilla.[18] The frontomaxillary facial angle is discussed in the next section.

## Frontomaxillary Facial Angle

The frontomaxillary facial (FMF) angle is the angle between the maxilla and forehead and in normal fetuses is quantified

at 85° (±10°) (Fig. 9.17A).[18] A wide FMF angle is reported in fetuses with trisomy 21[4,19] (Fig. 9.17B), whereas a narrow FMF angle is noted in fetuses with open spina bifida (Fig. 9.18).[20] Abnormal FMF angles are also reported in fetuses with trisomy 18 with midfacial hypoplasia and micrognathia[21] and in fetuses with trisomy 13 in association with holoprosencephaly.[22] Caution should be used, however, in the evaluation of the FMF angle because slightly oblique views will introduce false-positive and negative results. Measurement of the FMF angle using 3D multiplanar rendering has been shown to improve its accuracy.[18,23] The wide FMF angle in fetuses with aneuploidies is likely due to the short maxilla, whereas in spina bifida the narrow angle is probably due to the small flat head owing to the posterior shift of the brain and decreased fluid in the ventricles. Another facial angle is the maxilla–nasion–mandible (MNM) angle and uses the nasion as reference point of the intersection of the frontal and nasal bones.[8,24] The MNM angle is defined as the angle between the maxilla–nasion line and the mandible–nasion line in the midsagittal plane of the face and can be used to identify fetuses at high risk for aneuploidies, micrognathia, and clefts.[8]

## Prefrontal Space Distance

Prefrontal space distance (PSD) is obtained by drawing a line from the anterior aspect of both the mandible and maxilla and extended toward the fetal forehead (Fig. 9.19).[6,7] The

# Fronto-Maxillary-Facial Angle

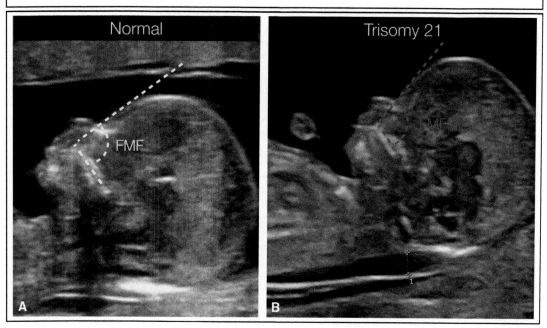

**Figure 9.17:** Midsagittal views of the fetal face showing the measurement of the fronto-maxillary-facial (FMF) angle in a normal fetus **(A)** and in a fetus with trisomy 21 **(B)**. The FMF angle is measured in the midsagittal view of the face between the maxilla and the forehead, as shown in **A** and **B**. In the normal fetus **(A)**, the angle is approximately 85° (*yellow lines*), whereas in the fetus with trisomy 21 **(B)**, the angle is wider than 85° (*red lines*). Nuchal translucency measurement is also seen in fetus **B**. See also Figure 9.18.

# Fronto-Maxillary-Facial Angle

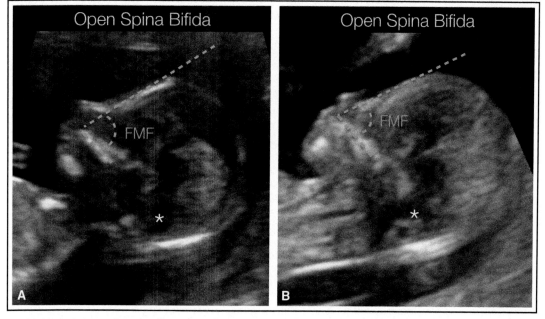

**Figure 9.18:** Midsagittal views of the fetal face showing the measurement of the fronto-maxillary-facial (FMF) angle in two fetuses **(A and B)** with open spina bifida. The FMF angle is typically smaller in fetuses with spina bifida due to a smaller head and decreased fluid in the ventricles, resulting in a flat face. Note the thickened brain stem (*asterisk*) and the almost-absent fluid in the intracranial translucency (IT).

# Prefrontal Space Distance

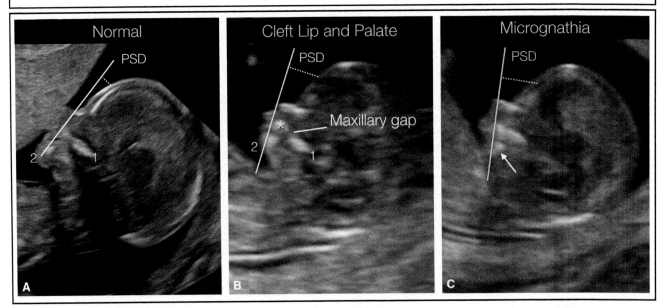

**Figure 9.19:** Midsagittal views of the fetal face showing the measurement of the prefrontal space distance in a normal fetus **(A)**, in a fetus with cleft lip and palate **(B)**, and in a fetus with micrognathia **(C)**. The prefrontal space distance (PSD) is the distance between the forehead and a line drawn from the anterior aspect of maxilla (*1*) and mandible (*2*). In the normal fetus **(A)**, the PSD is quite short. In the presence of a facial cleft (fetus **B**), there is a protrusion of the maxilla (*asterisk*), and the PSD is increased. In the presence of micrognathia (fetus **C**), the mandible is posteriorly shifted (*arrow*), leading to an increased PSD as well. Note in fetus **B** the presence of an interrupted maxilla, called maxillary gap, a midsagittal view sign for the presence of cleft lip and palate.

PSD is calculated by the distance of the prenasal skin to this extended line (Fig. 9.19). The distance can have positive or negative values.[6] PSD is abnormal in fetuses with aneuploidies, such as trisomies 21, 18, and 13,[6] as well as in fetuses with micrognathia and clefts[7] (Fig. 9.19).

## Orbit Size and Distances

To the best of our knowledge, no charts currently exist on the size of the orbit and the interorbital distances in the first trimester of pregnancy, and such measurements are not obtained routinely. Recently, a paper reported on the interlens distance, starting at 12 weeks of gestation.[25]

# FETAL FACIAL ABNORMALITIES IN ANEUPLOIDIES AND IN CNS MALFORMATIONS

## Fetal Profile in Aneuploidies

Trisomy 21 fetuses typically show an abnormal facial flat profile with an absent or hypoplastic nasal bone (Fig. 9.15), a short maxilla, an increased FMF angle (Fig. 9.17), and a thickened prenasal thickness (Fig. 9.16). Similar facial appearance can also be found in trisomy 18 fetuses, in addition to retrognathia

and facial clefts. Trisomy 13 fetuses show severe facial anomalies due to their association with holoprosencephaly (Fig. 9.20) and/or with facial clefts. Ultrasound markers of aneuploidies, including facial abnormalities in the first trimester, are discussed in detail in Chapter 6.

## Holoprosencephaly

Lobar and semilobar holoprosencephaly is often associated with facial abnormalities such as cyclopia, hypotelorism, proboscis, cebocephaly, agnathia-holoprosencephaly, nasal hypoplasia, and facial clefts.[26] In most cases, the profile is severely abnormal, in addition to the abnormal head shape and brain. **Figures 9.10** and **9.20** show abnormal profiles in fetuses with alobar holoprosencephaly. Holoprosencephaly is discussed in detail in Chapter 8.

## Acrania/Anencephaly/Exencephaly

In acrania/anencephaly/exencephaly, the profile and the frontal view of the face have characteristic abnormalities with the presence of large eyes and small face. Facial profile views in **Figure 9.21** show different aspects of the forehead region in acrania. Abnormalities in facial profiles in anencephaly/exencephaly are discussed in detail in Chapter 8.

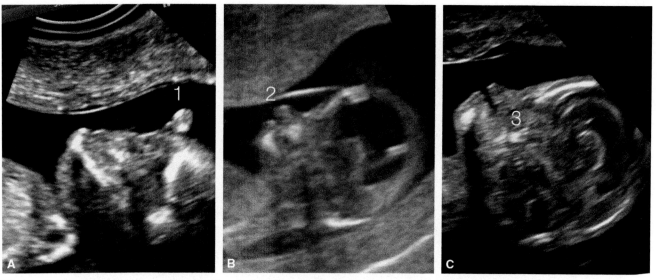

**Figure 9.20:** Midsagittal views of the fetal face in three fetuses **(A–C)** with alobar holoprosencephaly at 11, 12, and 13 weeks of gestation, respectively. In fetus **A**, no normal facial structures are identifiable, and a proboscis (*1*) can be seen in the midline. In fetus **B**, cebocephaly with an abnormal nose (*2*) is seen (compare with 3D image in Fig. 9.10). In fetus **C**, no maxilla (*3*) is seen in this midsagittal plane due to the presence of a large midline cleft.

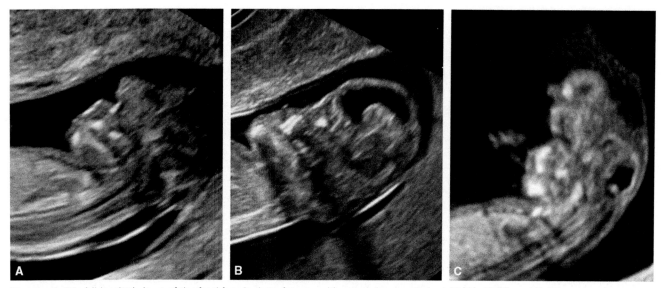

**Figure 9.21:** Midsagittal views of the fetal face in three fetuses with acrania/exencephaly at 10 **(A)**, 12 **(B)**, and 11 **(C)** weeks of gestation, respectively. Note the various aspects of acrania/exencephaly on ultrasound in early gestation. No normal-looking forehead can be seen, and the nasal region is abnormal as well.

## Open Spina Bifida

Open spina bifida is associated with reduced cerebrospinal fluid in the head, which results in a small head, with a small biparietal diameter (BPD) measurement.[27] The cerebrospinal fluid leakage leads to a flat forehead and a reduced FMF angle by about 10° in 90% of the cases.[20] **Figures 9.18A and B** show facial profiles with flat foreheads in two fetuses with open spina bifida in the first trimester of pregnancy.

## Epignathus

Epignathus is an oropharyngeal teratoma, generally originating from the oral cavity. Its origin can be the sphenoid bone, the palate, the tongue, or the pharynx.[28,29] The growth is usually out of the oral cavity,[28] but epignathus can also grow into the brain and face.[29] Reports of this very rare anomaly are generally from fetuses diagnosed in the second or third trimester, but similar to teratomas of other locations (see Chapter 14),

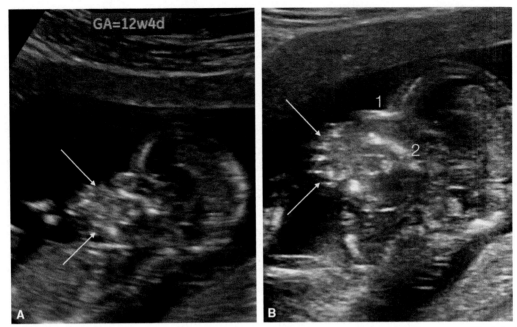

**Figure 9.22:** Midsagittal view of the face at 12 weeks of gestation in a fetus with epignathus. **B** represents a magnified view of **A**. Note the solid character of the tumor (*arrows*) arising from the fetal mouth. Nasal bone (*1*) and the maxilla (*2*) are identified in the midline.

its appearance can also be evident in the first trimester as well (Fig. 9.22). The typical appearance is a protrusion in the mouth region of irregular shape with a mixture of hyperechoic tissue with few cystic structures. If the protrusion is small, it can mimic bilateral facial clefting, but a detailed ultrasound reveals the irregular shape in epignathus, which is atypical for a cleft. Figure 9.22 shows an epignathus, evident in the midsagittal profile view of the face at 13 weeks of gestation.

## Frontal Cephalocele

As discussed in Chapter 8, most cephaloceles arise from the occipital region. Cephaloceles can also arise from the parietal or frontal regions of the head.[30] The frontal cephalocele, also called frontoethmoidal or anterior cephalocele, is less common than other cephalocele types. In the study by Sepulveda et al.[30] only 3 (9%) out of 25 cases of cephaloceles were frontal in location. The frontal cephalocele can be a meningocele with normal intracranial anatomy or an encephalocele with brain tissue protruding through the defect with resulting intracranial changes. In the first trimester, amniotic band syndrome should be considered a possible etiology when a frontal or parietal cephalocele is suspected (see Chapter 8). Differential diagnosis of frontal cephalocele includes the presence of proboscis in holoprosencephaly, nasal glioma, or teratoma. In holoprosencephaly, additional facial and intracerebral characteristic signs are present, which help to differentiate proboscis from cephalocele. Prognosis of frontal cephalocele cannot be predicted in the first trimester, but the earlier in gestation that frontal cephaloceles are detected, the worse is the prognosis. Figure 9.23 shows a fetus at 11 weeks of gestation with a frontal cephalocele.

## Posterior Fossa Disorders

Posterior fossa disorders with cerebellar abnormalities, increased fluid in the fourth ventricle, and/or compressed or abnormal kinking of the brain stem can be found in several conditions, including aneuploidies, syndromic conditions as Walker–Warburg syndrome, Joubert syndrome, or Dandy–Walker malformation, and as a normal variant with persistent Blake pouch cyst (see Chapter 8). Posterior fossa disorders are commonly seen in trisomies 18 and 13 or triploidy (Fig. 9.24). When Walker–Warburg syndrome is suspected, the eyes can be affected, and a targeted first-trimester transvaginal ultrasound examination of the eyes and lenses may show abnormalities that can be consistent with the diagnosis.[31] The presence of a prior history of Walker–Warburg syndrome is important as it targets the ultrasound examination in the first trimester. It is important to note, however, that the absence of cataract in the first trimester cannot rule out Walker–Warburg syndrome given that cataract may not be evident until later on in pregnancy.

# FETAL FACIAL ABNORMALITIES

## Cleft Lip and Palate

### Definition

Cleft lip and palate (CLP) is one of the most common congenital defects, with an incidence of 1/700 to 1/1,000 live births.[32,33] Given the high prevalence of CLP, imaging of the upper lip and philtrum is currently part of the basic obstetric ultrasound examination in the second trimester.[34] Among CLP cases, about a third affect the lip only, and two-thirds involve the lip and

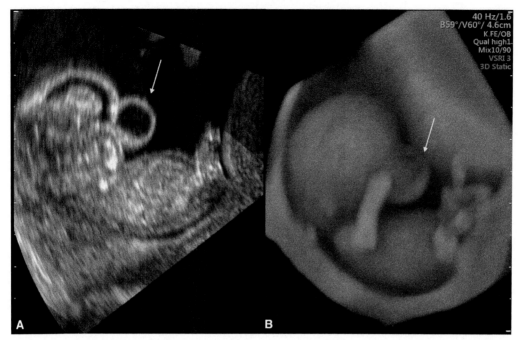

**Figure 9.23:** Fetus at 11 weeks of gestation with an anterior cephalocele, shown in a midsagittal 2D plane of the head in **A** and in three-dimensional ultrasound in surface mode in **B**. The completely cystic aspect of the defect suggests the diagnosis of cephalocele.

palate.[35] CLP can be either isolated or associated with a wide range of chromosomal anomalies and genetic syndromes. A family history of CLP is found in about one-third of patients with nonsyndromic CLP, and with recent genetic advancements, several novel loci that are significantly associated with CLP have been identified.[36] CLP occurs more frequently in males (male/female = 1.70), especially among isolated cases.[35] There are different classifications of facial clefts,[35,37,38] and it

is often difficult to collect all needed details for a precise classification of CLP in the first trimester of pregnancy. Prenatally, and especially in the first trimester, we recommend Nyberg's classification (Fig. 9.25) of CLP, with type 1 being the isolated cleft lip, type 2 with unilateral (or mediolateral) CLP, type 3 with bilateral CLP, type 4 with midline (or median) CLP, and type 5 with complete facial clefts, which is primarily seen in amniotic band syndrome.[38]

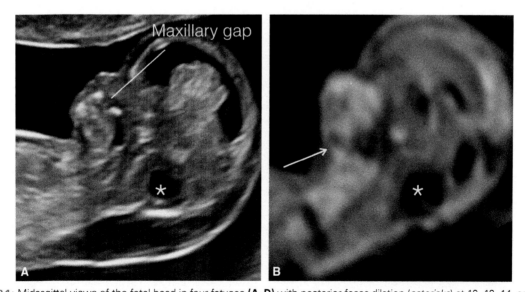

**Figure 9.24:** Midsagittal views of the fetal head in four fetuses **(A–D)** with posterior fossa dilation (*asterisks*) at 12, 12, 14, and 13 weeks of gestation, respectively. Fetus **A** has trisomy 18 with absent nasal bone and a cleft lip and palate recognized by the maxillary gap. Fetus **B** has trisomy 13 with micrognathia (*arrow*). Fetuses **C** and **D** had no abnormal facial findings in the profile views, and follow-up ultrasound examinations confirmed Dandy–Walker malformations in both.

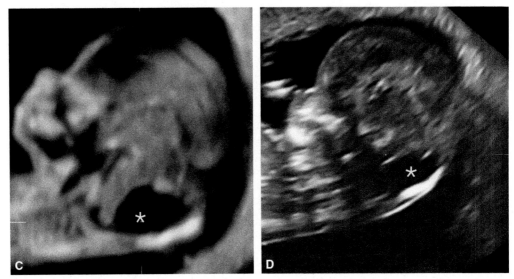

Figure 9.24: (continued)

## Cleft Types

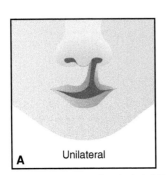

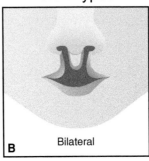

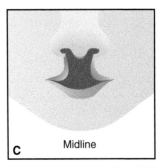

A　Unilateral　　　B　Bilateral　　　C　Midline

Figure 9.25: Schematic drawings of typical cleft lips and palates (CLP) observed by ultrasound in early gestation. CLP can be unilateral (mediolateral), either on the left or on the right side **(A)**. CLP can also be bilateral **(B)** with a pseudomass in the middle or midline, as shown in **C**. See text for details.

### Ultrasound Findings

The diagnosis of isolated CLP is often difficult in the first trimester, primarily related to the small size of facial structures.[39–41] Indeed, most cases of isolated CLP are not detected during the first-trimester ultrasound examination.[42,43] In the large study of Syngelaki et al.[42] (see Table 5.2 in Chapter 5), only 1 out of 20 fetuses (5%) with nonaneuploid clefts was detected in the first trimester, whereas in another recent study from two specialized referral centers, the detection rate of isolated clefts in early gestation was 24%.[43] The planes used for detecting CLP in the first trimester are similar to those used in the second-trimester ultrasound, but the visualization of the nose–lip region is not practical in the first trimester due to the low resolution and small size of these structures. For the identification of a CLP in the first trimester, we therefore recommend either an axial view of the maxilla or a more coronal oblique view of the retronasal triangle (Fig. 9.7).[9] In addition, in an ultrasound screening setting, our reported sign, called "maxillary gap sign" (Figs. 9.26 to 9.32) is fairly simple and can suspect the presence of CLP, which needs to be

confirmed in an axial plane of the maxilla or in the retronasal triangle view (Figs. 9.26 to 9.32). The maxillary gap sign is discussed in more detail later on in this section. The retronasal triangle (RNT) view, suggested by Sepulveda et al.,[9] is an oblique view of nose and anterior maxilla (Fig. 9.7) and is formed by the two nasal bones superiorly, the frontal processes of the maxilla laterally, and the alveolar ridge (primary palate) inferiorly[9] (Fig. 9.7). The RNT is obtained from the midsagittal view of the fetal face by rotating the transducer 90° with a slight tilt to bring the frontal processes of the maxilla and primary palate into the same plane.[44] The presence of CLP is reflected by a defect in the primary palate seen on the RNT view (Fig. 9.28A). In a prospective study using 3D ultrasound, the identification of CLP by visualization of the RNT in the first trimester has been shown to have a sensitivity of 87.5% and a specificity of 99.9%,[45] but it is still unknown if such a sensitivity can be reached with 2D screening ultrasound examinations. In difficult cases, 3D ultrasound can help in the display of the face and the RNT plane and thus plays an important role in confirming the presence of CLP in early

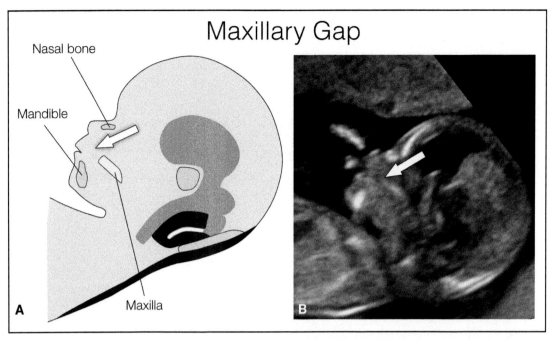

**Figure 9.26:** Schematic drawing of the midsagittal view of the fetal face **(A)** along with the corresponding ultrasound image **(B)** demonstrating the maxillary gap (*white arrows*) in a fetus with cleft lip and palate. Compare with the schematic drawing of a normal fetus in Figure 9.3. In this midsagittal view plane, the entire maxilla should be seen. The size and location of the maxillary gap vary according to the size and type of clefts. Compare with Figures 9.27 to 9.31.

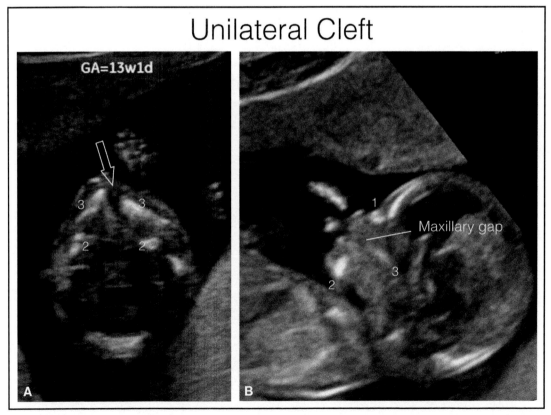

**Figure 9.27:** Axial **(A)** and midsagittal **(B)** views of the face at 13 weeks of gestation in a fetus with a unilateral cleft lip and palate. The cleft lip and palate is demonstrated in the axial view **(A)** (*open arrow*). Note the presence of a maxillary gap in the midsagittal view of the face **(B)**. The following facial structures are seen: nasal bone (*1*), mandible (*2*), and maxilla (*3*). In this fetus, the cleft was isolated, and the child was successfully operated on postnatally.

# Bilateral Cleft

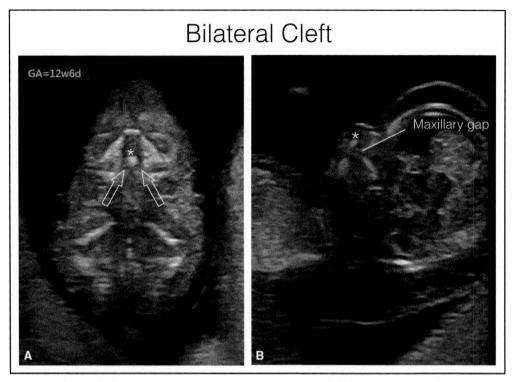

**Figure 9.28:** Retronasal triangle **(A)** and midsagittal **(B)** views of the face at 13 weeks of gestation in a fetus with bilateral cleft lip and palate. The bilateral clefts are demonstrated in the retronasal triangle view **(A)** (*open arrows*). Note the presence of a large maxillary gap in the midsagittal view of the face **(B)**. Also note the presence of a protrusion of a pseudomass (*asterisks*) in **A** and **B**, as is commonly seen in most fetuses with bilateral clefts in the first trimester. This fetus also had trisomy 18.

# Midline Cleft

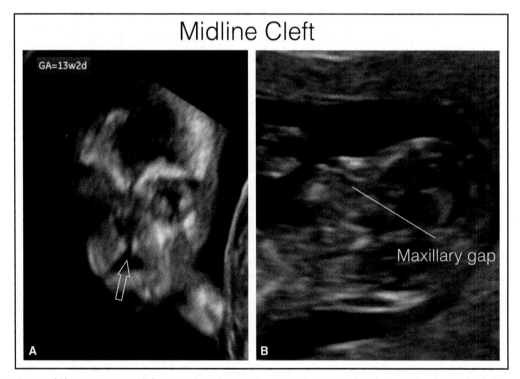

**Figure 9.29:** Coronal **(A)** and midsagittal **(B)** views of the face at 13 weeks of gestation in a fetus with a midline cleft. The midline cleft is demonstrated in the coronal view **(A)** (*open arrows*). Note the almost complete absence of the maxilla in the midsagittal view of the face **(B)**. In this fetus, holoprosencephaly was present along with trisomy 13.

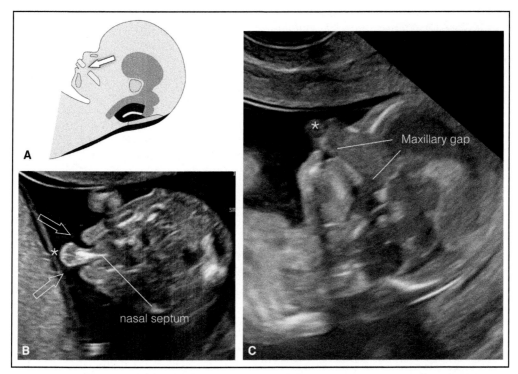

**Figure 9.30:** Schematic drawing of the midsagittal view of the fetal face **(A)** along with the corresponding axial **(B)** and sagittal **(C)** ultrasound images demonstrating the maxillary gap (*white arrow* in **A**, labeled in **C**) in a fetus with bilateral cleft lip and palate and trisomy 13. Note the presence in **B** and **C** of a protrusion of a pseudomass (*asterisks*) anterior to the maxillary region. The profile **(C)** is obviously abnormal in such cases. In this case, the maxillary gap is recognized (*white arrow* in **A**, labeled in **C**) as an interruption of the maxilla in its anterior part. Depending on the angle of insonation, the position of the gap may vary. In such cases, a strict midsagittal view may visualize the nasal septum and mimic a maxilla, but a slight parasagittal view reveals the maxillary gap.

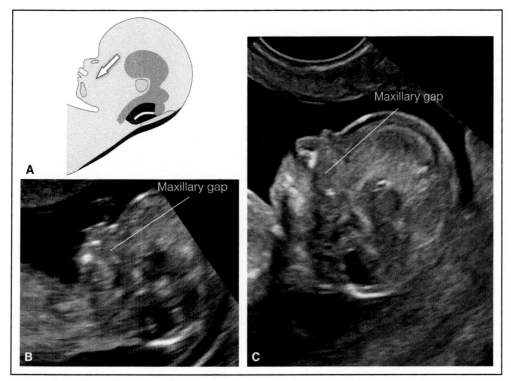

**Figure 9.31:** Schematic drawing of the midsagittal view of the fetal face **(A)** along with midsagittal views in two fetuses **(B and C)** with bilateral clefts and no obvious protrusion. Note the presence of a large maxillary gap in both fetuses. In such cases, the prefrontal space distance (see Fig. 9.19) will not be abnormal. Fetus **B** had trisomy 18, and fetus **C** had a syndromic condition. In both fetuses, the maxillary gap is recognized in the midsagittal view.

gestation (Fig. 9.11).[11,39,45,46] The RNT is probably the best view to detect or rule out CLP in the first trimester, but this additional plane is not always easy to obtain and is not part of screening ultrasound examinations. As previously stated and in our opinion, improved detection of CLP in the first trimester can be achieved if a sonographic marker can be integrated into the screening ultrasound. For this purpose, Chaoui et al.[43] reported on the first trimester presence of a maxillary gap in the midsagittal plane of the fetus as a clue for CLP (Fig. 9.26).[43] This finding is significant in the sense that the midsagittal plane of the fetus is routinely obtained for the assessment of NT, nasal bone, and posterior fossa. The maxillary gap is observed in 96% of nonisolated CLP and more than 65% of isolated CLP.[43] However, a small maxillary gap can be seen in 5% to 7% of normal fetuses and in this setting represents a false-positive diagnosis.[7,43] A possible reason for the presence of a small maxillary gap in normal fetuses is probably related to delayed ossification of the maxilla at 11 to 13 weeks of gestation. Indeed, a large maxillary gap of greater than 1.5 mm or complete absence of the maxilla in the midsagittal plane (Figs. 9.26 to 9.32) was seen in 69% of nonisolated CLP, in 35% of isolated CLP, and in none of the normal fetuses.[43] It is important to note, however, that the presence of a maxillary gap is a marker for CLP and the diagnosis has to be confirmed in the axial or frontal views with direct observation of the facial cleft. Furthermore, bilateral facial clefts typically show a premaxillary protrusion,[47] which can be easily seen in the midsagittal view of the face as a mass anterior to the mouth and nose region (Figs. 9.29 and 9.30). A more objective assessment is achieved by measuring the PSD[7] (Fig. 9.19) or the maxilla–nasion–mandible angle[8] as previously described in the Biometric Measurements of the Face section. With such measurements, cases with retrognathia associated with CLP can also be detected, and this is discussed in the next section.

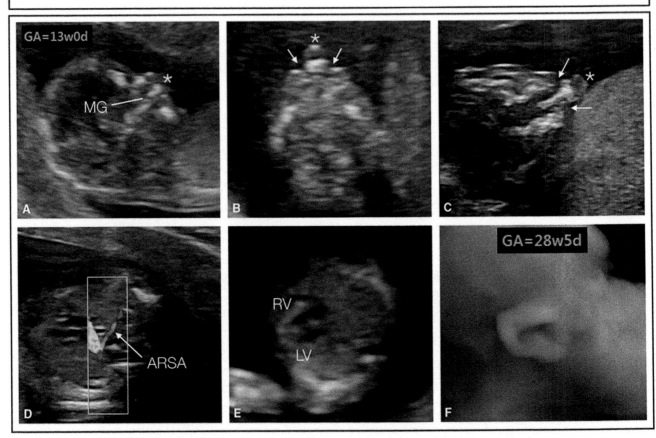

# CHARGE Syndrome

**Figure 9.32:** Ultrasound images of a fetus diagnosed with CHARGE syndrome. In the first trimester at 13 weeks of gestation, the following findings were noted: **A**, midsagittal view of the face showing a protrusion (*asterisk*) and a maxillary gap (MG) suggestive of the presence of a facial cleft. The bilateral facial clefts (*arrows*) along with the protrusion (*asterisks*) are demonstrated in an axial view of the maxilla in **B** on a convex transducer and in **C** on the linear transducer. **D:** An aberrant right subclavian artery (ARSA) with an otherwise normal heart (four-chamber view shown in **E**). Amniocentesis at 16 weeks of gestation revealed a normal karyotype and microarray. At 28 weeks of gestation, a perimembranous ventricular septal defect (not shown) in addition to the presence of a dysplastic ear (**F**) was noted, which led us to target molecular genetic testing for CHARGE syndrome, and a mutation on the *CHD7* gene was detected.

## Associated Malformations

CLP can be an isolated finding or associated with more than 100 genetic syndromes and aneuploidies[48] (see Chapter 6 and Table 9.2). In a large study involving 5,449 cases of CLP from the EUROCAT network in 14 European countries, a total of 3,860 CLP cases (70.8%) occurred as isolated anomalies, and 1,589 (29.2%) were associated with other defects such as multiple congenital anomalies of unknown origin and chromosomal and recognized syndromes.[35] Associated malformations were more frequent in infants who had CLP (34.0%) than in infants with cleft lip only (20.8%). This study confirmed that musculoskeletal, cardiovascular, and central nervous system defects are frequently associated with CLP.[35] The association of CLP with anomalies is highly dependent on the anatomic type of the cleft.[38,49] In a large study of 500 cases of CLP, Gillham et al.[49] found that unilateral CLP had 9.8%, bilateral CLP 25%, and median (or midline) CLP 100% association with other anomalies. Another study from a tertiary referral fetal center analyzed data from 70 fetuses with facial clefts and similarly found that all fetuses with midline clefts had associated anomalies.[50] In this study, however, the associated anomalies in the two other groups were higher, being 48% of fetuses with unilateral clefts and 72% with bilateral clefts, than in other studies.[50] Therefore, once a CLP is detected, detailed first-trimester ultrasound is recommended, looking for additional structural anomalies including facial, intracerebral, cardiac, and skeletal anomalies. Interestingly, almost all midline CLP, along with bilateral CLP but without premaxillary protrusion, are associated with intracerebral anomalies and aneuploidies.[49–51] On the other hand, CLP in combination with cardiac anomalies should raise the suspicion of deletion 22q11, deletion 4p− (Wolf–Hirschhorn

**Table 9.2 • Common Syndromic Conditions in Facial Clefts**

Numerical aneuploidies (trisomy 13, 18, triploidy, etc.)

Deletions and duplications (4p−, 22q11, 18p−, etc.)

CHARGE syndrome

Ectrodactyly–ectodermal dysplasia cleft (EEC) syndrome

Frontonasal dysplasia

Fryns syndrome

Goldenhar syndrome

Gorlin syndrome

Holoprosencephaly autosomal-dominant syndromes

Kallmann syndrome

Nager syndrome

Pierre Robin syndrome

Roberts syndrome

Treacher Collins syndrome

VACTERL sequence

van der Woude syndrome

syndrome), or CHARGE syndrome (Fig. 9.32). The presence of a CLP in the mother or father of an affected fetus should raise suspicion for an autosomal-dominant condition, such as Van der Woude syndrome. When a CLP is identified in the first trimester in our centers, we perform a detailed first-trimester ultrasound examination looking for additional abnormalities and offer the patient invasive diagnostic genetic testing for karyotype and microarray testing. A follow-up 2D and 3D ultrasound in the early second trimester is also performed for evaluation of fetal anatomy. Table 9.2 lists few of the numerous conditions associated with CLP.

## Micrognathia

### Definition

Micrognathia is the term used to describe a rare facial malformation that is characterized by a small, underdeveloped mandible. Retrognathia is a term used to describe a mandible that is receded in relation to the maxilla and is commonly present in association with the presence of micrognathia. Prenatally, both are commonly found concurrently and the terms are used interchangeably. In this chapter, we will use the term *micrognathia* to describe this condition because only severe findings may be detected in the first trimester.

### Ultrasound Findings

The presence of micrognathia is initially suspected in the mid-sagittal plane of the fetal face in the first trimester by noting that the mandible is not at the same level as the maxilla, but rather recessed posteriorly (Fig. 9.33). Unlike in normal facial anatomy, in the presence of micrognathia, a line drawn from the mandible toward the maxilla will not intersect the forehead (Fig. 9.19),[7,10] and this can be quantified by the FMF angle,[21] the PSD (Fig. 9.19),[7] or the MNM angle.[8] Often in the first trimester, the chin may appear impressively small in suspected micrognathia, but in follow-up ultrasound examination in the second and third trimesters, proportionate growth occurs and the fetal profile will look less abnormal (Fig. 9.34). In isolated cases, therefore, the severity of micrognathia cannot be predicted from the sole appearance of the profile view. An interesting observation is the assessment of the chin region in the coronal plane displayed by the RNT. In the normal fetus, facial anatomy of the RNT in the first trimester displays a characteristic gap between the right and left bodies of the mandible, referred to as the mandibular gap (Fig. 9.35).[10] This mandibular gap can be measured from the midpoint of the echogenic edge of one mandibular bone to the other and appears to increase linearly with increasing CRL.[10] Sepulveda et al.[10] observed that the absence of the mandibular gap or failure to identify the mandible in the RNT view is highly suggestive of micrognathia (Fig. 9.35). The absence of a mandibular gap in the coronal view of the face in the first trimester should therefore prompt the examiner to perform a detailed ultrasound in order to confirm micrognathia and to assess for the presence of other anomalies. Typically, micrognathia

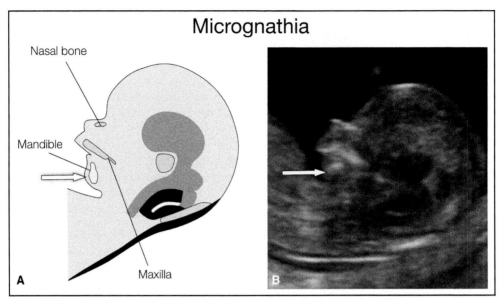

**Figure 9.33:** Schematic drawing of the midsagittal plane of the face **(A)** along with the corresponding midsagittal **(B)** ultrasound image of a fetus with micrognathia (*white arrows*). Compare with the schematic drawing of a normal fetus in Figure 9.3. Note that the mandibular tip does not reach the anterior aspect of the maxilla in **A** and **B**, but rather reaches the midportion of it. Micrognathia can be isolated as in the context of Pierre Robin sequence but also can be part of numerous syndromic conditions. Compare with Figures 9.34 to 9.37. See text for details.

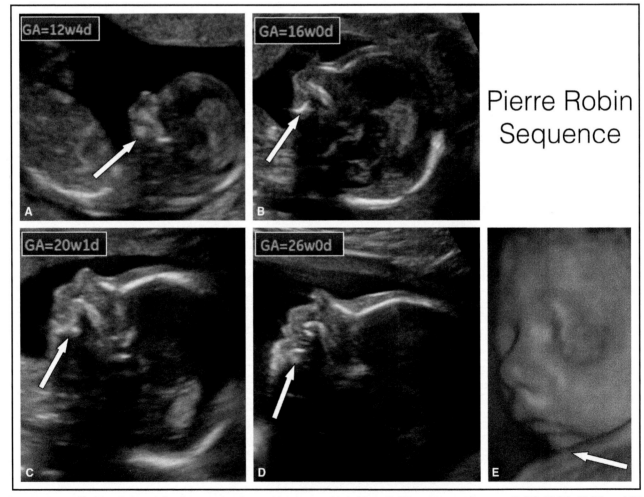

**Figure 9.34:** Facial growth and development in a fetus with micrognathia in Pierre Robin sequence, shown at 12 **(A)**, 16 **(B)**, 20 **(C)**, and 26 **(D)** weeks of gestation and in three-dimensional ultrasound in surface mode at 26 weeks of gestation **(E)**. *White arrows* point to the mandibles. Note that the micrognathia appears very pronounced (severe) in the first trimester **(A)**, but with the growth of the mandible the profile appears less abnormal in the second **(B–E)** and third trimesters. In this case, micrognathia was isolated, and a cleft palate was repaired after birth.

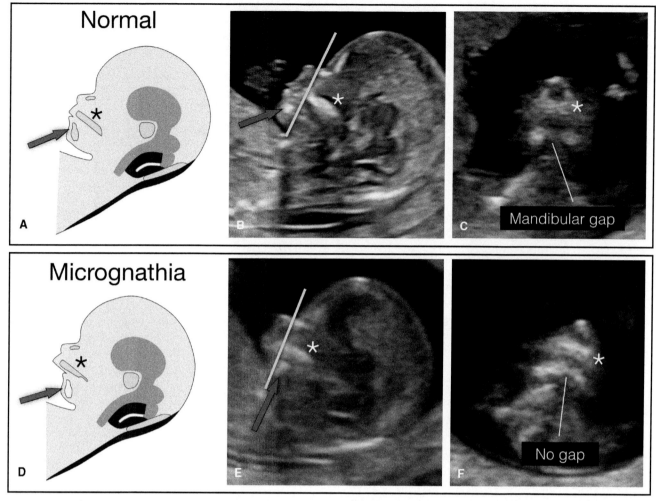

**Figure 9.35:** Schematic drawing of the midsagittal plane of the fetal face **(A, D)** along with the corresponding midsagittal **(B, E)** and retronasal triangle **(C, F)** ultrasound views in a normal fetus **(A–C)** and in a fetus with micrognathia **(D–F)**. Note in the normal fetus that the tip of the mandible (*red arrow*) reaches under the anterior aspect of the maxilla (*asterisk*), as shown in **A** and **B**. In the normal fetus, the retronasal triangle **(C)** demonstrates the normal mandibular gap. In the fetus with micrognathia **(D–F)**, the chin is receded behind the line (*red arrow*) **(E)**, and no mandibular gap is noted in the retronasal triangle view, as shown in **F**. See text for details.

leads to a small mouth space, and in these cases the tongue is shifted backward to what is called glossoptosis, which is almost always combined with a cleft of the posterior palate. Such a condition has already been reported in the early second trimester[52] and in our observation can also be seen in the first trimester. In suspected cases of micrognathia, we recommend a transvaginal ultrasound to visualize, if technically feasible, the posterior palate region (Fig. 9.5), as described by Wilhelm and Borgers,[53] for the demonstration of amniotic fluid in the pharynx, which is absent in micrognathia with glossoptosis. Since micrognathia is associated with many syndromic conditions (Fig. 9.36), the face, ears, and brain should be examined in detail in 2D and 3D ultrasound (Fig. 9.37).

### *Associated Malformations*

Micrognathia can be an isolated finding as in Pierre Robin sequence, commonly with a cleft palate and glossoptosis, but can also be associated with other chromosomal abnormalities,

including trisomies 18 and 13, triploidy, and numerous genetic syndromes.[8,54,55] Notably, the association of micrognathia with Pierre Robin sequence is well known and can be diagnosed in the first trimester[56] as shown in **Figure 9.35**. Low-set ears can be a marker for the possible association of micrognathia with syndromic conditions. The absence of a mandible or maxilla is observed in agnathia and is associated with otocephaly, a severe lethal condition.[26,57] In addition to these conditions, Goldenhaar syndrome and Treacher Collins syndrome should be considered. Prenatal management of the first-trimester diagnosis of micrognathia is similar to that of CLP.

### Anomalies of the Eyes

Anomalies of eyes and orbits are rarely detected in the first trimester except in the presence of other fetal anomalies or in a prior family history of such conditions (Figs. 9.38 to 9.40). Anomalies of eyes and orbits are typically found in association with

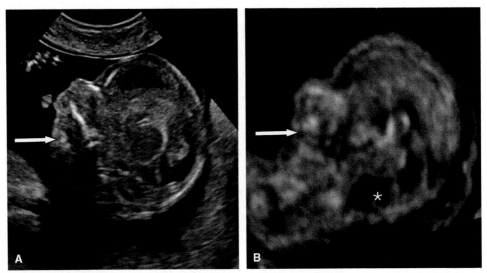

**Figure 9.36:** Midsagittal views of the face in two fetuses with trisomy 13 and micrognathia (*white arrows*) at 14 **(A)** and 12 **(B)** weeks of gestation, respectively. Note in fetus **B** the presence of dilated posterior fossa (*asterisk*). Figure 9.37 shows the 3D rendering of the face in fetus **B**.

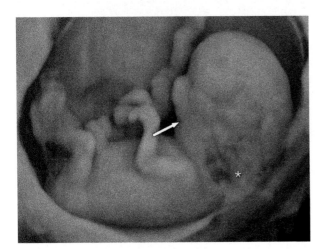

**Figure 9.37:** Three-dimensional ultrasound in surface mode of a fetus with trisomy 13 at 12 weeks of gestation (same as in Fig. 9.36B). Note the small, receded mandible (micrognathia) along with a thickened nuchal translucency (*asterisk*).

alobar holoprosencephaly, as in the presence of proboscis for instance (Figs. 9.10 and 9.39). Abnormal orbits, such as in hypotelorism or hypertelorism, are often subjectively assessed in the first trimester (Figs. 9.38 to 9.40), especially in syndromic conditions with facial dysmorphism. In general, trisomies 13 and 18 are the most common conditions detected in such cases (Figs. 9.38 and 9.39). Isolated anophthalmia is very rare, and microphthalmia can also be recognized when other fetal anomalies are present. Isolated microphthalmia or cataract can be difficult to diagnose at this early stage, as the anomaly itself may not be apparent in the first trimester of pregnancy. Fetal cataracts reported in the first trimester of pregnancy are commonly recurrent cases or present in suspected syndromes such as Walker–Warburg syndrome[31] or Warburg micro syndrome with microcephaly, which becomes apparent in the late second trimester. In high-risk patients, direct visualization of orbits and lenses with transvaginal ultrasound increases the reliability of demonstrating normal eyes and orbits. When

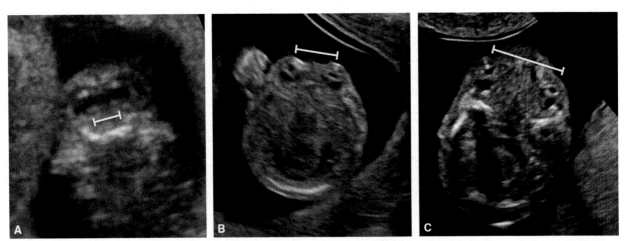

**Figure 9.38:** Axial views of the head at the level of the eyes in three abnormal fetuses. Fetus **A** has marked hypotelorism in association with holoprosencephaly and trisomy 13. Fetus **B** has hypotelorism in association with holoprosencephaly with normal chromosomes but with PlGF mutation. Fetus **C** has hypertelorism and abnormal orbital shape in association with trisomy 13 and odd facial features. Compare with normal orbital anatomy in Figure 9.8.

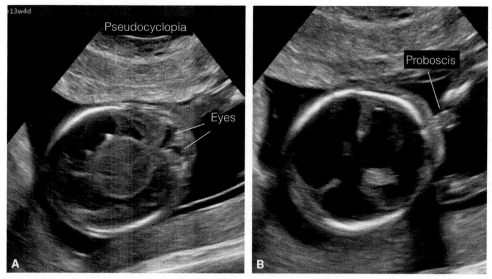

**Figure 9.39:** Axial views **(A and B)** of the head at the level of the eyes in a fetus with trisomy 13, holoprosencephaly, pseudocyclopia, and proboscis at 13 weeks of gestation. **A:** The plane at the level of the eyes with the almost fused eyes and no orbits. **B:** Is a more cranial plane showing the proboscis.

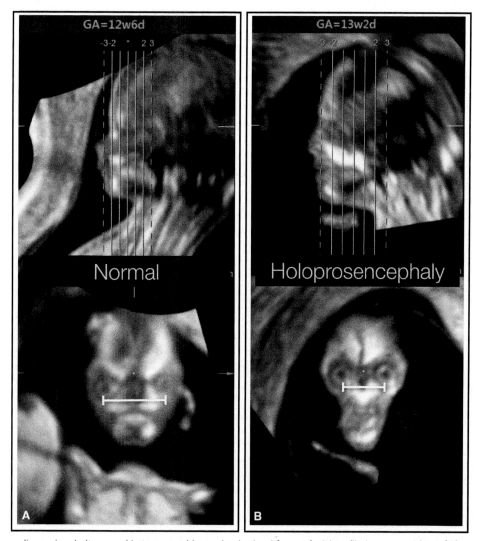

**Figure 9.40:** Three-dimensional ultrasound in tomographic mode obtained from a facial profile in a normal fetus **(A)** and in a fetus with holoprosencephaly **(B)**. Corresponding coronal views of the fetal face, showing the eyes are displayed in the lower images. Note the normal distance of the eyes (*white lines*) in the normal face in **A**, and narrowing of the orbits called hypotelorism in **B**.

suspected, a repeat ultrasound in the second trimester with the transvaginal approach, if feasible, will help to confirm or rule out abnormalities of eyes and orbits.

# FETAL NECK ABNORMALITIES

## Cystic Hygroma

### Definition

Cystic hygroma is a congenital abnormality involving the vascular lymphatic system in the fetus and is characterized by the presence of fluid-filled cystic spaces in the soft tissue, commonly in the posterolateral aspects of the neck or in other locations in the body (Figs. 9.41 to 9.44). Pathogenesis of cystic hygroma is thought to result from the abnormal connection between the lymphatic and vascular systems, primarily from failure of development of the communication between the jugular lymphatic sac and the jugular vein.[58] This may lead to progressive lymphedema and fetal hydrops. On occasion, however, a communication is established between the lymphatic and the vascular systems, resulting in resolution of the swelling. Cystic hygroma can be multiseptated and is thus classified as septated or nonseptated (Figs. 9.42 and 9.43). In some cases, a thick septum can be seen in the midline, corresponding to the presence of the nuchal ligament.[58] The prevalence of cystic hygroma is reported at 1:285 of first-trimester pregnancies.[59] There is currently a controversy on

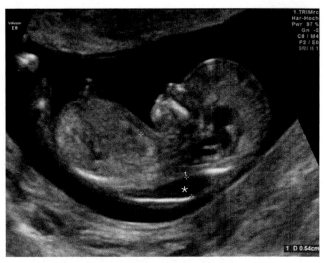

**Figure 9.41:** Midsagittal view of the fetus at 13 weeks of gestation showing a thickened nuchal translucency (NT) (*asterisk*). When the NT is septated, the diagnosis of cystic hygroma is made in some settings. The presence of NT septations is best assessed in the axial views.

whether cystic hygroma is an entity that is distinct from an enlarged NT, because septations can be seen in both conditions.[60] Irrespective of the designation of nuchal swelling as NT or cystic hygroma, the association of this finding with fetal anatomic and genetic abnormalities should be considered in pregnancy management.

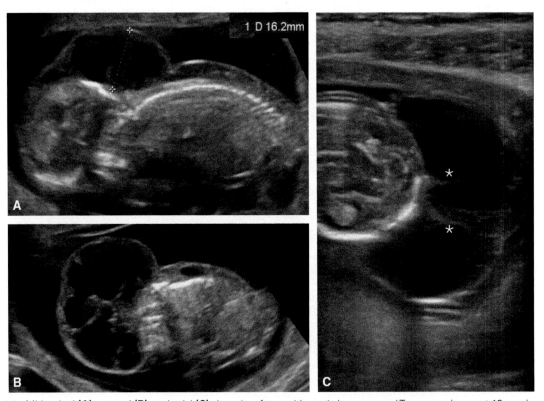

**Figure 9.42:** Midsagittal **(A)**, coronal **(B)**, and axial **(C)** views in a fetus with cystic hygroma and Turner syndrome at 13 weeks of gestation. Note the presence of NT thickening of 16 mm shown in **A** and NT septations (*asterisk*) shown in **B** and **C**.

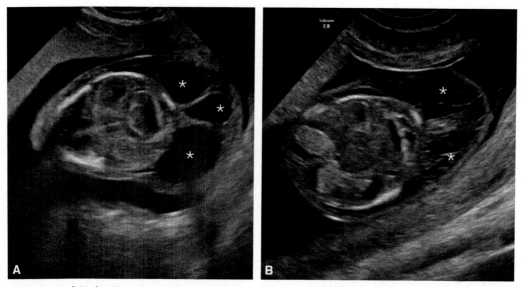

**Figure 9.43:** Axial views of the fetal head in two fetuses with cystic hygromas at 13 (**A**) and 12 (**B**) weeks of gestation, respectively. Note the presence of septations in both fetuses, and also note that the fluid within the septations (*asterisk*) is clear in **A** and echogenic, jelly-like in **B**.

## Ultrasound Findings

The presence of cystic masses on ultrasound in the posterolateral aspect of the fetal neck is suggestive of cystic hygroma. This is easily seen on an axial view of the neck (Figs. 9.42 and 9.43) and when extensive, cystic hygroma can be seen in the sagittal plane that is obtained for NT measurement (Figs. 9.41 and 9.42). The demonstration of the presence of septations is best done in the axial plane of the neck and upper chest (Fig. 9.44). A thick septum is commonly seen in the posterior midline neck region corresponding to the nuchal ligament (Fig. 9.43). When multiple septations are present, the ultrasound appearance resembles a honeycomb. Nonseptated cystic hygroma is seen as cystic spaces on either side of the fetal neck, representing dilated cervical lymphatics. Given the common association with other fetal malformations and chromosomal abnormalities, a comprehensive evaluation of the fetus by detailed ultrasound is warranted when a cystic hygroma is diagnosed in the first trimester.

## Associated Malformations

Cystic hygroma is associated with other fetal anatomic abnormalities in 60% of cases. Associated abnormalities commonly include cardiac, genitourinary, skeletal, and central nervous systems, and the majority can be seen on the first-trimester ultrasound. Chromosomal abnormalities are common, with trisomy 21 and Turner syndrome representing the two most

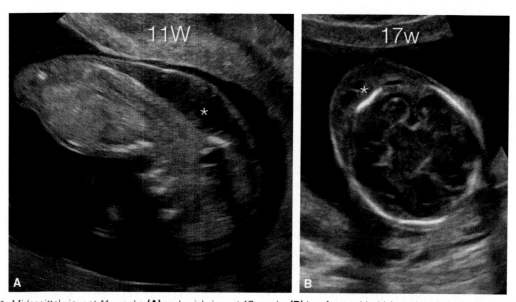

**Figure 9.44:** Midsagittal view at 11 weeks (**A**) and axial view at 17 weeks (**B**) in a fetus with thickened nuchal translucency (NT), diagnosed at 11 weeks, as shown in **A** (*asterisk*). In this fetus, nuchal edema persisted into the second trimester (**B**).

# Noonan Syndrome

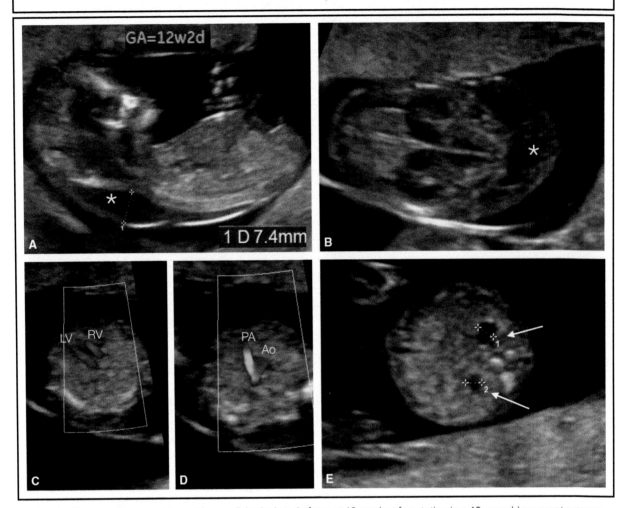

**Figure 9.45:** Ultrasound images obtained from a dichorionic twin fetus at 12 weeks of gestation in a 40-year-old pregnant woman presenting for genetic screening. Note in **A** and **B** the presence of an enlarged nuchal translucency (*asterisks*), measuring 7.4 mm. **C and D:** A normal four-chamber view and a normal three-vessel-trachea view, respectively. Mild urinary tract dilation is shown in **E**. Chorionic villous sampling revealed normal karyotype, but due to the ultrasound findings, molecular genetic examination for Noonan syndrome confirmed a mutation of the *PTPN11* gene, shown in 50% of affected cases.

common associated chromosomal findings, reported in more than 50% of cases.[59] A typical syndromic condition to be considered is the presence of Noonan syndrome (Fig. 9.45). Amniotic fluid abnormalities are common, but they are noted in the second and third trimesters of pregnancy. Generalized hydrops is also common and carries a poor prognosis.[61] The outcome is usually good when cystic hygroma resolves prenatally in the presence of a normal karyotype.

## Increased NT with Normal Karyotype

The relationship of an increased NT with chromosomal anomalies, especially Down syndrome, is currently well established. The detection of an increased NT currently leads to genetic counseling and options for additional screening workup, or invasive diagnostic testing. The presence of a thickened NT with normal karyotype represents a major challenge to counseling and for additional workup. Further management in that setting has been debated in the literature since the late 1990s.[62–69] The presence of a thickened NT is associated with aneuploidies (Fig. 9.46), and a thickened NT with a normal karyotype is associated with a wide spectrum of major and minor fetal anomalies, including genetic syndromes (Fig. 9.47) and an increased risk of in utero fetal demise (Fig. 9.48).[14,65,66,69,70] The risk of abnormal neurodevelopmental delay is currently unclear, and controversial observations are reported.[65] Despite normal ultrasound findings and a normal karyotype in the setting of a thickened NT, the birth of a "healthy" child without malformations decreases with increasing NT thickness

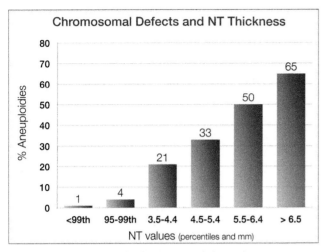

**Figure 9.46:** Relationship between nuchal translucency thickness (*x* axis) and prevalence of chromosomal defects (*y* axis). (Graph is based on data from Souka AP, von Kaisenberg CS, Hyett JA, et al. Increased nuchal translucency with normal karyotype. *Am J Obstet Gynecol.* 2005;192:1005–1021.)

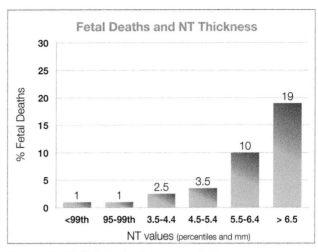

**Figure 9.48:** Relationship between nuchal translucency thickness (*x* axis) and prevalence of fetal deaths (*y* axis). (Graph is based on data from Souka AP, von Kaisenberg CS, Hyett JA, et al. Increased nuchal translucency with normal karyotype. *Am J Obstet Gynecol.* 2005;192:1005–1021.)

(Fig. 9.49). In this section, we present essential points and current literature related to this topic.

### Pathophysiology of Increased NT

Understanding the pathophysiology of increased neck fluid in fetuses with thickened NT is important as it allows for establishing associations with various abnormal fetal conditions.[14,65] This task, however, has not been proven to be easy, and it appears that a thickened NT can result from various conditions. A thickened NT can be caused by chromosomal anomalies, but can also be due to functional and structural cardiac abnormalities; disturbances in the lymphatic system;

disturbances in the collagen metabolism; mechanical causes such as intrathoracic compression, infection, metabolic and hematologic disorders; or a combination of some of these and others. The main types of anomalies associated with an increased NT in addition to aneuploidies[71] (Fig. 9.46) include cardiac defects[72] (Fig. 11.7 in Chapter 11), major malformations (Fig. 9.47) with specific syndromes (e.g., Noonan syndrome) (Fig. 9.45),[68,73] skeletal dysplasia,[74] syndromic and nonsyndromic diaphragmatic hernias, and complex syndromic conditions affecting brain, kidneys, and other organs.[65,66] The association of a thickened NT with these abnormalities increases with the NT thickness (Fig. 9.47).

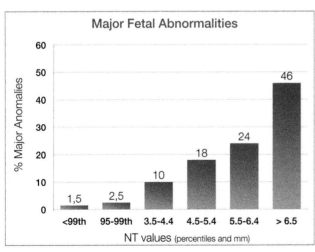

**Figure 9.47:** Relationship between nuchal translucency thickness (*x* axis) and prevalence of major anomalies (*y* axis). (Graph is based on data from Souka AP, von Kaisenberg CS, Hyett JA, et al. Increased nuchal translucency with normal karyotype. *Am J Obstet Gynecol.* 2005;192:1005–1021.)

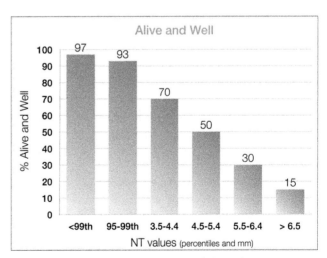

**Figure 9.49:** Relationship between nuchal translucency thickness (*x* axis) and prevalence of live birth of a child with no major anomalies (*y* axis). (Graph is based on data from Souka AP, von Kaisenberg CS, Hyett JA, et al. Increased nuchal translucency with normal karyotype. *Am J Obstet Gynecol.* 2005;192:1005–1021.)

## Congenital Cardiac Defects

The observation of Hyett et al.[72] that in fetuses with a thickened NT the prevalence of a cardiac anomaly is increased has been confirmed by other studies. A direct correlation exists between the size of the NT and the associated risk for cardiac defects (Fig. 11.7 in Chapter 11). In our centers, a thickened NT is an indication for an early ultrasound cardiac examination, even before performing an invasive procedure. A follow-up fetal echocardiogram is also performed at 16 to 22 weeks of gestation. Please refer to Chapter 11 for a detailed discussion of the evaluation of the fetal heart in the first trimester.

## Other Structural Anomalies and Genetic Syndromes

The list of reported structural anomalies and genetic syndromes in association with a thickened NT is quite long[66] (see Table 9.3). However, it is still unclear whether in all reported cases the relationship is causal or accidental.[65] Fetal anomalies

**Table 9.3 •** Some Fetal Abnormalities in Fetuses with Increased Nuchal Translucency Thickness

| Anomalies of CNS, Head and Neck | Thoracic and Abdominal Anomalies | Skeletal Anomalies | Genetic and Metabolic Diseases |
|---|---|---|---|
| Acrania/anencephaly | Ambiguous genitalia | Achondrogenesis | Beckwith–Wiedemann syndrome |
| Agenesis of the corpus callosum | Body stalk anomaly | Achondroplasia | CHARGE syndrome |
| Agnathia/micrognathia | Cardiac anomalies (all possible) | Asphyxiating thoracic dystrophy | Congenital lymphedema |
| Craniosynostosis | Cloacal exstrophy | Blomstrand osteochondrodysplasia | Cornelia de Lange syndrome |
| Cystic hygroma | Congenital adrenal hyperplasia | Campomelic dysplasia | Deficiency of the immune system |
| Neck lipoma | Congenital nephrotic syndrome | Cleidocranial dysplasia | DiGeorge syndrome |
| Dandy–Walker malformation | Cystic adenomatoid malformation | Hypochondroplasia | EEC syndrome |
| Diastematomyelia | Diaphragmatic hernia | Hypophosphatasia | Fetal akinesia deformation sequence |
| Encephalocele | Duodenal atresia | Jarcho–Levin syndrome | Fetal anemia (different etiologies) |
| Facial cleft | Esophageal atresia | Kyphoscoliosis | GM1 gangliosidosis |
| Fowler syndrome | Exomphalos | Limb reduction defect | Mucopolysaccharidosis type VII |
| Holoprosencephaly | Fryns syndrome | Nance–Sweeney syndrome | Myotonic dystrophy |
| Hydrolethalus syndrome | Gastroschisis | Osteogenesis imperfecta | Neonatal myoclonic encephalopathy |
| Iniencephaly | Hydronephrosis | Roberts syndrome | Noonan syndrome |
| Joubert syndrome | Hypospadias | Robinow syndrome | Perlman syndrome |
| Macrocephaly | Meckel–Gruber syndrome | Short-rib polydactyly syndrome | Severe developmental delay of unknown origin |
| Microcephaly | Megacystis | Sirenomelia | Smith–Lemli–Opitz syndrome |
| Microphthalmia | Multicystic dysplastic kidneys | Talipes equinovarus | Spinal muscular atrophy (SMA) type 1 |
| Spina bifida | Polycystic kidneys, infantile | Thanatophoric dwarfism | Stickler syndrome |
| Treacher Collins syndrome | Small bowel obstruction | VACTER association | Syndrome unspecified |
| Trigonocephaly C | | | Vitamin D–resistant rickets |
| Ventriculomegaly | | | Zellweger syndrome |

Modified from Souka AP, von Kaisenberg CS, Hyett JA, et al. Increased nuchal translucency with normal karyotype. *Am J Obstet Gynecol.* 2005;192:1005–1021. (Copyright Elsevier Ltd, with permission.)

such as omphalocele and diaphragmatic hernia, isolated or syndromic, are highly associated with a thickened NT (see case with Fryns syndrome in Fig. 10.20 in Chapter 10). Many syndromes are listed in series reporting on outcome of fetuses with thickened NT and normal chromosomes. It is, however, difficult to prove a causative relationship or a strong association between specific genetic syndromes and thickened NT because most syndromes have extremely low prevalence in the population.[65] In one study, genetic syndromes and single gene disorders were found in 12.7% of fetuses with thickened NT.[63] Noonan syndrome is currently accepted as the only molecular genetic condition with a clear association with a thickened NT in the first trimester (Fig. 9.45),[68] especially if nuchal edema persists into the second trimester. Skeletal dysplasias also have a strong association with thickened NT. In the list of first-trimester skeletal dysplasias reported by Khalil et al.,[74] most cases were associated with a thickened NT (see also Chapter 15 on skeletal anomalies). Table 9.3 summarizes some anomalies reported in the literature with a thickened NT.[66]

### Additional Genetic Evaluation

#### Comparative Genomic Hybridization Array

In a recent meta-analysis, an abnormal comparative genomic hybridization array (CGH) or microarray is present in about 5% of a thickened NT, with a range reaching 10% in some studies.[69] Offering CGH to pregnancies with a thickened NT thus appears to be warranted.

#### Monogenic Diseases

There are several studies reporting on the high prevalence of Noonan syndrome in fetuses with thickened NT,[68,73] especially when the thickened NT has persisted into the second trimester.[73] In one series of 120 fetuses, eight were shown to have Noonan syndrome.[68] Preliminary observations of a relationship between increased NT and the presence of spinal muscular atrophy (SMA-Type 1) was not confirmed on subsequent evaluation.[68] It is possible that in the future, whole genomic sequencing may be offered in these conditions, but the value of this approach has to be proven in large studies before wide implementation.

### Management and Follow-up of Thickened NT

Once a fetus is identified with a thickened NT, we recommend a detailed first-trimester ultrasound examination, including a transvaginal ultrasound if feasible. The components of the detailed first-trimester ultrasound examination are presented in Chapter 5. A follow-up ultrasound examination at 16 weeks of gestation is also warranted in order to reassess fetal anatomy.[75] Evaluation of the nuchal fold in the second trimester is also important because outcome is improved if the nuchal fold is normal (Fig. 9.49). A detailed second-trimester ultrasound examination at 18 to 22 weeks of gestation along with a fetal echocardiogram is also recommended. This approach will detect the majority of major malformations and syndromic conditions, many of which can be detected in the first and early second ultrasound examinations.

## REFERENCES

1. Chaoui R, Benoit B, Mitkowska-Wozniak H, et al. Assessment of intracranial translucency (IT) in the detection of spina bifida at the 11-13-week scan. *Ultrasound Obstet Gynecol.* 2009;34:249–252.
2. Cicero S, Curcio P, Papageorghiou A, et al. Absence of nasal bone in fetuses with trisomy 21 at 11-14 weeks of gestation: an observational study. *Lancet.* 2001;358:1665–1667.
3. Cicero S, Curcio P, Rembouskos G, et al. Maxillary length at 11-14 weeks of gestation in fetuses with trisomy 21. *Ultrasound Obstet Gynecol.* 2004;24:19–22.
4. Sonek J, Borenstein M, Dagklis T, et al. Frontomaxillary facial angle in fetuses with trisomy 21 at 11-136 weeks. *Amer J Obstet Gynecol.* 2007;196:271.e1–271.e4.
5. Manegold-Brauer G, Bourdil L, Berg C, et al. Prenasal thickness to nasal bone length ratio in normal and trisomy 21 fetuses at 11-14 weeks of gestation. *Prenat Diagn.* 2015;35:1079–1084.
6. Yazdi B, Riefler P, Fischmüller K, et al. The frontal space measurement in euploid and aneuploid pregnancies at 11-13 weeks' gestation. *Prenat Diagn.* 2013;33:1124–1130.
7. Hoopmann M, Sonek J, Esser T, et al. Frontal space distance in facial clefts and retrognathia at 11-13 weeks' gestation. *Ultrasound Obstet Gynecol.* 2016;48:171–176.
8. Bakker M, Pace M, de Jong-Pleij E, et al. Prenasal thickness, prefrontal space ratio and other facial profile markers in first-trimester fetuses with aneuploidies, cleft palate, and micrognathia. *Fetal Diagn Ther.* 2016. doi:10.1159/000449099.
9. Sepulveda W, Wong AE, Martinez-Ten P, et al. Retronasal triangle: a sonographic landmark for the screening of cleft palate in the first trimester. *Ultrasound Obstet Gynecol.* 2010;35:7–13.
10. Sepulveda W, Wong AE, Vinals F, et al. Absent mandibular gap in the retronasal triangle view: a clue to the diagnosis of micrognathia in the first trimester. *Ultrasound Obstet Gynecol.* 2012;39:152–156.
11. Chaoui R, Heling K-S. *3D Ultrasound in Prenatal Diagnosis: A Practical Approach.* 1st ed. Berlin, New York: DeGruyter; 2016.
12. Guis F, Ville Y, Vincent Y, et al. Ultrasound evaluation of the length of the fetal nasal bones throughout gestation. *Ultrasound Obstet Gynecol.* 1995;5:304–307.
13. Nicolaides KH. Screening for fetal aneuploidies at 11 to 13 weeks. *Prenat Diagn.* 2011;31:7–15.
14. Nicolaides KH. Nuchal translucency and other first-trimester sonographic markers of chromosomal abnormalities. *Am J Obstet Gynecol.* 2004;191:45–67.
15. Maymon R, Levinsohn-Tavor O, Cuckle H, et al. Second trimester ultrasound prenasal thickness combined with nasal bone length: a new method of Down syndrome screening. *Prenat Diagn.* 2005;25:906–911.
16. Persico N, Borenstein M, Molina F, et al. Prenasal thickness in trisomy-21 fetuses at 16-24 weeks of gestation. *Ultrasound Obstet Gynecol.* 2008;32:751–754.
17. Miron J-P, Cuckle H, Miron P. Prenasal thickness in first-trimester screening for Down syndrome. *Prenat Diagn.* 2012;32:695–697.
18. Borenstein M, Persico N, Kaihura C, et al. Frontomaxillary facial angle in chromosomally normal fetuses at 11 + 0 to 13 + 6 weeks. *Ultrasound Obstet Gynecol.* 2007;30:737–741.
19. Borenstein M, Persico N, Kagan KO, et al. Frontomaxillary facial angle in screening for trisomy 21 at 11 + 0 to 13 + 6 weeks. *Ultrasound Obstet Gynecol.* 2008;32:5–11.
20. Lachmann R, Picciarelli G, Moratalla J, et al. Frontomaxillary facial angle in fetuses with spina bifida at 11-13 weeks' gestation. *Ultrasound Obstet Gynecol.* 2010;36:268–271.

21. Borenstein M, Persico N, Strobl I, et al. Frontomaxillary and mandibulo-maxillary facial angles at 11 + 0 to 13 + 6 weeks in fetuses with trisomy 18. *Ultrasound Obstet Gynecol*. 2007;30:928–933.

22. Borenstein M, Persico N, Dagklis T, et al. Frontomaxillary facial angle in fetuses with trisomy 13 at 11 + 0 to 13 + 6 weeks. *Ultrasound Obstet Gynecol*. 2007;30:819–823.

23. Plasencia W, Dagklis T, Pachoumi C, et al. Frontomaxillary facial angle at 11 + 0 to 13 + 6 weeks: effect of plane of acquisition. *Ultrasound Obstet Gynecol*. 2007;29:660–665.

24. de Jong-Pleij EAP, Ribbert LSM, Manten GTR, et al. Maxilla-nasion-mandible angle: a new method to assess profile anomalies in pregnancy. *Ultrasound Obstet Gynecol*. 2011;37:562–569.

25. Kivilevitch Z, Salomon LJ, Benoit B, et al. Fetal interlens distance: normal values during pregnancy. *Ultrasound Obstet Gynecol*. 2010;36:186–190.

26. Blaas HGK, Eriksson AG, Salvesen KÅ, et al. Brains and faces in holoprosencephaly: pre- and postnatal description of 30 cases. *Ultrasound Obstet Gynecol*. 2002;19:24–38.

27. Karl K, Benoit B, Entezami M, et al. Small biparietal diameter in fetuses with spina bifida on 11-13-week and mid-gestation ultrasound. *Ultrasound Obstet Gynecol*. 2012;40:140–144.

28. Tonni G, Centini G, Inaudi P, et al. Prenatal diagnosis of severe epignathus in a twin: case report and review of the literature. *Cleft Palate-Craniofac J*. 2010;47:421–425.

29. Gull I, Wolman I, Har-Toov J, et al. Antenatal sonographic diagnosis of epignathus at 15 weeks of pregnancy. *Ultrasound Obstet Gynecol*. 1999;13:271–273.

30. Sepulveda W, Wong AE, Andreeva E, et al. Sonographic spectrum of first-trimester fetal cephalocele: review of 35 cases. *Ultrasound Obstet Gynecol*. 2015;46:29–33.

31. Ashwal E, Achiron A, Gilboa Y, et al. Prenatal ultrasonographic diagnosis of cataract: in utero manifestations of cryptic disease. *Ultraschall Med*. 2016. doi:10.1055/s-0042-120841.

32. Vanderas AP. Incidence of cleft lip, cleft palate, and cleft lip and palate among races: a review. *Cleft Palate J*. 1987;24:216–225.

33. IPDTOC Working Group. Prevalence at birth of cleft lip with or without cleft palate: data from the International Perinatal Database of Typical Oral Clefts (IPDTOC). *Cleft Palate Craniofac J*. 2011;48:66–81.

34. American Institute of Ultrasound in Medicine. AIUM practice guideline for the performance of obstetric ultrasound examinations. *J Ultrasound Med*. 2013;32:1083–1101.

35. Calzolari E, Pierini A, Astolfi G, et al. Associated anomalies in multi-malformed infants with cleft lip and palate: an epidemiologic study of nearly 6 million births in 23 EUROCAT registries. *Am J Med Genet A*. 2007;143A:528–537.

36. Dixon MJ, Marazita ML, Beaty TH, et al. Cleft lip and palate: understanding genetic and environmental influences. *Nat Rev Genet*. 2011;12:167–178.

37. Kernahan DA. The striped Y—a symbolic classification for cleft lip and palate. *Plast Reconstr Surg*. 1971;47:469–470.

38. Nyberg DA, Sickler GK, Hegge FN, et al. Fetal cleft lip with and without cleft palate: US classification and correlation with outcome. *Radiology*. 1995;195:677–684.

39. Ghi T, Arcangeli T, Radico D, et al. Three-dimensional sonographic imaging of fetal bilateral cleft lip and palate in the first trimester. *Ultrasound Obstet Gynecol*. 2009;34:119–120.

40. Gullino E, Serra M, Ansaldi C, et al. Bilateral cleft lip and palate diagnosed sonographically at 11 weeks of pregnancy. *J Clin Ultrasound*. 2006;34:398–401.

41. Picone O, De Keersmaecker B, Ville Y. Ultrasonographic features of orofacial clefts at first trimester of pregnancy: report of two cases [in French]. *J Gynéco Obstétr et Biol Reprod*. 2003;32:736–739.

42. Syngelaki A, Chelemen T, Dagklis T, et al. Challenges in the diagnosis of fetal non-chromosomal abnormalities at 11-13 weeks. *Prenat Diagn*. 2011;31:90–102.

43. Chaoui R, Orosz G, Heling KS, et al. Maxillary gap at 11-13 weeks' gestation: marker of cleft lip and palate. *Ultrasound Obstet Gynecol*. 2015;46:665–669.

44. Sepulveda W, Cafici D, Bartholomew J, et al. First-trimester assessment of the fetal palate: a novel application of the Volume NT algorithm. *J Ultrasound Med*. 2012;31:1443–1448.

45. Li W-J, Wang X-Q, Yan R-L, et al. Clinical significance of first-trimester screening of the retronasal triangle for identification of primary cleft palate. *Fetal Diagn Ther*. 2015;38(2):135–141.

46. Tonni G, Grisolia G, Sepulveda W. Early prenatal diagnosis of orofacial clefts: evaluation of the retronasal triangle using a new three-dimensional reslicing technique. *Fetal Diagn Ther*. 2013;34:31–37.

47. Nyberg DA, Hegge FN, Kramer D, et al. Premaxillary protrusion: a sonographic clue to bilateral cleft lip and palate. *J Ultrasound Med*. 1993;12:331–335.

48. Jones MC. Facial clefting. Etiology and developmental pathogenesis. *Clin Plast Surg*. 1993;20:599–606.

49. Gillham JC, Anand S, Bullen PJ. Antenatal detection of cleft lip with or without cleft palate: incidence of associated chromosomal and structural anomalies. *Ultrasound Obstet Gynecol*. 2009;34:410–415.

50. Bergé SJ, Plath H, Van de Vondel PT, et al. Fetal cleft lip and palate: sonographic diagnosis, chromosomal abnormalities, associated anomalies and postnatal outcome in 70 fetuses. *Ultrasound Obstet Gynecol*. 2001;18:422–431.

51. Gabrielli S, Piva M, Ghi T, et al. Bilateral cleft lip and palate without premaxillary protrusion is associated with lethal aneuploidies. *Ultrasound Obstet Gynecol*. 2009;34:416–418.

52. Bronshtein M, Blazer S, Zalel Y, et al. Ultrasonographic diagnosis of glossoptosis in fetuses with Pierre Robin sequence in early and mid pregnancy. *Am J Obstet Gynecol*. 2005;193:1561–1564.

53. Wilhelm L, Borgers H. The "equals sign": a novel marker in the diagnosis of fetal isolated cleft palate. *Ultrasound Obstet Gynecol*. 2010;36:439–444.

54. Bianchi DW. Micrognathia. In: Bianchi DW, Crombleholme TM, D'Alton M, eds. *Fetology: Diagnosis and Management of the Fetal Patient*. New York, NY: McGraw-Hill Medical Pub. Division; 2010: 233–238.

55. Paladini D. Fetal micrognathia: almost always an ominous finding. *Ultrasound Obstet Gynecol*. 2010;35:377–384.

56. Teoh M, Meagher S. First-trimester diagnosis of micrognathia as a presentation of Pierre Robin syndrome. *Ultrasound Obstet Gynecol*. 2003;21:616–618.

57. Chaoui R, Heling KS, Thiel G, et al. Agnathia-otocephaly with holoprosencephaly on prenatal three-dimensional ultrasound. *Ultrasound Obstet Gynecol*. 2011;37:745–748.

58. Chervenak FA, Isaacson G, Blakemore KJ, et al. Fetal cystic hygroma. Cause and natural history. *N Engl J Med*. 1983;309:822–825.

59. Malone FD, Ball RH, Nyberg DA, et al. First-trimester septated cystic hygroma: prevalence, natural history, and pediatric outcome. *Obstet Gynecol*. 2005;106:288–294.

60. Molina FS, Avgidou K, Kagan K-O, et al. Cystic hygromas, nuchal edema, and nuchal translucency at 11-14 weeks of gestation. *Obstet Gynecol*. 2006;107:678–683.

61. Johnson MP, Johnson A, Holzgreve W, et al. First-trimester simple hygroma: cause and outcome. *Am J Obstet Gynecol*. 1993;168:156–161.

62. Souka AP, Snijders RJ, Novakov A, et al. Defects and syndromes in chromosomally normal fetuses with increased nuchal translucency thickness at 10-14 weeks of gestation. *Ultrasound Obstet Gynecol*. 1998;11:391–400.

63. Bilardo CM, Pajkrt E, de Graaf I, et al. Outcome of fetuses with enlarged nuchal translucency and normal karyotype. *Ultrasound Obstet Gynecol*. 1998;11:401–406.

64. Bilardo CM. Increased nuchal translucency and normal karyotype: coping with uncertainty. *Ultrasound Obstet Gynecol*. 2001;17:99–101.

65. Hyett JA. Increased nuchal translucency in fetuses with a normal karyotype. *Prenat Diagn*. 2002;22:864–868.

66. Souka AP, Kaisenberg von CS, Hyett JA, et al. Increased nuchal translucency with normal karyotype. *Am J Obstet Gynecol*. 2005;192:1005–1021.

67. Bakker M, Pajkrt E, Bilardo CM. Increased nuchal translucency with normal karyotype and anomaly scan: what next? *Best Pract Res Clin Obstet Gynaecol*. 2014;28:355–366.

68. Pergament E, Alamillo C, Sak K, et al. Genetic assessment following increased nuchal translucency and normal karyotype. *Prenat Diagn.* 2011;31:307–310.

69. Grande M, Jansen FAR, Blumenfeld YJ, et al. Genomic microarray in fetuses with increased nuchal translucency and normal karyotype: a systematic review and meta-analysis. *Ultrasound Obstet Gynecol.* 2015;46:650–658.

70. Hyett J, Perdu M, Sharland G, et al. Using fetal nuchal translucency to screen for major congenital cardiac defects at 10-14 weeks of gestation: population based cohort study. *BMJ (Clin Res Ed).* 1999;318:81–85.

71. Snijders RJ, Noble P, Sebire N, et al. UK multicentre project on assessment of risk of trisomy 21 by maternal age and fetal nuchal-translucency thickness at 10-14 weeks of gestation. Fetal Medicine Foundation First Trimester Screening Group. *Lancet.* 1998;352:343–346.

72. Hyett JA, Perdu M, Sharland GK, et al. Increased nuchal translucency at 10-14 weeks of gestation as a marker for major cardiac defects. *Ultrasound Obstet Gynecol.* 1997;10:242–246.

73. Bakker M, Pajkrt E, Mathijssen IB, et al. Targeted ultrasound examination and DNA testing for Noonan syndrome, in fetuses with increased nuchal translucency and normal karyotype. *Prenat Diagn.* 2011;31: 833–840.

74. Khalil A, Pajkrt E, Chitty LS. Early prenatal diagnosis of skeletal anomalies. *Prenat Diagn.* 2011;31:115–124.

75. Le Lous M, Bouhanna P, Colmant C, et al. The performance of an intermediate 16th-week ultrasound scan for the follow-up of euploid fetuses with increased nuchal translucency. *Prenat Diagn.* 2016;36: 148–153.

# CHAPTER 10

# The Fetal Chest

## INTRODUCTION

The examination of the fetal chest in the first trimester includes the assessment of the right and left lung, the bony and cartilaginous thoracic cage, the diaphragm, and the heart with surrounding vasculature. Because of the importance and prevalence of cardiac anomalies, normal and abnormal anatomy of the heart and surrounding vasculature are presented in Chapter 11. Normal and abnormal appearance of lungs, diaphragm, and rib cage in the first trimester are discussed in this chapter. Pentalogy of Cantrell, involving a sternal defect, and ectopia cordis are discussed in Chapter 12.

## EMBRYOLOGY

The respiratory diverticulum or lung bud is first seen around day 22 from fertilization as a ventral outgrowth of the primitive foregut. As the lung bud grows, it is surrounded by mesoderm, which gives rise to the lung vasculature, connective tissue, and muscle within the bronchial tree. The lengthening lung bud bifurcates on day 28 into the right and left lung buds, which gives rise to the right and left lung, respectively. Growth and bifurcation of the lung buds along with the surrounding mesenchyme continues throughout pregnancy. The terminal bronchioles are seen by the 28th week of gestation (menstrual) and the terminal sacs are formed by the 36th week of gestation. Maturation of the alveoli occurs between the 36th week of gestation and term. Alveolar growth continues into early childhood.

The four embryonic structures—septum transversum, pleuroperitoneal membranes, mesoderm of body wall, and the esophageal mesoderm—coalesce to form the diaphragm (Fig. 10.1). The central tendon of the diaphragm is primarily formed from the septum transversum. The diaphragm is completely formed by the end of the 10th to 11th week of gestation.

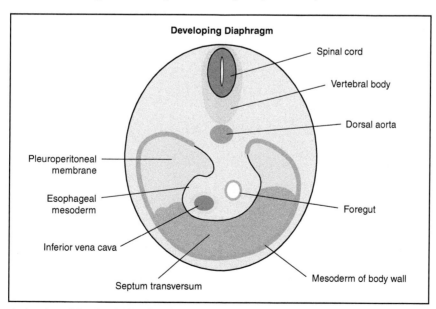

**Figure 10.1:** Schematic drawing of the developing diaphragm. Note that the diaphragm is formed by the fusion of the septum transversum, the pleuroperitoneal membranes, the mesoderm of body wall and the esophageal mesoderm, with the central tendon being primarily formed from the septum transversum.

In the sixth week of embryogenesis, the sternum arises from the somatic mesoderm as paired longitudinal sternal bars. These bars fuse in the midline to form a cartilaginous sternum at around the 10th week. Sternal ossification starts at day 60 in a segmental arrangement. The xiphoid process does not ossify until after birth. The vertebral bodies and ribs are also derived from the paraxial mesoderm.

## NORMAL SONOGRAPHIC ANATOMY

The systematic visualization of the fetal chest in the first trimester is generally achieved from multiple sonographic planes. Axial views, at the level of the upper abdomen (Fig. 10.2A), the chest (Figs. 10.2B, 10.3, and 10.4A), and mediastinum

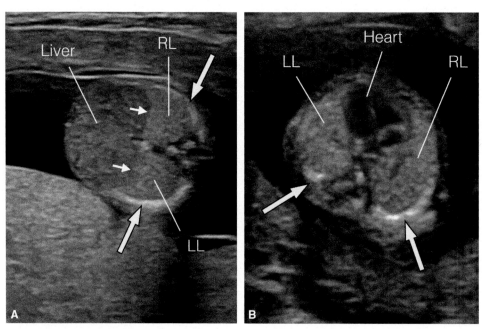

Figure 10.2: **A:** Axial plane of the upper abdomen in a fetus at 13 weeks of gestation showing the right (RL) and left (LL) lungs and the diaphragm (*white arrows*), separating the lungs from the liver. Note that the lungs are slightly more echogenic than the liver. **B:** Axial view of the thorax at the level of the four-chamber view in the same fetus. Note the position of the heart in the left hemithorax surrounded by the RL and LL. The ribs (*yellow arrows*) are seen laterally in both **A** and **B**.

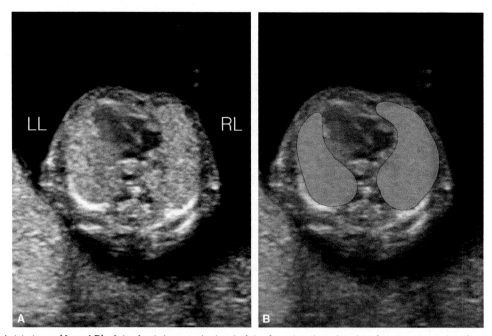

Figure 10.3: Axial planes **(A and B)** of the fetal chest at the level of the four-chamber view in a fetus at 12 weeks of gestation. The four-chamber view plane is optimal for the visualization of the right (RL) and left (LL) lungs. The lungs are highlighted in **B**.

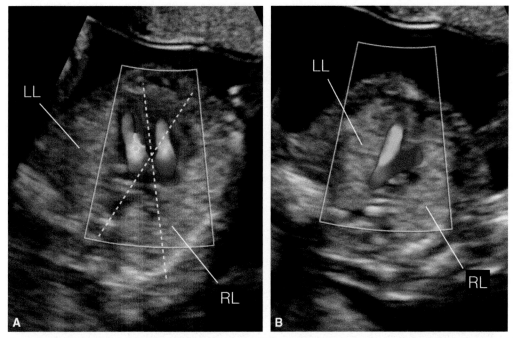

**Figure 10.4:** Axial views in color Doppler at the four-chamber view **(A)** and the three-vessel-trachea view **(B)** in a fetus at 13 weeks of gestation. Note that the right (RL) and left (LL) lungs are seen in both planes **(A and B)**. Comprehensive evaluation of the fetal lungs in axial views requires an evaluation at the level of the four-chamber view **(A)** and the three-vessel-trachea view **(B)**. The cardiac axis and position as evaluated in the four-chamber plane **(A)** is not only important for detecting cardiac abnormalities, but also for suspecting lung anomalies.

(Fig. 10.4B), allow for the evaluation of the diaphragm, right and left lungs, midline structures such as the esophagus, trachea/bronchi, and the thymus gland. In the normal fetus, the lungs appear slightly more echogenic than the liver and cardiac muscle (Fig. 10.2). At the four-chamber view plane, the right and left lungs are seen and the rib cage assessed (Figs. 10.2B, 10.3 and 10.4A). Comprehensive evaluation of the lungs in axial views requires the assessment at the level

of the four-chamber view (Figs. 10.2B, 10.3 and 10.4A) and superiorly into the upper mediastinum at the three-vessel-trachea view (Fig. 10.4B). Assessment of cardiac position and axis in the chest (Fig. 10.4A) is helpful in the identification of lung abnormalities.

The right (Fig. 10.5A) and left (Fig. 10.5B) parasagittal views of the fetal chest are important for assessment of individual lung lobes, the diaphragm, and the rib cage (Fig. 10.6A). The

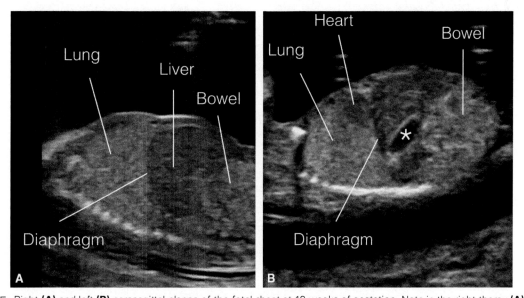

**Figure 10.5:** Right **(A)** and left **(B)** parasagittal planes of the fetal chest at 13 weeks of gestation. Note in the right thorax **(A)** the slightly hyperechoic lung as compared to the liver and the diaphragm in between. The bowel has the same echogenicity as the lung. The parasagittal view on the left **(B)** shows the lung, portion of the heart, the diaphragm, and the stomach (*asterisk*).

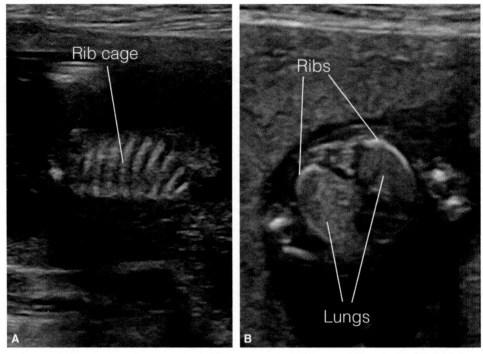

**Figure 10.6: A:** A parasagittal plane of the thorax at the lateral chest wall in a fetus at 12 weeks of gestation showing the rib cage laterally with the normal arrangement of the ribs. **B:** An axial plane of the chest at the level of the four-chamber view in the same fetus demonstrating the ribs laterally.

ribs can also be assessed from an axial plane of the chest at the level of the four-chamber view (Fig. 10.6B). In our opinion, the evaluation of the diaphragm is best achieved in coronal views (Fig. 10.7), starting from the posterior coronal view of the spine and moving more anteriorly toward the sternum.

In these planes the diaphragm muscle and tendon on the right and left chest can be well visualized. The transvaginal approach improves visualization of all chest structures due to higher resolution (Fig. 10.7B). Three-dimensional ultrasound in a surface (Fig. 10.8) or tomographic display (Fig. 10.9)

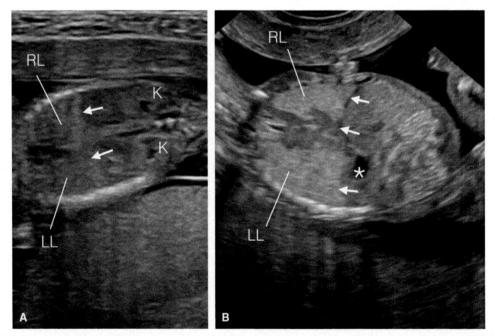

**Figure 10.7:** Coronal views of the fetal abdomen and chest at 13 weeks of gestation obtained by the transabdominal **(A)** and transvaginal **(B)** approach in the same fetus. Note in **A**, the right (RL) and left (LL) lung seen in a coronal view with the diaphragm (*arrows*) separating the chest from the abdomen. The kidneys (K) are seen in the abdomen in **A**. In the transvaginal approach **(B)**, the borders of the RL and LL are better seen and the diaphragm is clearly delineated (*arrows*). The stomach is also seen in **B** as an anechoic structure in the abdomen (*asterisk*).

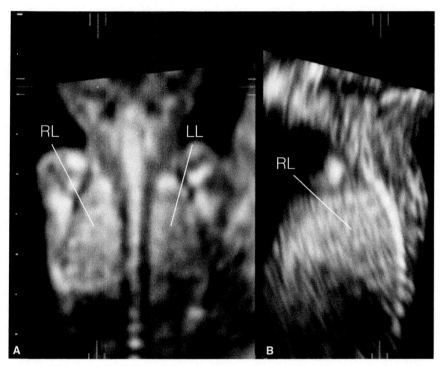

**Figure 10.8:** Surface display of a three-dimensional transvaginal ultrasound volume of the chest in a fetus at 13 weeks of gestation showing the posterior coronal plane **(A)** and right parasagittal plane **(B)**. Note the full display of the right (RL) and left (LL) lungs in **A** and the RL in **B**.

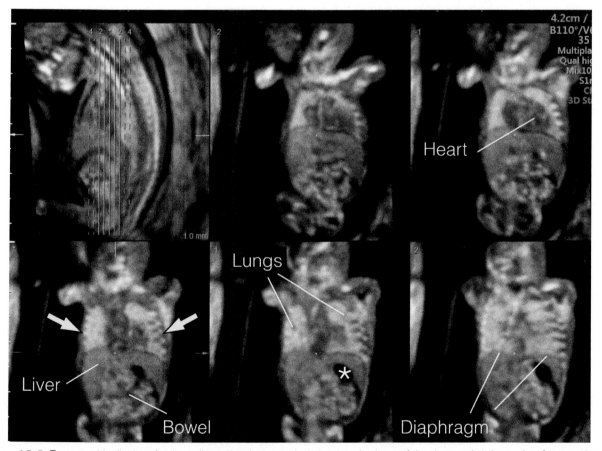

**Figure 10.9:** Tomographic display of a three-dimensional transvaginal ultrasound volume of the chest and abdomen in a fetus at 13 weeks of gestation. The volume displays the coronal planes of the fetus showing in the chest the thoracic cage with ribs (*yellow arrows*), lungs, heart, diaphragm, and in the abdomen the stomach (*asterisk*), liver, and bowel.

can help in demonstrating various chest structures, especially in transvaginal scanning where transducer manipulation is limited. Clear visualization of the lungs can be achieved from about the 12th week of gestation onward.

## CHEST ABNORMALITIES

### Hydrothorax/Pleural Effusion

#### Definition

Hydrothorax (pleural effusion) is the accumulation of fluid in the pleural space between the lungs and the thoracic cage. Hydrothorax may occur unilaterally or bilaterally and may be primary or secondary. Primary hydrothorax is a diagnosis made after excluding causes of hydrothorax, which are many, and involve fetal lung or cardiovascular malformations, fetal arrhythmias, infections, chromosomal aneuploidy, and others. In a prospective study between 7 and 10 weeks of gestation, hydrothorax was found in 1.2% of embryos.[1] The presence of bilateral hydrothorax in the first trimester is associated with a poor prognosis. Follow-up of 14 fetuses with bilateral hydrothorax diagnosed in the first trimester showed only one survivor. A high incidence of chromosomal aneuploidy, including monosomy X, was also reported.[1] Isolated unilateral hydrothorax with no other fetal abnormality may be a transient finding with disappearance of the effusion upon follow-up ultrasound in the second trimester.

#### Ultrasound Findings

Accumulation of fluid around the lungs is relatively easy to detect on ultrasound on axial (Figs. 10.10, 10.11, and 10.12A), coronal, or sagittal views (Fig. 10.12B). A typical sign for hydrothorax involves the presence of fluid between the lateral borders of the lungs and the ribs (Figs. 10.10 to 10.12). This sign allows for differentiating hydrothorax from pericardial effusion, which can be difficult in some cases. In pericardial effusion, the fluid surrounds the heart and is on the medial aspects of the lungs (Fig. 10.13). The presence of severe hydrothorax results in lung compression with the typical "butterfly" appearance of the lungs. The association of hydrothorax with fetal hydrops is easily seen and is commonly noted with increased nuchal translucency (NT) and genetic abnormalities (Figs. 10.10 and 10.11). Diagnostic or therapeutic thoracocentesis is typically reserved for the second or third trimester of pregnancy. Figure 10.12 shows a fetus with an isolated unilateral hydrothorax that resolved by the second trimester of pregnancy.

#### Associated Abnormalities

Associated abnormalities are many and include cardiovascular and skeletal malformations, fetal arrhythmias, chromosomal abnormalities including monosomy X, trisomy 21, Noonan syndrome, and hematologic conditions. Persistence of hydrothorax is later associated with pulmonary hypoplasia due to compression of lungs. Increased pressure in the thoracic cavity, associated with bilateral hydrothorax, may lead in the second trimester to reduction in venous return to the heart, resulting in fetal hydrops and polyhydramnios due to compression of the esophagus.

### Congenital Diaphragmatic Hernia

#### Definition

Congenital diaphragmatic hernia (CDH) results from a defect in the diaphragm with protrusion of the abdominal organs into the thoracic cavity. The diaphragmatic defect is most commonly located in the posterolateral part of the diaphragm (Bochdalek

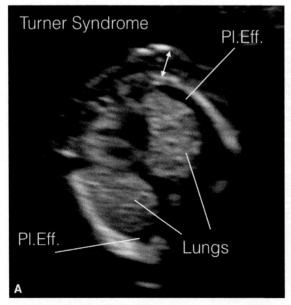
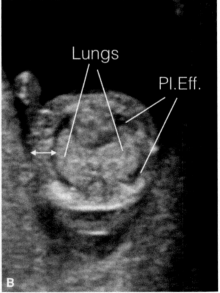

**Figure 10.10:** Axial views of the fetal chest in a fetus at 12 weeks **(A)** and another fetus at 11 weeks **(B)** of gestation with pleural effusions (Pl.Eff.). Note the location of pleural effusion on the lateral aspects of the lungs. Also note the presence of skin edema in both fetuses (*double headed arrows*). Turner's syndrome was confirmed in both cases.

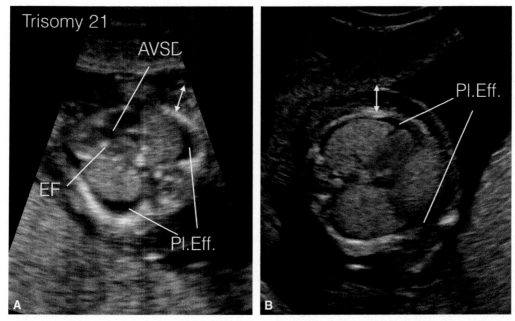

**Figure 10.11:** Bilateral mild pleural effusions (Pl.Eff.) in two fetuses with trisomy 21 at 12 **(A)** and 13 **(B)** weeks of gestation demonstrated in the axial plane of the chest. Note in **A** that the heart shows a large atrioventricular septal defect (AVSD), an echogenic focus (EF), and a shifted cardiac axis to the left. Also note the presence of skin edema (*double headed arrows*) in both fetuses. Both fetuses also had thickened nuchal translucencies (data not shown).

type). Other types of diaphragmatic defects include the parasternal region of the diaphragm (Morgagni type) located in the anterior portion of the diaphragm, the central tendinous region of the diaphragm located in the central septum transversum region of the diaphragm, and hiatal hernias occurring through a defective esophageal orifice. The Bochdalek type is the most common and accounts for about 80% to 90% of CDHs. CDHs are left-sided in about 85%, right-sided in about 13%, and

bilateral in about 2%. CDH is a fairly common malformation occurring in about 1:2,000 to 1:3,000 pregnancies.

The embryologic development of the diaphragm is typically completed by the 12th week of gestation (see section on Embryology) and thus CDH can be diagnosed in the first trimester. It is reasonable to assume however that the timing of herniation of intraabdominal content into the chest can be delayed to the second trimester or beyond, as it is

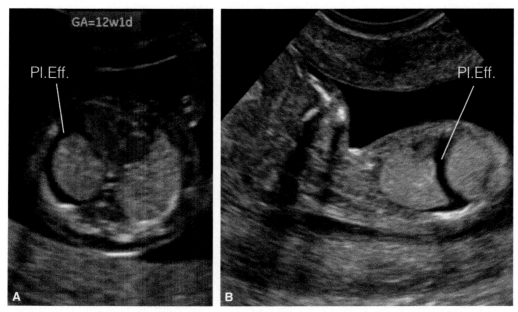

**Figure 10.12:** Axial **(A)** and left parasagittal **(B)** planes of a fetus with isolated pleural effusion (Pl.Eff.) in the left hemithorax at 12 weeks of gestation. Note in **A** that the effusion is on the lateral aspect of the lung. Compare with Figures 10.10 and 10.11. This effusion spontaneously resolved on follow-up ultrasound in the second trimester of pregnancy.

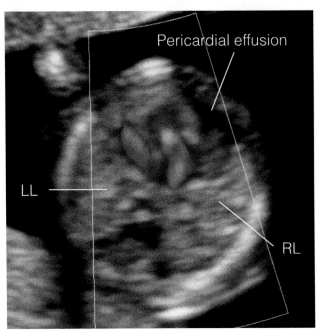

**Figure 10.13:** Axial plane of the chest at the level of the four-chamber view in a fetus with pericardial effusion at 12 weeks of gestation. Note that the pericardial effusion is located on the medial aspect of the lungs. Compare with Figure 10.12. RL, right lung; LL, left lung.

dependent upon the size of the diaphragmatic defect and intraabdominal pressure. A normal ultrasound examination of the chest in the first trimester therefore does not rule out the presence of a CDH.

### Ultrasound Findings

CDH is first suspected on ultrasound in the first trimester by the presence of an abnormal cardiac axis and mediastinal shift on the axial four-chamber view plane of the chest (Figs. 10.14 and 10.15). The demonstration of the herniated stomach and other intraabdominal organs into the chest confirms the diagnosis (Fig. 10.14), and this is ideally visualized in a coronal view (Fig. 10.16). The diagnosis of CDH in the first trimester is challenging, especially in isolated cases, as the typical signs of mediastinal shift and the demonstration of intraabdominal content in the chest may not be evident. In our experience, mild shifting of cardiac position in the four-chamber-view (Figs. 10.14 and 10.15), abnormal course of the ductus venosus in the abdomen, or a more cranial position of the stomach in coronal views of the chest and abdomen (Fig. 10.16) provide clues to the diagnosis. Polyhydramnios, a common association with CDH in the second and third trimesters, is not seen in the first trimester. Observed/expected lung-to-head ratio and liver herniation into the chest are ultrasound parameters that can stratify severity of CDH in the second and third trimesters of pregnancy. In the first trimester, the presence of associated anomalies is most important for assessing prognosis. Interestingly, the ipsilateral lung in CDH can be well identified in the first trimester (Figs. 10.15 and 10.16), but the dynamics of its slow growth is not predictable. Follow-up ultrasound examination in the second trimester of pregnancy often reveals increased severity of the diaphragmatic hernia with more herniation of abdominal content into the chest (Fig. 10.17). Furthermore, the presence of severe CDH in the first trimester is more commonly associated with chromosomal abnormalities (Fig. 10.18) and a thickened NT.[2] Some cases of CDH are not detectable in the first trimester due to delayed organ herniation into the chest.[3] In one study, only 50% of the CDH cases were identified on first trimester ultrasound[2] (see Table 5.2).

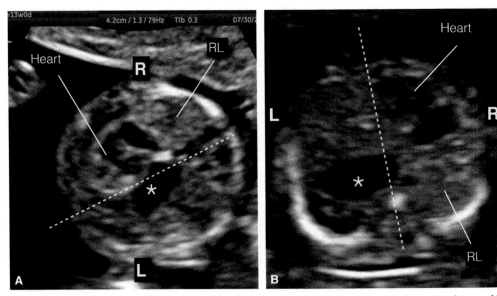

**Figure 10.14:** Axial planes of the chest at the level of the four-chamber view at 13 weeks of gestation in two fetuses **(A,B)** with left-sided congenital diaphragmatic hernias. Note that the heart is shifted to the right chest in both fetuses. Also note that the stomach (*asterisk*) is in the left hemithorax and the right lung (RL) is compressed. R, right; L, left.

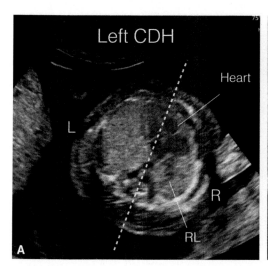

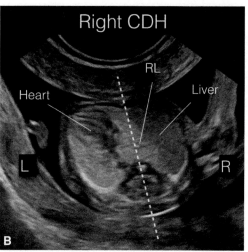

**Figure 10.15:** Axial planes of the chest at the level of the four-chamber view at 13 weeks of gestation in a fetus **(A)** with left-sided congenital diaphragmatic hernia (CDH) and another fetus **(B)** with right-sided CDH. Note that the heart is shifted to the right in **A** and to the left in **B**. The liver is seen in the right hemithorax in **B**. The right lung (RL) is seen compressed in both fetuses. R, right; L, left.

## Associated Abnormalities

CDH can be an isolated finding (60%) or can be associated with fetal structural and genetic abnormalities (40%). The association with an enlarged NT is estimated to be between 12%[4] and 46%.[5] The association of enlarged NT and CDH in the first trimester suggests a poor neonatal outcome even after ruling out chromosomal or genetic defects.[3,4] CDH is considered a

major fetal abnormality with postnatal mortality in the range of 30% to 40% in isolated cases. Typical syndromes with CDH include trisomy 18 (Fig. 10.16), tetrasomy 12p (Pallister–Killian syndrome) (Fig. 10.19), Fryns syndrome (Fig. 10.20), Cornelia de Lange syndrome, and other syndromic conditions.

### Pallister–Killian Syndrome

Pallister–Killian syndrome is a mosaic of tetrasomy for chromosome 12p, where in addition to the two copies of chromosome 12, an extra isochromosome is present, made from two p arms of chromosome 12 (see upper panel in Fig. 10.19). Typical anomalies found in tetrasomy 12p include diaphragmatic hernia, facial dysmorphism, rhizomelic limb shortening, and abdominal defects (omphalocele and anal atresia). The patient in Figure 10.19 was referred due to advanced maternal age and the detection on ultrasound of a thickened NT (Fig. 10.19A) and omphalocele (Fig. 10.19B), which was initially suggestive of trisomy 18. Biometric assessment showed a normal crown-rump length, head and abdominal circumference, and a short femur (Fig. 10.19C). Detailed first trimester ultrasound examination revealed a left-sided CDH (Fig. 10.19D and E) with polydactyly (Fig. 10.19F), in addition to the short femur (Fig. 10.19C). CVS revealed the presence of Pallister–Killian syndrome.

### Fryns Syndrome

Fryns syndrome is an autosomal recessive disease with currently no identifiable gene locus. Typical features include a diaphragmatic hernia in 90% of cases with multiple anomalies including a coarse face with facial clefts, micrognathia, large mouth, hypertelorism with occasionally microphthalmia and nuchal edema. In addition, cerebral anomalies mainly of the posterior fossa (50% of cases), short hands, dysplastic kidneys, and others are present. Figure 10.20 is a first trimester ultrasound of a patient with a prior history of a fetus with

**Figure 10.16:** Coronal view of the chest and abdomen in a fetus at 13 weeks of gestation with left-sided congenital diaphragmatic hernia and trisomy 18. The stomach (*asterisk*) is seen herniated through the diaphragm (*arrows*) into the left hemithorax, with no associated shift in the heart. At this early gestation, the left lung (LL) appears normal in size and with advancing gestation; lung compression and hypoplasia will develop. R, right; RL, right lung; L, left.

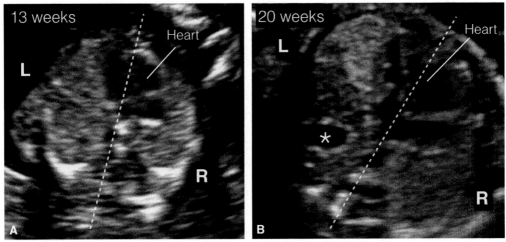

**Figure 10.17:** Axial planes of the chest at the level of the four-chamber view at 13 **(A)** and 20 **(B)** weeks of gestation in the same fetus. Note in **A** that the heart is shifted to the right, suggesting the presence of a left-sided congenital diaphragmatic hernia (CDH). The stomach is not yet visible in the chest at this early gestation in **A**. At 20 weeks of gestation **(B)**, the stomach (*asterisk*) is clearly seen in the left chest, confirming the presence of a CDH with more cardiac shifting into the right hemithorax. R, right; L, left.

multiple anomalies suggestive of Fryns syndrome. Because of the autosomal recessive inheritance of Fryns syndrome, a detailed first trimester ultrasound was performed and revealed the presence of a thickened NT (Fig. 10.20A and B), a dilated posterior fossa (Fig. 10.20B), abnormal profile with maxillary gap, suggestive of facial clefting (Fig. 10.20B), short hands (Fig. 10.20C), hyperechogenic kidneys with urinary tract dilation (Fig. 10.20D), and a left-sided CDH (Fig. 10.20E and F). These findings were suggestive of recurrence of Fryns syndrome.

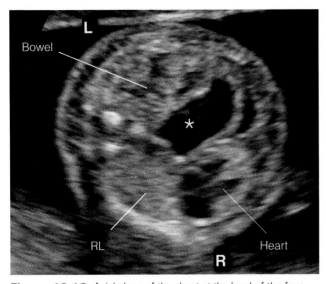

**Figure 10.18:** Axial plane of the chest at the level of the four-chamber view at 14 weeks of gestation in a fetus with left-sided congenital diaphragmatic hernia (CDH) and chromosomal aneuploidy (trisomies 9 and 10). Note the severity of the CDH with the heart severely shifted to the right hemithorax and the stomach (*asterisk*) and abdominal content occupying the majority of the right chest. The right lung (RL) is compressed. R, right; L, left.

## Pulmonary Agenesis and Pulmonary Hypoplasia

Unilateral or bilateral agenesis of the lung(s) is an extremely rare condition that is amenable to first trimester diagnosis. The true etiology is unknown and sporadic occurrence is assumed in most cases; however, a genetic cause can also be present. Several recurrences of bilateral pulmonary agenesis were reported in a single family.[6] In this report, the diagnosis was performed in the second and third trimesters in two fetuses and at 12 weeks of gestation in the third fetus.[6] The authors reported that the heart occupied almost the entire chest, whereas the thymus occupied the remaining space, mimicking lung tissue.[6] Agenesis of branching pulmonary arteries may be an important clue to the presence of lung agenesis.

Unilateral lung agenesis can also be diagnosed in the first trimester as the heart is shifted toward the empty hemithorax (Fig. 10.21). The diagnosis is first suspected by the presence of dextrocardia or levocardia. Typically, the first impression is that a CDH is present but the demonstration of normal liver, bowel, and diaphragm with high-resolution transvaginal ultrasound can be of help in achieving the diagnosis of unilateral lung agenesis. In right lung agenesis, there is absence of the right bronchus and right pulmonary artery and upon follow-up ultrasound examinations, associated cardiac anomalies as well as tracheoesophageal fistula with esophageal atresia can be associated findings. Outcome can be good provided no additional anomalies are found. Figure 10.21 shows a case with an absent right lung with the heart completely positioned in the right chest. The patient was referred to us at 14 weeks of gestation with the suspected diagnosis of dextrocardia performed at 12 weeks by the referring physician.

Unilateral pulmonary hypoplasia can be suggestive for the presence of Scimitar syndrome with partial anomalous venous drainage into the inferior vena cava.[7,8] The diagnosis, similar to other venous anomalies, is very difficult to make in the first trimester and a follow-up is recommended in the second trimester.

# Pallister-Killian Syndrome (Tetrasomy 12p)

12

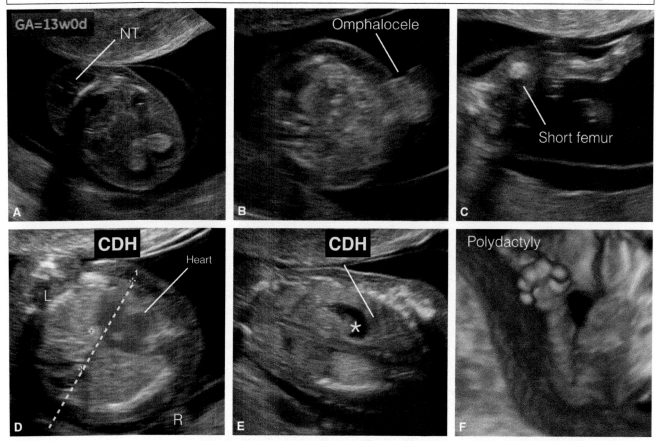

**Figure 10.19:** Fetus at 13 weeks of gestation with a tetrasomy 12p, also called Pallister–Killian syndrome with a thickened nuchal translucency (NT) **(A)**, an omphalocele **(B)**, a short femur **(C)**, a left-sided diaphragmatic hernia (CDH) **(D and E)** with the heart shifted to the right hemithorax and the stomach (*asterisk*) seen in the chest **(E)**. In addition, polydactyly is present **(F)**. R, right; L, Left. See text for more details.

Bilateral pulmonary hypoplasia is a challenging diagnosis to make prenatally and is typically associated with other serious conditions such as preterm premature rupture of membranes, bilateral renal agenesis or dysplasia, CDH, bilateral pleural effusions, lethal skeletal dysplasia with thoracic hypoplasia, and others.[7] In all these conditions, the lungs may appear normal in the first trimester and the prediction of lung hypoplasia cannot be performed in early gestation. Follow-up ultrasound examinations in the second and third trimesters are recommended in order to suspect the presence of pulmonary hypoplasia.

## Lung Abnormalities That are Not Detectable in the First Trimester

In addition to bilateral pulmonary hypoplasia, several lung abnormalities that are commonly seen in the second and third trimesters of pregnancy are currently not detectable in the first trimester. These include bronchopulmonary sequestration (BPS), cystic congenital adenomatoid malformation (CCAM) of the lung either with macrocystic or microcystic lesions, isolated bronchogenic cyst and chronic high airway obstructions.[7] The diagnosis of these lung abnormalities is typically performed around 16 to 17 weeks of gestation.[9] In a first trimester study on fetal malformations, CCAM and BPS cases were not diagnosed in the first trimester[2] (see Table 5.2) and the authors thus classified these lesions in the group of "not detectable" anomalies. The authors postulate that the production of pulmonary fluid and its retention within the abnormally developed lung tissue occur after the onset of the canalicular phase of lung development, typically at 16 weeks of gestation.[2] This is possibly the reason why these lung abnormalities are not visible in early gestation.

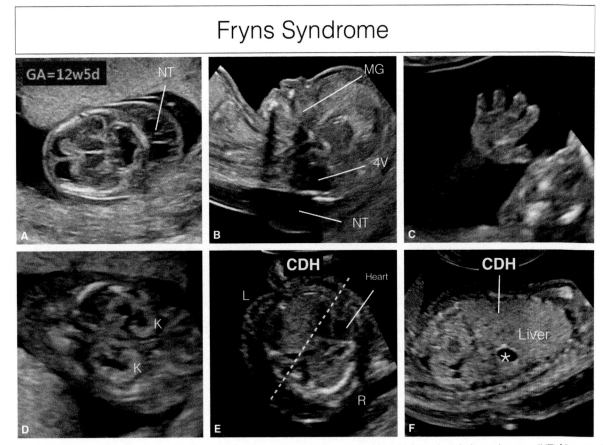

**Figure 10.20:** Fetus at 12 weeks of gestation with Fryns syndrome, presenting with a thickened nuchal translucency (NT) **(A and B)**, a dilated fourth ventricle (4V) and facial cleft with a maxillary gap (MG) in **(B)**, short hand **(C)**, hyperechogenic kidneys (K) with renal track dilation **(D)**, and the typical diaphragmatic hernia (CDH) **(E and F)**, with the heart shifted into the right hemithorax **(E)** and liver and stomach (*asterisk*) shifted in the upper thorax (F). R, right; L, Left. See text for more details.

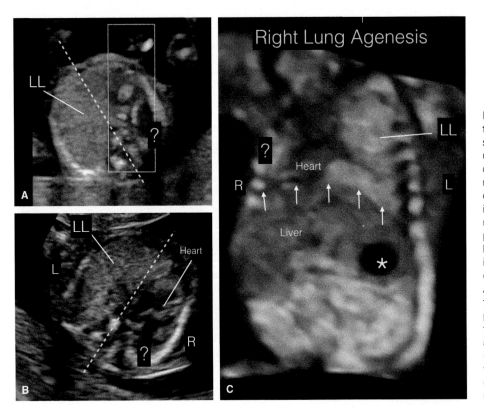

**Figure 10.21:** Axial views of the chest in color Doppler **(A)**, gray scale **(B)**, and three-dimensional (3D) ultrasound of a coronal view of the chest and abdomen **(C)** in a fetus with right pulmonary agenesis at 14 weeks of gestation. The heart is completely in the right chest **(A and B)** with normal diastolic filling **(A)**. Note the presence in **A–C** of a large-appearing left lung (LL) with no right lung seen in the right hemithorax (?). There is no evidence of a stomach in the chest in **A** and **B**. Note on the 3D ultrasound that the liver is in its normal anatomic position in the right (R) abdomen and the stomach (*asterisk*) in the left (L) abdomen. A well-delineated diaphragm (*arrows*) is also seen in **C**. This patient was referred due to the presence of dextrocardia detected at 12 weeks of gestation. See text for details.

# REFERENCES

1. Hashimoto K, Shimizu T, Fukuda M, et al. Pregnancy outcome of embryonic/fetal pleural effusion in the first trimester. *J Ultrasound Med.* 2003;22:501–505.

2. Syngelaki A, Chelemen T, Dagklis T, et al. Challenges in the diagnosis of fetal non-chromosomal abnormalities at 11-13 weeks. *Prenat Diagn.* 2011;31:90–102.

3. Sepulveda W, Wong AE, Casasbuenas A, et al. Congenital diaphragmatic hernia in a first-trimester ultrasound aneuploidy screening program. *Prenat Diagn.* 2008;28:531–534.

4. Spaggiari E, Stirnemann J, Ville Y. Outcome in fetuses with isolated congenital diaphragmatic hernia with increased nuchal translucency thickness in first trimester. *Prenat Diagn.* 2012;32:268–271.

5. Sebire NJ, Snijders RJ, Davenport M, et al. Fetal nuchal translucency thickness at 10-14 weeks' gestation and congenital diaphragmatic hernia. *Obstet Gynecol.* 1997;90:943–946.

6. Ramanah R, Martin A, Guigue V, et al. Recurrent prenatally diagnosed isolated bilateral pulmonary agenesis. *Ultrasound Obstet Gynecol.* 2012;40:724–725.

7. Karl K, Chaoui R. Pulmonary abnormalities. In: Coady AM, Bower S, eds. *Twining's Textbook of Fetal Abnormalities.* New York, NY: Elsevier Health Sciences; 2014:397–419.

8. Abuhamad A, Chaoui R. *A Practical Guide to Fetal Echocardiography: Normal and Abnormal Hearts.* 3rd ed. Philadelphia, PA: Wolters Kluwer Health/Lippincott Williams & Wilkins; 2015.

9. Cavoretto P, Molina F, Poggi S, et al. Prenatal diagnosis and outcome of echogenic fetal lung lesions. *Ultrasound Obstet Gynecol.* 2008;32:769–783.

# CHAPTER 11

# The Fetal Heart and Great Vessels

## INTRODUCTION

Fetal cardiac examination in the first trimester focuses in general on the evaluation of body situs, the four chambers, and the great vessels in order to confirm normal anatomy and to rule out complex congenital heart defects (CHDs). Many CHDs can be detected in the first trimester and are discussed in this chapter. First trimester ultrasound evaluation of the fetal heart can also assess for the presence of indirect markers such as tricuspid regurgitation (TR), abnormal cardiac axis, or an aberrant right subclavian artery (ARSA), which can be clues to CHD or fetal aneuploidy. Ultrasound examination of the fetal heart and great vessels can be a challenge in the first trimester as it requires high-resolution images in two-dimensional (2D) gray scale and color Doppler and often needs a combined transabdominal and transvaginal approach. In this chapter, embryology of the fetal heart is first presented along with normal fetal cardiac anatomy by ultrasound. Various fetal cardiac malformations that can be detected in the first trimester are then presented. For a more comprehensive discussion on the sonographic cardiac examination technique and a wide range of normal and abnormal fetal hearts, we recommend our textbook "Practical Guide to Fetal Echocardiography: Normal and Abnormal Hearts."[1]

## EMBRYOLOGY

The spectrum of congenital cardiac malformations is wide and is better understood with a basic knowledge of cardiac embryology.

Starting in the third week postconception, clusters of angiogenic cardiac precursor cells develop in the lateral splanchnic mesoderm and migrate anteriorly toward the midline to fuse into a single heart tube. Heart tube pulsations are first recognized around day 21 to 22 postconception (day 35 to 36 menstrual age, end fifth gestational week). The heart develops according to well-defined major steps, namely (1) the formation of the primitive heart tube; (2) the looping of the heart tube; and (3) the septation of atria, ventricles, and outflow tracts (Fig. 11.1). The primitive heart tube is anchored caudally by the vitello-umbilical veins and cranially by the dorsal aortae and pharyngeal arches, and shows transitional folding zones such as the primary fold at the arterial pole and the atrioventricular (AV) ring at the venous pole (Fig. 11.1). These transitional zones later form the cardiac septa and valves. Figure 11.1 illustrates these developmental steps.[1] With looping and bulging, the primitive ventricle moves downward to the right, whereas the primitive atrium moves upward and to the left behind the ventricle. Within this tube and at different sites, septations occur to differentiate the two atria, two ventricles, two AV valves, and two separate outflow tracts. The paired branchial arteries with two aortae progressively regress, resulting in a left aortic arch with its corresponding bifurcations. On the venous side, different paired veins regress and fuse to develop the systemic venous system with the hepatic veins and superior and inferior venae cavae.

The primitive atrium is divided into two by the formation of two septa, the septum primum and the septum secundum. Both septa fuse except for the foramen primum, which remains patent and becomes the foramen ovale with blood shunting from the right to the left atrium. The formation of the ventricular septum is more complex and consists of the fusion of septae of different spatial cardiac regions (interventricular septum, inlet septum, and conal septum), thus explaining that ventricular septal defects (VSDs) are by far the most common cardiac abnormalities (isolated and combined). The separation of the outflow tracts involves a spiral rotation of nearly 180 degrees, leading to the formation of a spiral aortopulmonary septum. This septum, resulting from the complete fusion of both bulbus and truncus ridges, separates the outflow tract into two arterial vessels, the aorta and pulmonary artery. Because of the spiraling of this septum, the pulmonary artery appears to twist around the ascending aorta. The bulbar development is responsible for incorporating the great vessels within their corresponding ventricle. In the right ventricle, the bulbus cordis is represented by the conus arteriosus, which is the infundibulum and in the left ventricle the bulbus cordis forms

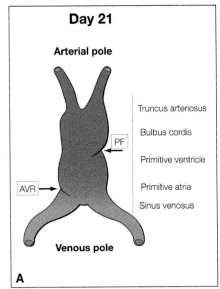 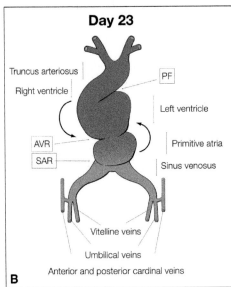 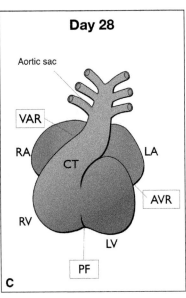

**Figure 11.1:** Frontal views of the different stages of the developing heart: in **A** the primitive heart tube stage, in **B** cardiac looping stage and in **C** view of the looped heart during septation of atria, ventricles and great vessels. **A:** Two transitional zones are identifiable: the atrioventricular ring (AVR) forming the future atrioventricular valves and the primary fold (PF) forming the future interventricular septum. **B:** The cardiac tube starts to loop with folding along the long axis and rotation to the right and ventral, resulting in a D-looped heart. Primitive cardiac chambers are better identified and are separated by transitional zones as the sinoatrial ring (SAR), the AVR, and the PF. **C:** After looping, several transitional zones can be identified separating the primitive cardiac chambers, the AVR between the common atrium (*blue*) and common ventricle (*red*), the PF between the primitive left (LV) and right (RV) ventricle, and the VAR in the conotruncus (CT) region of the outflow tract of the heart. RA, right atrium; LA, left atrium.

the walls of the aortic vestibule, which is the septo-aortic and mitral-aortic continuity.[1] For more details on cardiac embryogenesis, we recommend monographs and review articles on this subject.[1–4]

## NORMAL SONOGRAPHIC ANATOMY AND EXAMINATION TECHNIQUE

The steps for the examination of the fetal heart in the first trimester are no different from the cardiac examination in the second and third trimesters. It is recommended to follow a systematic step-by-step segmental approach to cardiac imaging. Although in the second trimester the screening cardiac examination can be performed with gray-scale ultrasound alone, in the first trimester, gray-scale ultrasound should be complemented by color Doppler, especially for the evaluation of the great vessels.[1] 2D ultrasound imaging with high resolution can now be achieved with transabdominal linear or transvaginal transducers. In our experience, the transvaginal ultrasound approach is recommended when the fetus is in transverse position low in the uterus, which provides for the closest distance from the transvaginal transducer to the fetal chest (see Chapter 3). Furthermore, the transvaginal approach is helpful in fetuses at less than 13 weeks of gestation or in the presence of suspected cardiac malformations.

The basic approach to fetal cardiac imaging by ultrasound is first performed in gray-scale 2D ultrasound, with a focus on the fetal situs and the apical and transverse views of the four-chamber heart (4CV) (Fig. 11.2). Ultrasound system optimization for the gray-scale cardiac examination in the first trimester is shown in Table 11.1. Although the fetal abdomen and the 4CV can be reliably imaged in gray scale in the first trimester, the anatomic orientation of the right and left ventricular outflow tracts is not commonly seen in fetuses at less than 14 weeks of gestation because of their small size. We therefore recommend the use of color or high-definition (power) Doppler as an adjunct to gray-scale imaging for cardiac evaluation in the first trimester. Color Doppler in the first trimester is therefore mostly used to indirectly evaluate the shape and size of cardiac chambers and great vessels. The optimization of color Doppler is summarized in Table 11.2. Color Doppler application at the level of the four-chamber view (Fig. 11.3) is an important step for identifying normal and abnormal cardiac anatomy, especially for fetuses at less than 14 weeks of gestation. Color Doppler demonstration of the upper transverse views in the chest including the three-vessel-trachea (3VT) and the transverse ductal views (Fig. 11.4) is essential for imaging of the great vessels and is far superior to what can be achieved by gray-scale evaluation alone. Several cardiac abnormalities involving the outflow tracts can be recognized in the first trimester in the 3VT view. The location, size, patency, and blood flow directions of the aortic and ductal arches are more easily recognized in the first trimester on color Doppler ultrasound (Fig. 11.4).

All ultrasound planes recommended for cardiac anatomic evaluation in the second and third trimesters of pregnancy

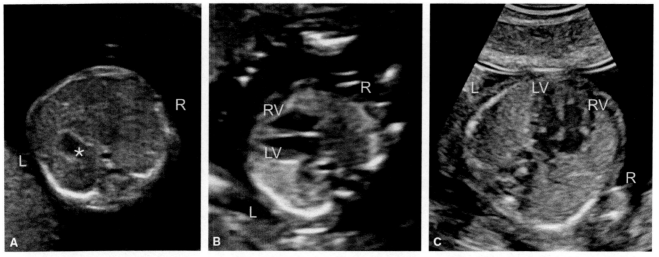

**Figure 11.2:** Typical planes displayed in gray scale during the first trimester cardiac examination include the visualization of the abdominal situs **(A)** with stomach (*asterisk*) and the four-chamber view, displayed in a transverse **(B)** or in an apical view **(C)**. LV, left ventricle; RV, right ventricle; R, right; L, Left.

| **Table 11.1 • Optimization of the gray-scale cardiac examination in the first trimester** | **Table 11.2 • Optimization of Color Doppler Cardiac Examination in the First Trimester** |
|---|---|
| Fetus in dorsoposterior position (NT-position) | Optimize the gray-scale image before activating color Doppler |
| Image magnified | Narrow color Doppler box |
| Narrow sector width | Mid-velocity color Doppler range |
| Fetal thorax to occupy one-third of ultrasound image | Mid-filter levels |
| High contrast image settings | Mid-to-high persistence |
| Mid- to high-resolution transducers | Low color Doppler gain |
| Ultrasound insonation from apical to right lateral of the fetal heart | Low power output |
| | Bidirectional color Doppler if available |
| NT-nuchal translucency | |

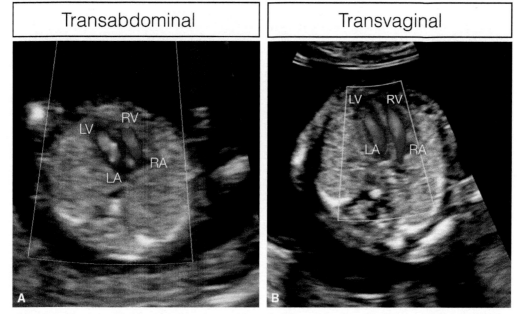

**Figure 11.3:** Color Doppler of an apical four-chamber view at 12 weeks of gestation by transabdominal **(A)** and transvaginal **(B)** ultrasound examination demonstrating diastolic flow from both right (RA) and left (LA) atrium into right (RV) and left (LV) ventricle, respectively. Note that the heart in **B** is displayed with a higher resolution due to the transvaginal approach.

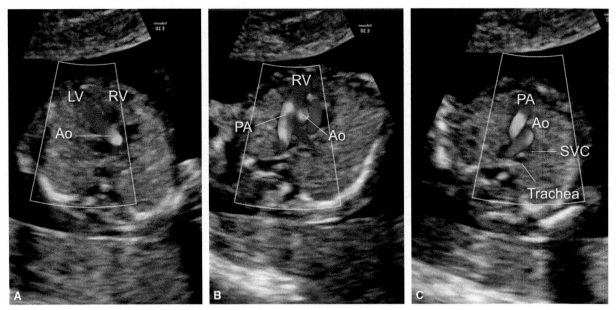

**Figure 11.4:** Transvaginal ultrasound of the outflow tracts in color Doppler in a fetus at 13 weeks of gestation showing the five-chamber view **(A)**, the short axis view of the right ventricle (RV) **(B)**, and the three-vessel-trachea view **(C)**. Ao, aorta; LV, left ventricle; PA, pulmonary artery; SVC, superior vena cava.

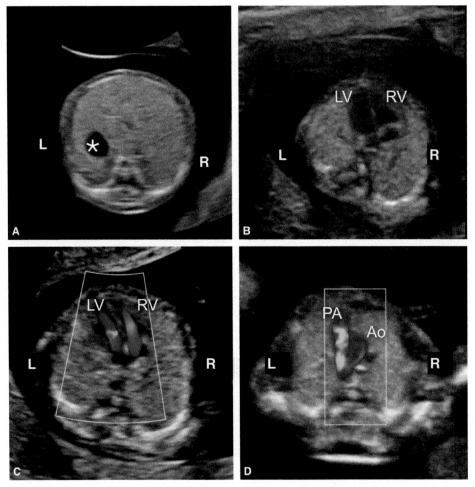

**Figure 11.5:** Four essential planes in the first trimester cardiac examination include the plane at the abdominal circumference level **(A)** to visualize abdominal situs with the stomach (*asterisk*) on the left side, the four-chamber view **(B)** in gray scale, as well as the four-chamber view in color Doppler in diastole **(C)** and the three-vessel-trachea view in color Doppler in systole **(D)**. LV, left ventricle; RV, right ventricle; PA, pulmonary artery; Ao, aorta; R, right; L, Left.

can be obtained in the first trimester under optimal scanning conditions. Based upon our experience however, visualization in the first trimester of four essential planes—(1) the axial view of the upper abdomen, (2) the 4CV in gray scale, (3) the 4CV in color Doppler, and (4) the 3VT in color Doppler (Fig. 11.5)—provides enough information to rule out most major cardiac malformations.

## CONGENITAL HEART DISEASE IN THE FIRST TRIMESTER

Congenital heart disease (CHD) is the most common severe congenital abnormality.[5,6] About half of the cases of CHD are severe and account for over half of deaths from congenital abnormalities in childhood.[5] Moreover, CHD results in the most costly hospital admissions for birth defects in the United States.[7] The incidence of CHD is dependent on the age at which the population is initially examined and the definition of CHD used. An incidence of 8 to 9 per 1,000 live births has been reported in large population studies.[5,6] It is generally accepted that in the first trimester of pregnancy the prevalence of CHD is higher, as many fetuses with complex anomalies die in utero, especially when associated with extracardiac malformations or early hydrops. One of the poor prognostic signs of CHD is its association with extracardiac anomalies including genetic diseases. The detection of a fetal anomaly is therefore an indication for fetal echocardiography. Even when isolated, CHD can be associated with aneuploidy or syndromic conditions. Prenatal diagnosis of CHD in the first trimester allows for pregnancy counseling and provides enough time for diagnostic options and decision-making.[1] CHD can be suspected in the first trimester by the presence of indirect signs such as a thickened nuchal translucency (NT), by the presence of extracardiac malformations, or by the direct observation of cardiac and great vessel anatomic abnormalities.

## ASSOCIATED EXTRACARDIAC MALFORMATIONS

Cardiac anomalies are often associated with extracardiac malformations either as part of a defined genetic disease or in isolation. Cardiac anomalies may be found in association with brain, abdominal, urogenital, or skeletal anomalies among others. Even if CHD appears isolated, a careful follow-up should be performed in the second trimester to look for associated extracardiac anomalies. Either isolated or in combination with other extracardiac anomalies, the detection of a CHD is a major hint for a possible association with aneuploidy or other syndromic conditions. The true incidence of CHD association with aneuploidy is unknown but more than 20% of all CHD detected in the first trimester are associated with chromosomal numeric aberrations. This may represent an overestimation given that a significant percentage of CHD in the first trimester is detected after a thickened NT is diagnosed. Aneuploidies associated with CHD in the first trimester include

trisomies 21, 18, and 13, as well as with Turner syndrome and triploidy (see Chapter 6 for more details). Other chromosomal anomalies are possible but rather accidental. One major chromosomal anomaly is the association with deletion 22q11, testing for which has to be offered when invasive procedure is performed, especially when a conotruncal anomaly is detected (see below). Deletions and duplications are more commonly detected nowadays given the widespread use of microarray as a diagnostic test following chorionic villous sampling when CHD is diagnosed in the first trimester. Monogenic diseases associated with cardiac defects are usually not detected in early gestation. For more details on genetics of cardiac anomalies, we recommend monographs and review articles on this subject.[1,8]

### Deletion 22q11.2 Syndrome (DiGeorge Syndrome)

Deletion 22q11.2 syndrome (also called DiGeorge syndrome or CATCH 22) is the most common deletion in humans and is the second most common chromosomal anomaly in infants with CHD (second to trisomy 21). It has an estimated prevalence of 1:2,000 to 1:4,000 live births.[9] The acronym CATCH-22 was used to describe features of DiGeorge syndrome to include **C**ardiac anomalies, **A**bnormal facies, **T**hymus hypoplasia, **C**left palate, **H**ypocalcemia, and the microdeletion on chromosome 22.[8] Phenotypic abnormalities include cardiac anomalies, mainly outflow tract abnormalities in combination with thymus hypoplasia or aplasia, cleft palate, velopharyngeal insufficiency, and dysmorphic facial features.[9] Disorders of the skeleton can affect the limbs and the spine. Mental disorders are found in 30% of the adults with this deletion.[8] Diagnosis of this deletion can be achieved by fluorescence in situ hybridization (FISH) technique or with microarray analysis. In an affected fetus or infant, the parental examination reveals, in approximately 6%, an affected parent with subtle signs of this syndrome with a 50% transmission to future offspring.[8] Cardiac anomalies that are found in deletion 22q11.2 syndrome primarily include conotruncal anomalies such as an interrupted aortic arch, common arterial trunk (CAT), absent pulmonary valve syndrome, pulmonary atresia with VSD, tetralogy of Fallot (TOF), and conoventricular septal defects.[8,10,11] The presence of a right aortic arch either in isolation or in combination with a cardiac anomaly increases the risk for deletion 22q11.2.[12] Reports on the detection of deletion 22q11.2 in the first trimester are scarce, but in our opinion, this is primarily due to missed diagnosis of cardiac and extracardiac abnormalities rather than due to the inability to make the diagnosis in the first trimester. Several ultrasound features of deletion 22q11.2 that are seen in the second trimester such as a small thymus,[10] a dilated cavum septi pellucidi,[13] or polyhydramnios[14] are not seen in the first trimester. Facial dysmorphism, as another feature of deletion 22q11.2, is too subtle to be a reliable sonographic feature, even in the second trimester. In the presence of a first trimester cardiac or extracardiac abnormality in the fetus, genetic counseling for invasive diagnostic testing with chorionic villous sampling or amniocentesis is recommended and with the widespread use of microarray, deletion 22q11.2 will be more commonly detected

# Deletion 22q11 (DiGeorge Syndrome)

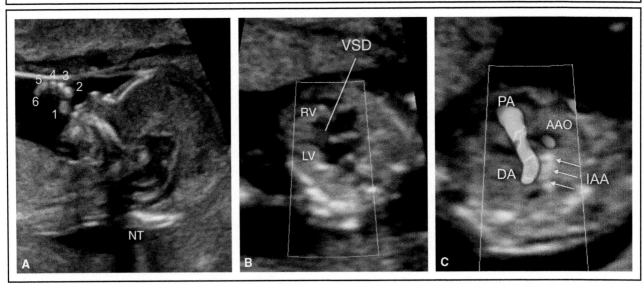

**Figure 11.6:** Fetus at 13 weeks of gestation with deletion 22q11. Note in **A** the presence of a normal facial profile with normal nuchal translucency (NT). Also note in **A** the presence of hexadactyly (numbers 1–6), shown in hand. In **B**, the four-chamber view demonstrates a ventricular septal defect (VSD). **C:** Obtained at the three-vessel-trachea view and shows an interrupted aortic arch (IAA) (*arrows*). Chorionic villous sampling with targeted FISH confirmed the suspected deletion 22q11. AAO, ascending aorta; DA, ductus arteriosus; LV, left ventricle; PA, pulmonary artery; RV, right ventricle.

in early gestation. **Figure 11.6** shows a fetus at 13 weeks of gestation with deletion 22q11.2 detected with targeted FISH performed due to the presence of polydactyly and an interrupted aortic arch seen on the first trimester ultrasound.

## INDIRECT SIGNS OF CARDIAC ANOMALIES IN THE FIRST TRIMESTER

Several ultrasound markers associated with an increased risk for CHD have been described in the first trimester and are today part of the indications for an early fetal echocardiography as listed in **Table 11.3**. Four of these common ultrasound markers are discussed in the following section.

### Increased Nuchal Translucency Thickness

In addition to chromosomal anomalies, several reports have noted an association between increased NT and major fetal malformations including cardiac defects (**Fig. 11.7**). Prospective studies in mixed low- and high-risk screening populations showed a sensitivity of about 21% for a NT >99th percentile. Studies on the association of NT with CHD have shown that the prevalence of major cardiac defects increases exponentially with fetal NT thickness, without an obvious predilection to a specific CHD.[15,16] The underlying pathophysiologic mechanism

| **Table 11.3 • Suggested Indications for Fetal Cardiac Imaging in the First Trimester** | |
|---|---|
| Maternal indications | Increased risk for aneuploidy (including maternal or paternal balanced translocations) |
| | Maternal poorly controlled diabetes mellitus |
| | Maternal cardiac teratogen exposure |
| | Previous child with complex cardiac malformation |
| Fetal indications | Thickened nuchal translucency |
| | Abnormal cardiac axis |
| | Reverse flow in A-wave of ductus venosus |
| | Tricuspid regurgitation |
| | Extracardiac fetal malformations |
| | Fetal hydrops in the first trimester |

relating the presence of a thickened NT to fetal cardiac defect is not fully understood.

### Reversed A-Wave in Ductus Venosus

Under normal conditions, ductus venosus (DV) waveforms show a biphasic pattern throughout the cardiac cycle. Abnormal DV waveform pattern is typically characterized by

## Prevalence CHD/1000 against NT measurement

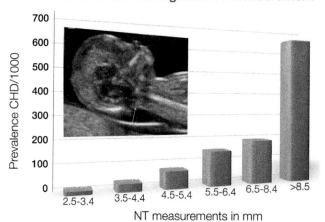

Figure 11.7: Relationship between increased nuchal translucency (NT) thickness and risk of congenital heart disease (CHD) based on a meta-analysis of 12 studies. Note that the prevalence of CHD increases with increased NT thickness. (Adapted from Clur SA, Ottenkamp J, Bilardo CM. The nuchal translucency and the fetal heart: a literature review. *Prenat Diagn.* 2009;29:739–748; copyright John Wiley & Sons, Ltd., with permission.)

an absent or reversed A-wave during the atrial contraction phase of diastole (Fig. 11.8A). This flow pattern in the first trimester has been associated with an increased risk of aneuploidy. In chromosomally normal fetuses, abnormal DV waveforms have also been shown to be associated with structural cardiac anomalies.[17] The underlying pathophysiologic mechanism linking the reversed DV A-wave to fetal CHD is unclear, but an increased right atrial preload as a result of an increase in volume, pressure, or both in CHD could be one of the underlying mechanisms. Detecting a reversed A-wave in the DV increases the risk for the presence of CHD in the fetus.[16]

## Tricuspid Regurgitation

TR can occur in the fetus at all gestational ages and can be transient. TR at 11 to 13 weeks of gestation is a common finding in fetuses with trisomies 21, 18, and 13, and in those with major cardiac defects.[16] TR is found in about 1% of euploid fetuses, in 55% of fetuses with trisomy 21, in one-third of fetuses with trisomy 18 and trisomy 13, and in one-third of those with complex cardiac defects.[18] A standardized approach to the diagnosis of TR is important and includes the following (see also Chapter 1): the image is magnified, an apical four-chamber view of the fetal heart is obtained, pulsed-wave Doppler sample volume of 2.0 to 3.0 mm is positioned across the tricuspid valve, and the angle to the direction of flow is less than 30 degrees from the direction of the interventricular septum. A TR is thus diagnosed when it is seen for at least half of systole with a velocity of over 60 cm per second. The detection of TR (Fig. 11.8B) increases the risk for the presence of a complex cardiac defect.

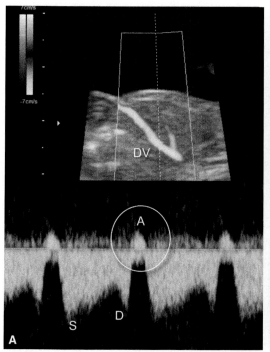

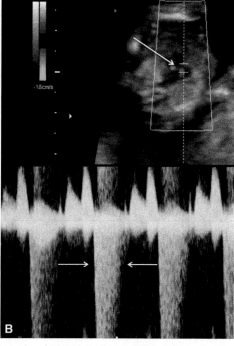

Figure 11.8: **A:** Pulsed Doppler of ductus venosus (DV) in a fetus at 13 weeks of gestation with a cardiac defect, showing reversed flow in the A-waves (*open circle*) during atrial contractions. The presence of this pattern suggests an increased risk for associated cardiac abnormalities. **B:** Pulsed Doppler of the tricuspid valve (*long arrow*) in a fetus with a tetralogy of Fallot. Note the presence of tricuspid regurgitation on pulsed Doppler (*opposing arrows*). The presence of tricuspid regurgitation increases the risk for the presence of cardiac abnormalities. S, peak systolic velocity; D, peak diastolic velocity.

## Cardiac Axis in Early Gestation

Several studies have established an association between an abnormal cardiac axis and CHD in mid-second and third trimesters of pregnancy and also recently in early gestation. Cardiac axis measurement in the first trimester can be challenging and requires the use of high-definition color in order to clearly delineate the ventricular septum (Fig. 11.9). In a case–control study design, we have recently reported on the fetal cardiac axis in 197 fetuses with confirmed CHD between 11 0/7 and 14 6/7 weeks of gestation, matched with a control group.[19] In the control group, the mean cardiac axis was 44.5 ± 7.4 degrees and did not significantly change in early pregnancy.[19] In the CHD group, 25.9% of fetuses had cardiac axis measurements within normal limits.[19] In 74.1%, the cardiac axis was abnormal. The performance of cardiac axis measurement in detection of major CHD was significantly better than enlarged NT, TR, or reversed A-wave in DV used alone or in combination.[19]

## COMMON FETAL CARDIAC ANOMALIES

In the following sections, we will present CHD that can be diagnosed in the first trimester of pregnancy. For each fetal cardiac abnormality, we will define the abnormality, describe sonographic findings along with optimal planes for diagnosis in the first trimester, and briefly list associated cardiac and extracardiac malformations. Table 11.4 lists abnormal ultrasound findings and corresponding cardiac anomalies in the first trimester of pregnancy. For more detailed information on prenatal cardiac imaging and CHD in the first, second, and third trimesters of pregnancy, we refer the readers to our book on this subject.[1]

## Hypoplastic Left Heart Syndrome

### Definition

Hypoplastic left heart syndrome (HLHS) is a group of complex cardiac malformations involving significant underdevelopment of the left ventricle and the left ventricular outflow tract, resulting in an obstruction to systemic cardiac output. In general, two main classic forms of HLHS can be observed in the first trimester: one form involves atresia of both the mitral and aortic valves, with practically no communication between the left atrium and left ventricle and a nearly absent or severely hypoplastic left ventricle (Fig. 11.10A), and the other form involves a visible left ventricle, with hyperechoic wall, globular shape, and poor contractility in association with severely dysplastic mitral valve combined with a severe aortic stenosis or aortic atresia (Fig. 11.10B). The reported birth incidence of HLHS is 0.1 to 0.25 per 1,000 live births.[6]

### Ultrasound Findings

In HLHS, the four-chamber view appears abnormal in gray scale and in color Doppler. Cases with a combined mitral and aortic atresia show an absent left ventricle, and can be detected at 12 to 13 weeks of gestation (Figs. 11.11A and 11.12A). In gray scale, the left ventricle appears small or absent in the 4CV (Figs. 11.11A and 11.12A), and color Doppler shows an absence of flow into the left ventricle (Figs. 11.11B and 11.12B). The classic appearance of a single ventricle on gray scale and color Doppler in the first trimester is thus suggestive of HLHS. When suspected on the 4CV in the first trimester, HLHS should be confirmed in the 3VT view, which reveals an enlarged pulmonary artery with a small aortic arch with

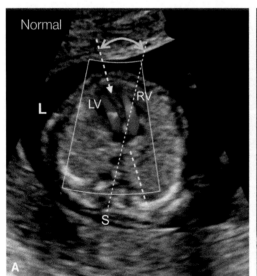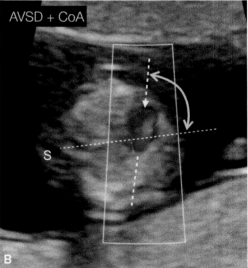

**Figure 11.9:** Cardiac axis (*blue arrows*) measurement in two fetuses at 13 weeks of gestation in color Doppler. In fetus **A** with a normal heart anatomy, the cardiac axis is normal. In fetus **B** with an atrioventricular septal defect (AVSD) and ventricle disproportion with aortic coarctation (CoA), the cardiac axis is deviated with a wide angle. Cardiac axis is measured in a four-chamber view of the heart by the angle of two lines; the first line starts at the spine (S) posteriorly and ends in mid-chest anteriorly, bisecting the chest into two equal halves, the second line runs through the ventricular septum. RV, right ventricle; LV, left ventricle; L, left.

**Table 11.4 •** Abnormal Ultrasound Findings and Suspected Cardiac Anomalies in the First Trimester

| | |
|---|---|
| Four-chamber view in gray scale and color Doppler | Abnormal cardiac axis (left-sided in TOF, CAT—mesocardia in TGA, DORV, dextrocardia in heterotaxy) |
| | Severe tricuspid insufficiency in Ebstein anomaly |
| | Single ventricle in AVSD, univentricular heart, HLHS, tricuspid atresia with VSD |
| | Ventricle disproportion in coarctation of the aorta, HLHS, HRHS, pulmonary atresia with VSD, mitral atresia and tricuspid atresia |
| Three-vessel-trachea view in color Doppler | Discrepant great vessel size with forward flow in the small vessel in TOF, coarctation of the aorta, Tricuspid atresia with VSD |
| | Discrepant great vessel size with reversed flow in the small vessel in HLHS, HRHS, PA with VSD |
| | Single large great vessel in CAT, PA with VSD |
| | Single great vessel of normal size in TGA or DORV |
| | Interrupted aortic isthmus in interrupted aortic arch |
| | Aortic arch right-sided to the trachea in right-sided aortic arch with left ductus arteriosus, right-sided aortic arch with right ductus arteriosus, and double aortic arch |

TOF, tetralogy of Fallot; CAT, common arterial trunk; TGA, transposition of the great arteries; DORV, double outlet right ventricle; AVSD, atrioventricular septal defect; HLHS, hypoplastic left heart syndrome; VSD, ventricular septal defect; HRHS, hypoplastic right heart syndrome; PA, pulmonary atresia.

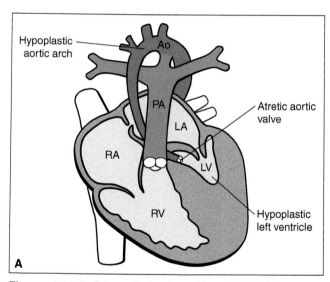 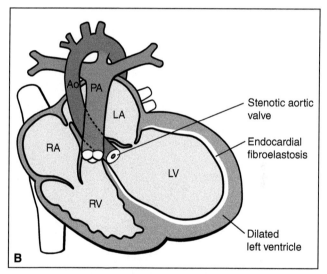

**Figure 11.10:** Schematic drawings of hypoplastic left heart syndrome (HLHS). Note in **A** the typical features of hypoplastic hypokinetic left ventricle (LV), dysplastic mitral valve, atretic aortic valve, and hypoplastic aorta (Ao). **B:** The infrequent type of HLHS in the first trimester with dilated, hyperechogenic left ventricle (fibroelastosis), narrowing at the aortic valve level and obstruction to left ventricular outflow, in association with critical aortic stenosis. RA, right atrium; RV, right ventricle; PA, pulmonary artery; LA, left atrium.

reverse flow on color Doppler (Figs. 11.11C and 11.12C). An echogenic globular left ventricle can occasionally be seen in the first trimester in HLHS (Fig. 11.13) and represents left ventricular changes (fibroelastosis), similar to that noted in the second and third trimesters of pregnancy. Of note is that the presence of a "normal" four-chamber view in the first trimester cannot rule out HLHS, as it has been shown to develop between the first and second trimesters of gestation.

### Associated Malformations

HLHS is associated with a 4% to 5% incidence of chromosomal abnormalities,[20] such as Turner syndrome, trisomies 13 and 18, and others, and when HLHS is suspected in the first trimester, counseling with regard to genetic testing should be performed. Extracardiac malformations have been reported in 10% to 25% of infants with HLHS[21] with

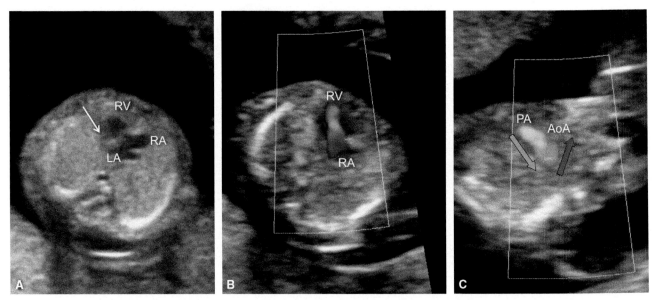

**Figure 11.11:** Hypoplastic left heart syndrome in a fetus at 13 weeks of gestation demonstrated by transabdominal ultrasound. Note in **A** the absence of a left ventricle (*arrow*) in the four-chamber view. In **B**, color Doppler shows diastolic flow between right atrium (RA) and right ventricle (RV) with absent left ventricular flow. In **C**, three-vessel-trachea view in color Doppler shows antegrade flow in the pulmonary artery (PA) (*blue arrow*) and retrograde flow into the aortic arch (AoA) (*red arrow*). LA, left atrium.

associated genetic syndromes, such as Turner syndrome, Noonan syndrome, Smith–Lemli–Opitz syndrome, and Holt–Oram syndrome.[21] Fetuses with HLHS may develop growth restriction in the late second and third trimesters of pregnancy probably due to a 20% reduction in combined cardiac output.[22] When HLHS is diagnosed in the first trimester, follow-up ultrasound examinations are recommended.

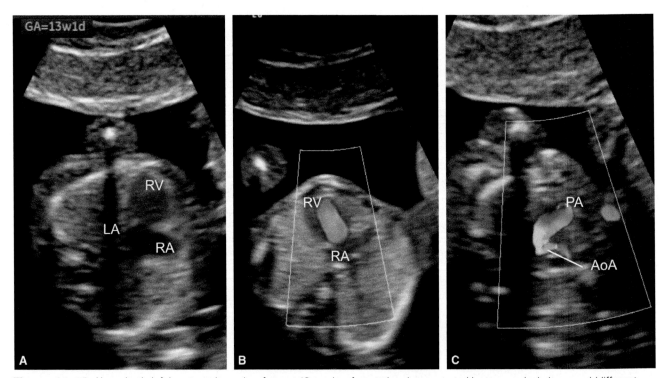

**Figure 11.12:** Hypoplastic left heart syndrome in a fetus at 13 weeks of gestation demonstrated by transvaginal ultrasound (different fetus than in Fig. 11.11). Note in **A** the absence of a left ventricle (LV) in the four-chamber view. In **B**, color Doppler shows diastolic flow between right atrium (RA) and right ventricle (RV) with absent left ventricular flow. In **C**, three-vessel-trachea view in color Doppler shows antegrade flow in the pulmonary artery (PA) and retrograde flow into the small aortic arch (AoA). Note the increased resolution in the ultrasound images as compared to Figure 11.11 obtained transabdominally. Compare with Figure 11.11. LA, left atrium.

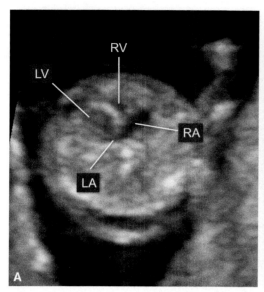
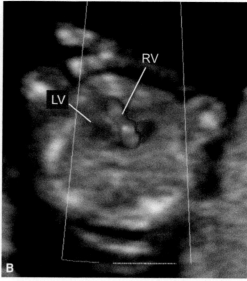

**Figure 11.13:** Four-chamber view in a fetus with hypoplastic left heart syndrome (HLHS) at 13 weeks of gestation with gray-scale **(A)** and color Doppler **(B)** imaging. Note the presence in **A** of a relatively small echogenic left ventricular (LV) cavity. Color Doppler in **B** shows absence of mitral inflow during diastole. The presence of an echogenic LV is unusually found in HLHS in the first trimester in comparison with the second trimester. RA, right atrium; RV, right ventricle; LA, left atrium.

## Coarctation of the Aorta

### Definition

Coarctation of the aorta (CoA) involves narrowing of the aortic arch, typically located at the isthmic region, between the left subclavian artery and the ductus arteriosus (Fig. 11.14). CoA is a common anomaly, found in about 5% to 8% of newborns and infants with CHD.[6,23] CoA can be classified as simple when it occurs without important intracardiac lesions and complex when it occurs in association with significant intracardiac pathology.

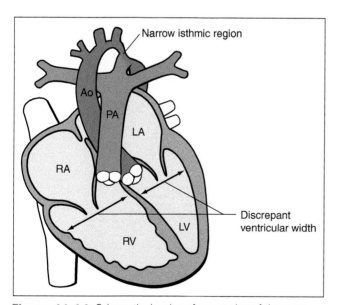

**Figure 11.14:** Schematic drawing of coarctation of the aorta. See text for details. RA, right atrium; RV, right ventricle; LA, left atrium; LV, left ventricle; PA, pulmonary artery; Ao, aorta.

### Ultrasound Findings

The presence of ventricular disproportion with a small left ventricle in the first trimester is one of the markers for the presence of CoA. In gray scale, the ventricular disproportion can be best demonstrated in a transverse view of the heart (Fig. 11.15). Color Doppler demonstrates a difference in ventricular filling in the 4CV by showing increased flow across the right ventricle when compared with the left ventricle (Fig. 11.15B). The diagnosis of CoA is confirmed in the 3VT by revealing a small aortic arch in comparison with the pulmonary artery (Fig. 11.16). Typically, the aortic arch shows antegrade flow in CoA (Fig. 11.16B), which enables its distinction from HLHS where reversal flow is demonstrated on color Doppler (Fig. 11.12C). When the aortic arch does not appear to be continuous with the descending aorta, the diagnosis of an interrupted aortic arch should be suspected. It has to be borne in mind that confirming the presence of CoA in the second trimester is critical because ventricular discrepancies found in the first trimester of pregnancy may resolve with advancing gestation. Making an accurate diagnosis of CoA is difficult in the first trimester and commonly leads to false-positive diagnoses.

### Associated Malformations

The most common associated cardiac abnormalities in complex CoA include large VSD, bicuspid aortic valve, aortic stenosis at the valvular and subvalvular levels, mitral stenosis, and persistent left superior vena cava.[24,25] These associated cardiac abnormalities are difficult, if not impossible, to see on the first trimester ultrasound. Chromosomal abnormalities are commonly associated with CoA, with Turner syndrome representing the most common abnormality.[26] If CoA is suspected in the presence

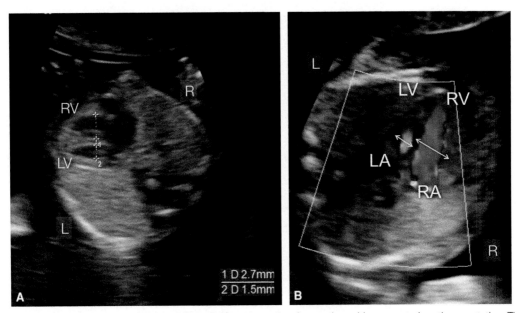

**Figure 11.15:** Four-chamber views in two fetuses **(A and B)** at 13 weeks of gestation with suspected aortic coarctation. The axial gray-scale four-chamber view in **A** and the apical color Doppler four-chamber view in **B** are abnormal and show discrepant ventricular chamber size with a diminutive left ventricle (LV). RV, right ventricle; L, left; R, right; LA, left atrium; RA, right atrium.

of other findings such as cystic hygroma and/or early fetal hydrops, Turner syndrome should be considered in the diagnosis. CoA can also be found in association with other chromosomal aberrations, such as trisomy 13 or trisomy 18, especially in the presence of multiple extracardiac malformations. The presence of CoA with tachycardia, impaired fetal growth, and/or multiple structural anomalies is suggestive of trisomy 13.

## Pulmonary Atresia with Intact Ventricular Septum

### Definition

Pulmonary atresia with intact ventricular septum (PA-IVS) is a group of cardiac malformations having in common absent communication between the right ventricle and the pulmonary

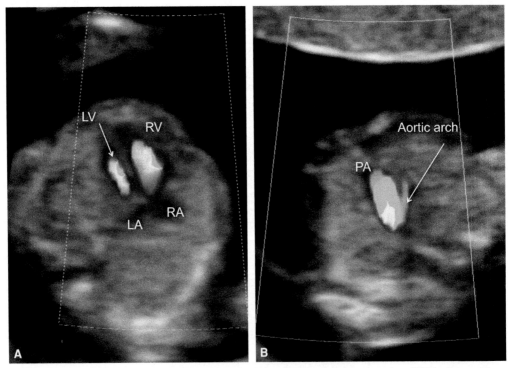

**Figure 11.16:** Color Doppler at the level of the four-chamber view **(A)** and three-vessel-trachea view **(B)** in a fetus with coarctation of the aorta at 14 weeks of gestation. A diminutive left ventricle (LV) is noted in the four-chamber view **(A)**, and a small aortic arch is noted in the three-vessel-trachea view **(B)**. RV, right ventricle; RA, right atrium; LA, left atrium; PA, pulmonary artery.

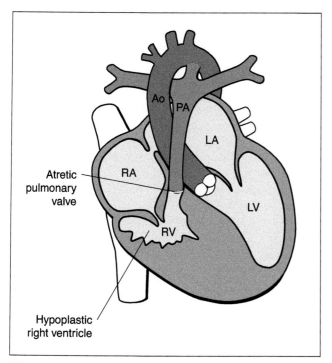

**Figure 11.17:** Schematic drawing of pulmonary atresia with intact ventricular septum (PA-IVS). See text for details. RA, right atrium; RV, right ventricle; LV, left ventricle; LA, left atrium; Ao, aorta; PA, pulmonary artery.

arterial circulation (pulmonary atresia) in combination with an intact ventricular septum. The right ventricular cavity is either hypoplastic with thickened right ventricular myocardium (Fig. 11.17), or dilated with significant tricuspid valve regurgitation and a dilated right atrium. A hypoplastic right ventricle occurs in the majority of cases.[27] PA-IVS is a rare condition with a prevalence of 0.042 to 0.053 per 1,000 live births.[28]

### Ultrasound Findings

PA-IVS can be suspected in the first trimester with the detection of a small hypoplastic, hypokinetic right ventricle at the 4CV (Fig. 11.18A). The anatomic depiction of the right ventricle is similar to that of the left ventricle in HLHS. In most cases, this finding is supported by color Doppler showing lack of right ventricular filling in the 4CV (Fig. 11.18B) and reverse flow in the ductus arteriosus and pulmonary artery in the 3VT view (Fig. 11.18C). Often the dysplastic tricuspid valve is insufficient, and valvular regurgitation can be demonstrated with color and pulsed Doppler.

### Associated Malformations

One of the major associated findings in hearts with PA-IVS and hypoplastic right ventricles is an anomaly of the coronary circulation, namely ventriculo-coronary arterial communication, found in about one-third of cases of PA-IVS but typically

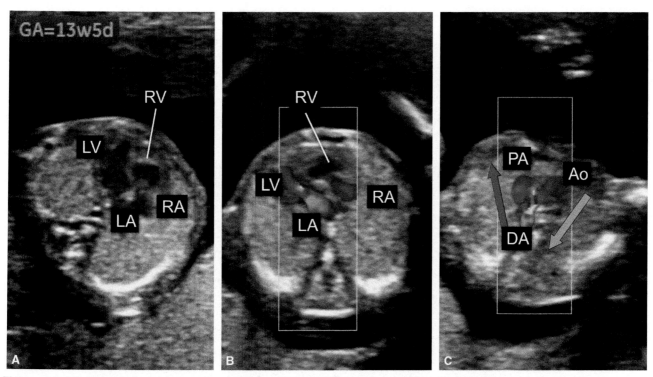

**Figure 11.18:** Four-chamber view in gray scale **(A)**, color Doppler **(B)**, and three-vessel-trachea view **(C)** in a fetus with pulmonary atresia with intact ventricular septum (PA-IVS) at 13 weeks of gestation. **A:** Gray scale of a diminutive right ventricle (RV) with bulging of the interventricular septum into the left ventricle (LV). **B:** Diastole in color Doppler in the absence of diastolic flow into the right ventricle. **C:** The three-vessel-trachea view in color Doppler indicates the typical pattern of antegrade flow in the aortic arch (Ao) (*blue arrow*) in comparison with the retrograde flow across the ductus arteriosus (DA) into the pulmonary artery (PA) (*red arrow*). RA, right atrium; LA, left atrium.

not seen in early gestation. Other associated cardiac findings include right atrial dilation, tricuspid valve abnormalities, subvalvular obstruction of the aortic valve, atrial septal defects, dextrocardia, and transposition of great arteries. Sequential evaluation into the second trimester should be performed to rule out the association with heterotaxy, especially with situs abnormalities. Extracardiac anomalies may be found but without an organ-specific pattern. Chromosomal aberrations such as trisomy 21 or 22q11 microdeletion are rare.

## Tricuspid Atresia with Ventricular Septal Defect

### Definition

Tricuspid atresia with ventricular septal defect (TA-VSD) is characterized by the absence of the right AV connection,

resulting in lack of communication between the right atrium and ventricle. The right ventricle is therefore diminutive in size. An inlet-type VSD, typically perimembranous, is always present, and the size of the right ventricle is related to the size of the VSD. A large interatrial communication, in the form of a widely patent foramen ovale or atrial septal defect, is necessary given an obstructed tricuspid valve. TA-VSD is classified into three types based on the spatial orientation of the great vessels.[29] TA-VSD type 1 occurs in 70% to 80% of cases and is associated with normally oriented great arteries. TA-VSD type 2 occurs in 12% to 25% of cases and is associated with D-transposition of the great vessels. TA-VSD type 3, an uncommon malformation, is seen in the remainder of TA cases and usually denotes complex great vessel abnormalities such as truncus arteriosus or L-transposition. TA-VSD is rare, with an incidence of 0.08 per 1,000 live births[30] Figure 11.19 represents a schematic drawing of type 1 TA-VSD.

### Ultrasound Findings

TA-VSD can be detected in the first trimester on gray scale and color Doppler of the 4CV. Typically an enlarged left ventricle and a hypoplastic right ventricle is noted on gray scale at the 4CV and color Doppler on transabdominal ultrasound reveals what appears to be a single ventricular heart. With high-resolution transabdominal and transvaginal transducers, the hypoplastic right ventricle is seen and the VSD is shown with blood flow from the left to the right ventricle (Fig. 11.20A). In type 1 TA-VSD at the 3VT view, the pulmonary artery is smaller than the aorta with antegrade flow in both great arteries (Fig. 11.20B). TA-VSD has been associated with an enlarged NT in the first trimester.[31] Because reversed A-wave in the DV has been reported in the second and third trimesters in association with TA-VSD, this finding may be present in the first trimester and may represent an early sign of right atrial increased preload.[32]

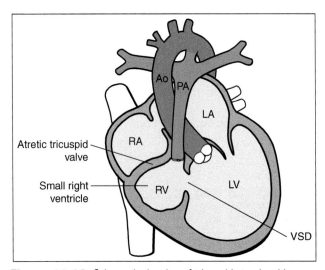

**Figure 11.19:** Schematic drawing of tricuspid atresia with ventricular septal defect (TA-VSD). See text for details. RA, right atrium; RV, right ventricle; LV, left ventricle; LA, left atrium; Ao, aorta; PA, pulmonary artery.

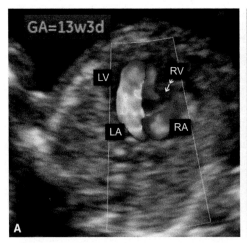
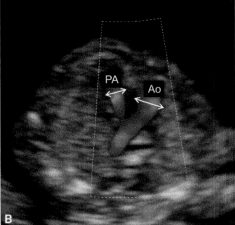

**Figure 11.20:** Transvaginal ultrasound of tricuspid atresia with ventricular septal defect (TA-VSD) in color Doppler in a fetus at 13 weeks of gestation. **A:** Obtained at the four-chamber view and shows blood inflow through the mitral valve into the left ventricle (LV), with blood reaching the right ventricle (RV) through the VSD (*arrow*). **B:** The three-vessel-trachea view with a narrow pulmonary artery (PA) (associated pulmonary stenosis) as compared to the aorta (Ao). LA, left atrium; RA, right atrium.

## Associated Malformations

Associated cardiac findings include a large interatrial communication such as a patent foramen ovale or an atrial septal defect, a VSD, transposition of the great vessels, and various degrees of right ventricular outflow obstruction. Extracardiac anomalies can also be found and fetal karyotyping should be offered despite a rare association with chromosomal aberration including 22q11 microdeletion.[33]

## Atrioventricular Septal Defect

### Definition

Atrioventricular septal defect (AVSD) represents a cardiac abnormality characterized by a deficient AV septation and abnormalities

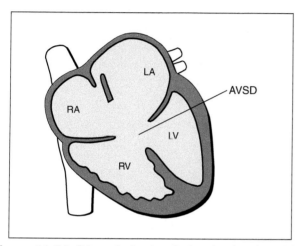

**Figure 11.21:** Schematic drawing of a four-chamber view with a complete atrioventricular septal defect (AVSD). LA, left atrium; RA, right atrium; LV, left ventricle; RV, right ventricle.

of the AV valves, primarily resulting in the presence of a common AV junction. Common synonyms to AVSD include AV canal defect or endocardial cushion defect. In the *complete form* of an AVSD, there is a combination of an atrial septum primum defect and an inlet VSD with an abnormal common AV valve, which connects to the right and left ventricles (Fig. 11.21). The common AV valve usually has five leaflets. *Partial AVSD* includes an atrial septum primum defect and a cleft in the mitral valve with two distinct mitral and tricuspid valve annuli that attach at the same level on the interventricular septum. Partial AVSD is difficult to detect in the first trimester. AVSDs can also be classified as balanced or unbalanced. In unbalanced AVSD, the AV connection predominantly drains to one of the two ventricles, resulting in ventricular size disproportion. Unbalanced AVSD is typically found in association with heterotaxy syndrome. AVSDs are common cardiac malformations found in 4% to 7.4% of all infants with CHD.[34]

### Ultrasound Findings

AVSD may be recognized in the first trimester by demonstrating the defect in the center of the heart during diastole on gray-scale ultrasound at the 4CV (Fig. 11.22A). In an apical insonation of the 4CV in systole, the linear insertion of the AV valves can be seen, albeit quite difficult in the first trimester. Color Doppler reveals the classic single channel of blood flow entering the common AV (Figs. 11.22B and 11.23) instead of two distinct channels over the tricuspid and mitral valves as is shown in normal hearts (Fig. 11.3). Occasionally, the defect is so large that the image resembles a univentricular heart. A typical finding is the presence of valve regurgitation on color Doppler at the common AV valve (Fig. 11.24). Often a thickened NT is found in association with AVSD and this combination suggests the presence of trisomy 21 or trisomy 18. The combination of

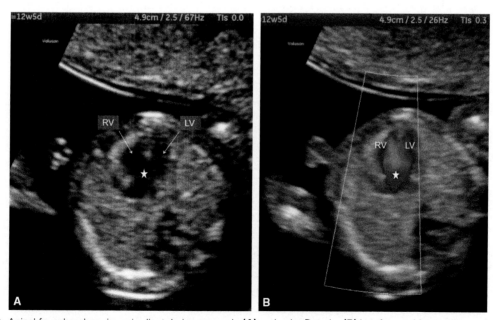

**Figure 11.22:** Apical four-chamber views in diastole in gray scale **(A)** and color Doppler **(B)** in a fetus with complete atrioventricular septal defect (AVSD) at 12 weeks of gestation. AVSD is demonstrated by the star in **A** and **B**. Note the presence in **B** of a single channel of blood on color Doppler entering the ventricles over a common atrioventricular valve. LV, left ventricle; RV, right ventricle.

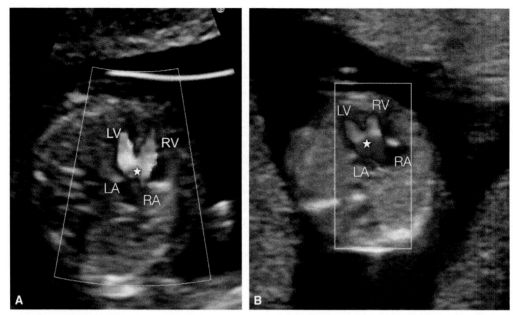

**Figure 11.23:** Apical four-chamber views during diastole in color Doppler in two fetuses with complete atrioventricular septal defect (AVSD) at 12 weeks of gestation. AVSD is demonstrated by the star in **A** and **B**. Note the presence in diastole of a single channel of blood entering the ventricles over a common atrioventricular valve. LA, left atrium; RA, right atrium; LV, left ventricle; RV, right ventricle.

AVSD with heart block or a right-sided position of the stomach raises the suspicion of isomerism and heterotaxy syndrome.

### Associated Malformations

Associated cardiac abnormalities in AVSD include TOF, double outlet ventricle, right aortic arch, and other conotruncal anomalies. Extracardiac anomalies in AVSD primarily include chromosomal abnormalities, mainly trisomy 21 and much less commonly trisomies 18 and 13. About 40% to 45% of children with Down syndrome have CHD and of these, 40% are AVSD, commonly of the complete type.[34] Antenatal diagnosis of AVSD, when isolated, is associated with trisomy 21 in 58% of cases.[35] When AVSD is associated with heterotaxy, the risk of chromosomal abnormality is virtually absent, but the outcome is worsened due to the severity of the cardiac and extracardiac malformations.

## Ventricular Septal Defect

### Definition

VSD is an opening in the ventricular septum, leading to a hemodynamic communication between the left and right ventricles. VSDs are common CHDs, second only to bicuspid aortic valve.[36] Typically VSDs are reported based on their anatomic locations on the septum. In prenatal series, muscular VSDs are most common and account for about 80% to 90%, with perimembranous VSDs being the second most common.[37] VSDs are frequently associated with various cardiac anomalies.

### Ultrasound Findings

VSDs are generally too small to be reliably detected as isolated anomalies in the first trimester. Caution should be made in diagnosing VSDs in early gestation given a significant

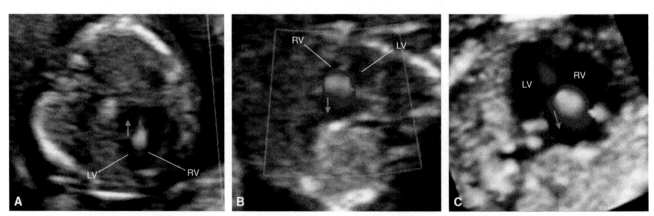

**Figure 11.24: A–C:** Four-chamber views in color Doppler and during systole in three fetuses with complete atrioventricular septal defect at 12, 13, and 14 weeks, respectively. Note the presence of valve regurgitation (*faint arrows*) across the common atrioventricular valve in the three fetuses. LV, left ventricle; RV, right ventricle.

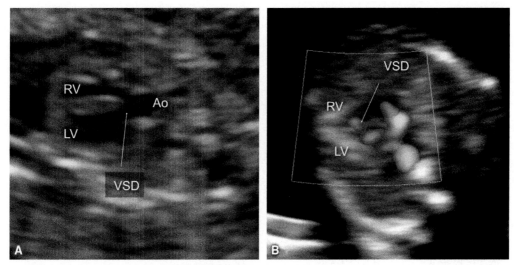

**Figure 11.25: A:** A five-chamber view in a fetus with tetralogy of Fallot at 13 weeks of gestation. Note the presence of a perimembranous ventricular septal defect (VSD). **B:** A transverse four-chamber view in color Doppler at 12 weeks of gestation with a muscular VSD. Note the presence of blood flow across the VSD documented by color Doppler. LV, left ventricle; RV, right ventricle; Ao, aorta.

false-positive diagnosis resulting from echo dropout in 2D ultrasound and color overlapping when using color Doppler. In most cases, the VSD is reliably demonstrated when it is associated with another cardiac anomaly (Fig. 11.25A) or when the four-chamber view anatomy is abnormal. The presence of blood flow shunting across the VSD confirms its presence in the first trimester (Fig. 11.25B). When a VSD is suspected but cannot be confirmed in the first trimester, a follow-up examination is recommended after 16 weeks of gestation with careful evaluation of the ventricular septum.

### Associated Malformations

Associated cardiac anomalies are common and are typically diagnosed prior to the diagnosis of VSD in the first trimester. The association of an extracardiac abnormality with a VSD increases the risk for the presence of a syndrome or chromosomal

aberration. VSDs are the most common abnormalities in many chromosomal defects, such as trisomies 21, 18, and 13.[36] An isolated muscular VSD has a risk of chromosomal abnormalities similar to that of normal pregnancy.[37]

## Ebstein Anomaly

### Definition

In Ebstein anomaly, the septal and posterior leaflets of the tricuspid valve are displaced inferiorly from the tricuspid valve annulus, toward the apex of the heart, and originate from the right ventricular myocardium (Fig. 11.26). The anterior tricuspid leaflet maintains its normal attachment to the tricuspid valve annulus. The proximal portion of the right ventricle is then continuous with the true right atrium and forms an "atrialized" portion of the right ventricle (Fig. 11.26).

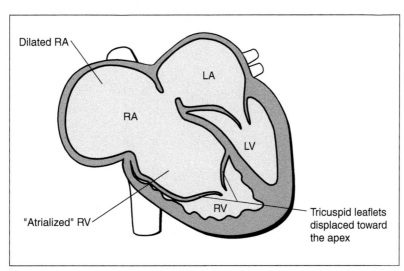

**Figure 11.26:** Schematic drawing of Ebstein anomaly. See text for details. LA, left atrium; RA, right atrium; LV, left ventricle; RV, right ventricle.

The spectrum of Ebstein anomaly is wide and varies from a minor form, with minimal displacement of the tricuspid valves with mild TR, to a severe form, with the "atrialization" of the entire right ventricle. Ebstein anomaly is one of the less common cardiac abnormalities occurring in about 0.5% to 1% of CHD in live births.[6]

### Ultrasound Findings

Ebstein anomaly is detected in the first trimester by the presence of significant TR. Other main findings of Ebstein anomaly such as cardiomegaly and a dilated right atrium are typically seen later in gestation. The displaced apical attachment of the tricuspid valve in the right ventricle can be seen on gray-scale ultrasound in an apical or axial 4CV (Fig. 11.27A). Severe TR originating near the apex of the RV can be clearly demonstrated on color and pulsed Doppler (Fig. 11.27B and C). In severe Ebstein anomaly in the first trimester, the presence of cardiomegaly may be associated with a thickened NT and fetal hydrops, a sign of impending fetal demise. Although some severe cases of Ebstein anomalies may be suspected in the first trimester, mild Ebstein cases can be missed and only detected in the second trimesters of pregnancy. The presence of significant TR in the first trimester can be a marker of Ebstein anomaly, which is typically confirmed in the second trimester of pregnancy.

## Associated Malformations

Associated cardiac abnormalities include an obstruction of the right ventricular outflow tract as pulmonary stenosis or atresia in more than 60% of fetuses diagnosed with Ebstein anomaly prenatally.[38] Atrial septal defect, which is not evident in the first trimester, represents another common association and has been reported in up to 60% of children with Ebstein anomaly. Most cases of Ebstein anomaly are isolated findings, but an association with chromosomal anomalies, such as trisomy 21 or trisomy 13, has been reported in addition to familial cases. Long-term complications of Ebstein include pulmonary hypoplasia in neonates and rhythm disorders in children.

## Univentricular Heart

### Definition

Univentricular heart or univentricular AV connection describes a group of cardiac malformations where the AV connection is completely or predominantly to a single ventricular chamber. Embryologically, this malformation is thought to result from failure of the development of the bulboventricular loop stage. From a clinical point of view, a CHD with a univentricular heart describes a heart with one functioning ventricle with inflow from one or both atria. Within univentricular heart,

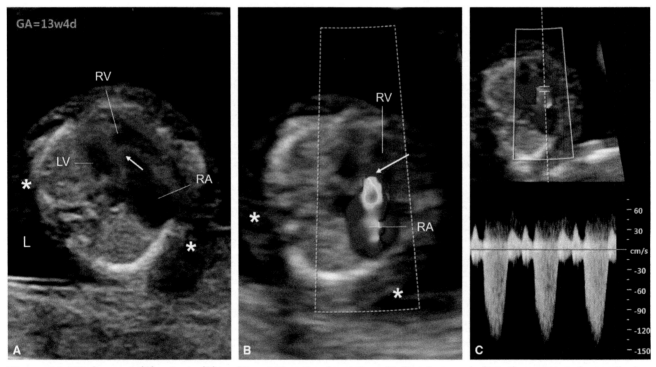

**Figure 11.27:** Gray scale **(A)** and color **(B)** in a fetus at 13 weeks of gestation with Ebstein anomaly. Note the presence of generalized hydrops (*asterisks*) in **A** and **B**. The displaced apical attachment of the tricuspid valve in the right ventricle (RV) is shown in **A** (*arrow*). Severe tricuspid regurgitation originating near the apex of the RV is shown in **B** (*arrow*). **C:** Pulsed Doppler of the regurgitant jet across the dysplastic tricuspid valve. RA, right atrium; LV, left ventricle; L, left.

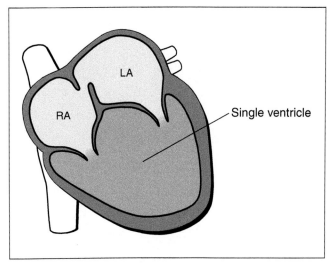

**Figure 11.28:** Schematic drawing of double inlet univentricular heart. See text for details. LA, left atrium; RA, right atrium.

three subgroups can be identified: double inlet, where two atria connect to a single ventricle through two patent AV valves; single inlet, where one atrium connects to a single ventricle through a single AV valve; and common inlet, where both atria connect to a single ventricle through a single AV valve. The morphology of the ventricle is generally a left ventricular morphology with a rudimentary right chamber. Figure 11.28 represents a schematic drawing of a univentricular heart with double inlet ventricle.

## Ultrasound Findings

The detection of a univentricular heart in the first trimester is fairly common, not because the condition itself is common, but rather because several severe cardiac anomalies appear as a single ventricle on gray scale and color Doppler. Interestingly, the classic univentricular heart is rarely detected in the first trimester and as shown in Figure 11.29, this anomaly commonly escapes detection given the presence of two inflow streams on color Doppler. Given the small size of the first trimester fetal heart, several cardiac malformations such as HLHS, tricuspid atresia, mitral atresia, large AVSD, and severe CoA may present as a single ventricle heart, especially on transabdominal scanning with color Doppler (Figs. 11.11, 11.12, and 11.22). When a single ventricle heart is suspected on color Doppler in the first trimester, a thorough evaluation of the fetal heart with transvaginal ultrasound is recommended in order to delineate the specific cardiac abnormality. It is preferred in such situations to examine the fetal heart on transvaginal ultrasound in gray scale first and to assess in detail the anatomy of the cardiac chambers and great vessels before switching to color Doppler. Figure 11.30 shows other cardiac malformations that were initially suspected as univentricular hearts on color Doppler evaluation.

## Associated Malformations

Associated malformations in univentricular heart are atresia, hypoplasia, or straddling of the AV valves, pulmonary (or subpulmonic) outflow obstruction, aortic (or subaortic) outflow obstruction, and conduction abnormalities, primarily due to the anatomic disruption of the conduction system.[39] Many of these associated cardiac malformations may not be evident or are difficult to detect in the first trimester of pregnancy.

The most important extracardiac abnormality to rule out is the presence of right or left isomerism, especially in the presence of a common inlet ventricle.[40] Chromosome anomalies and other extracardiac anomalies are possible but rather unusual.

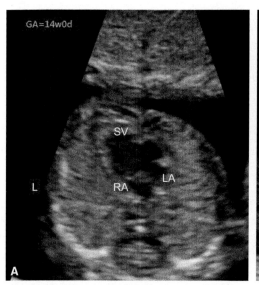
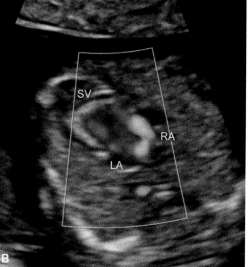

**Figure 11.29:** Fetus at 14 weeks of gestation with a double inlet univentricular heart. Note that on gray-scale ultrasound **(A)** and color Doppler **(B)**, both right (RA) and left atrium (LA) drain through two atrioventricular valves into a single ventricle (SV). Interestingly, in color Doppler **(B)**, this can be easily misdiagnosed as two-ventricular heart. L, left.

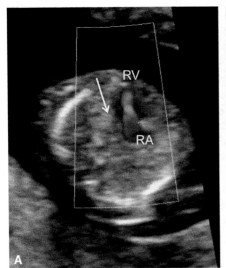 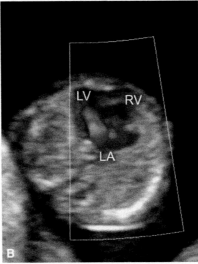 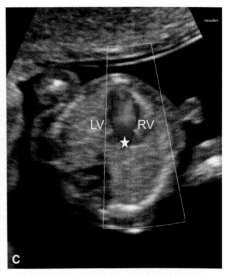

**Figure 11.30:** Abnormal apical four-chamber views in color Doppler in three fetuses **(A–C)** with cardiac anomalies suspicious for a "univentricular heart" at 12 to 13 weeks of gestation. In fetus **A**, a single chamber (right ventricle) is perfused on color Doppler in a case of hypoplastic left heart syndrome (*arrow points* to the absent left ventricle). Fetus **B** shows flow into one ventricle, which is the left ventricle (LV), with absence of diastolic flow into the hypoplastic right ventricle (RV) in a fetus with pulmonary atresia and dysplastic tricuspid valve. In fetus **C**, a defect is seen in the center of the heart (*star*) (single color channel) in a case of a large atrioventricular septal defect. RA, right atrium; LA, left atrium.

## Heterotaxy Syndrome, Atrial Isomerism, and Situs Inversus

### Definition

*Heterotaxy Syndrome* (in Greek, heteros means different and taxis means arrangement) is a general term that is used to describe the complete spectrum of abnormal organ arrangement.[41] The term right and left atrial isomerism (in Greek, iso means same and meros means turn) has been suggested and used in heterotaxy syndrome as the atrial morphology best describes organ arrangement.[42] Isomerism of the thoracic organs is characterized by a rather symmetric arrangement of the otherwise asymmetric structures including the atria and lungs,[43] thus allowing a classification into two main groups: bilateral left-sidedness, also called left atrial isomerism and bilateral right-sidedness, also called right atrial isomerism. Heterotaxy syndrome including right and left atrial isomerism is found in between 2.2% and 4.2% of infants with CHD.[6]

*Situs inversus* is defined as a mirror-image arrangement of the thoracic and abdominal organs to situs solitus (normal anatomy). Partial situs inversus can be either limited to the abdominal organs and is generally called situs inversus with levocardia or limited to the chest and is called dextrocardia.

### Ultrasound Findings

Right and left isomerism can be detected in the first trimester, owing to a thickened NT in combination with cardiac anomaly or in the presence of hydrops with complete heart block.[43,44] Abnormal situs on ultrasound in the first trimester may represent the first clue to the presence of right or left isomerism (Figs. 11.31 and 11.32). The cardiac axis can be shifted thus revealing a suspicion for the presence of cardiac abnormality (Fig. 11.31).[19] The presence of complete heart block in the first trimester should raise suspicion for left atrial isomerism, as Sjögren antibodies are not typically associated with bradyarrhythmia before 16 weeks. The detection of AVSD and univentricular heart is feasible in the first trimester and the suspicion of such an anomaly, especially in combination with a right-sided stomach, should suggest the presence of heterotaxy (Fig. 11.31). The arrangement of the abdominal vessels either as juxtaposition of the aorta and inferior vena cava (right isomerism) or as interruption of the inferior vena cava with azygos continuity (left isomerism) is difficult to diagnose in the first trimester. The addition of color Doppler, however, may assist in the diagnosis of abnormalities in the abdominal vessels. The assessment of pulmonary venous connections is also possible but rather difficult in early gestation.

Partial and complete situs inversus can be detected in the first trimester. The transvaginal approach to determining fetal situs may be challenging given the difficulty inherent in the transvaginal probe orientation. Suspected situs abnormalities should be confirmed at a later gestation.

### Associated Malformations

Associated cardiac malformations are numerous in heterotaxy and primarily include AVSD and univentricular heart. Associated extracardiac anomalies in heterotaxy are typically not detected in the first trimester and include various gastrointestinal anomalies and extrahepatic biliary atresia.[45]

Associated cardiac anomalies in situs inversus are on the order of 0.3% to 5% and include VSD, TOF, double outlet right

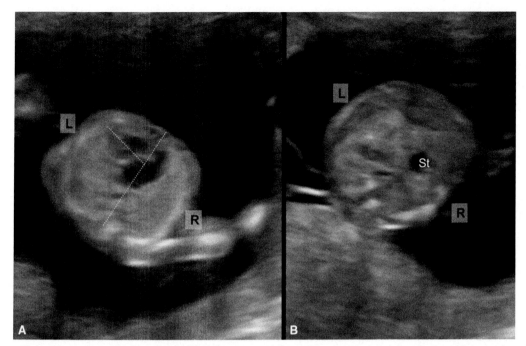

**Figure 11.31:** Transverse views of the fetal chest **(A)** and abdomen **(B)** in a fetus at 13 weeks of gestation with isomerism, first suspected by the discrepant positions of the heart in the left chest **(A)** and the stomach (*St*) in the right abdomen **(B)**. Note the presence of an abnormal cardiac axis and an abnormal four-chamber view in **A**. L, left; R, right.

ventricle (DORV), and complete or corrected transposition of the arteries.[1] The presence of primary ciliary dyskinesia has also been demonstrated in patients with heterotaxy and patients with complete situs inversus.[46] Interestingly, chromosomal aberrations such as trisomies are nearly absent in this group.

## Tetralogy of Fallot

### Definition

TOF is characterized by a subaortic (malaligned) VSD, an aortic root that overrides the VSD, and infundibular

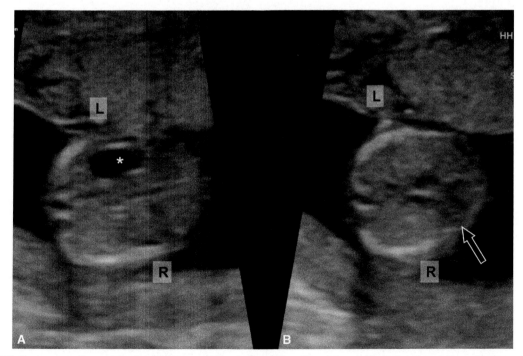

**Figure 11.32:** Transverse views of the fetal abdomen **(A)** and chest **(B)** and in a fetus at 13 weeks of gestation with isomerism, first suspected by the discrepant positions of the heart in the right chest (dextrocardia) **(A)** and the stomach (*asterisk*) in the left abdomen **(B)**. L, left; R, right.

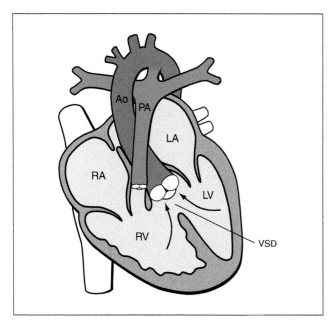

**Figure 11.33:** Schematic drawing of tetralogy of Fallot. See text for details. LA, left atrium; RA, right atrium; LV, left ventricle; RV, right ventricle; VSD, ventricular septal defect; PA, pulmonary artery; Ao, aorta.

pulmonary stenosis (Fig. 11.33). Right ventricular hypertrophy, which represents the fourth anatomic feature of the "tetralogy," is typically not present prenatally. TOF with pulmonary stenosis is the classic form, but the spectrum of TOF includes severe forms, such as TOF with pulmonary atresia and TOF with absent pulmonary valve. TOF is one of the most common forms of cyanotic CHD and is found in about 1 in 3,600 live births.[5] The classic form of TOF with pulmonary stenosis accounts for about 80% of all newborns with TOF.

### *Ultrasound Findings*

In its classic form, TOF may be difficult to diagnose in the first trimester. The sonographic anatomy of the four-chamber view in TOF can appear normal in the first trimester, unless in association with cardiac axis deviation (Fig. 11.34A and B). Clues to the diagnosis of TOF include a large aortic root in the five-chamber view on gray scale and color Doppler ultrasound (Figs. 11.34C and 11.35A) with a small pulmonary artery (Figs. 11.34D and 11.35B). Although the aortic override may not be easily noted on the five-chamber view, the small pulmonary artery can be easily detected in

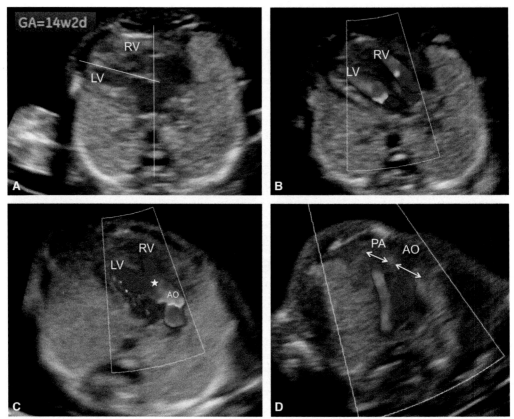

**Figure 11.34:** Tetralogy of Fallot at 14 weeks of gestation examined transvaginally. **A and B:** Axial planes of the chest at the four-chamber view in gray scale and color Doppler, respectively. In **A** and **B**, the four-chamber view appears normal with an axis deviation to the left **(A)** and with normal filling during diastole **(B)**. **C:** The five-chamber view in color Doppler. Note in **C** overriding of the dilated aorta over the ventricular septal defect (*star*). **D:** The three-vessel-trachea view in color Doppler. Note in **D** the discrepant vessel size with a small pulmonary artery (PA) as compared to the dilated overriding aorta (AO). Antegrade flow is noted in both great vessels in **D**. LV, left ventricle; RV, right ventricle.

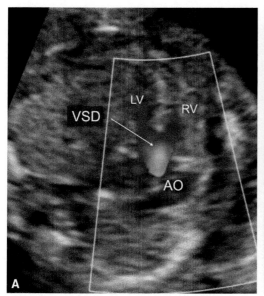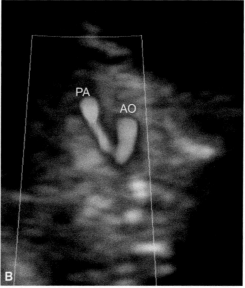

**Figure 11.35:** Tetralogy of Fallot at 13 weeks of gestation. **A:** An axial plane at the level of the five-chamber view in color Doppler. Note in **A**, the large ventricular septal defect (VSD) with the overriding aorta (AO). **B:** The three-vessel-trachea view in color Doppler. Note in **B** the discrepant vessel size with a small pulmonary artery (PA) as compared to the AO. Antegrade flow is noted in both great vessels in **B**. LV, left ventricle; RV, right ventricle.

the 3VT in color Doppler (Figs. 11.34D and 11.35B). The discrepant size between the aorta and pulmonary artery in the 3VT view with antegrade flow in both vessels on color Doppler is an important sign for TOF in the first trimester (Figs. 11.34D and 11.35B). In our experience, TOF in the first trimester is more commonly detected by the abnormal 3VT view than by the five-chamber view demonstrating aortic override.

### Associated Malformations

Associated cardiac abnormalities with TOF include a right aortic arch, found in up to 25% of the cases or occasionally, an AVSD, which increases the risk of chromosomal abnormalities. There is a high association of TOF with extracardiac malformations, chromosomal anomalies, and genetic syndromes.[47] The rate of chromosomal abnormalities is around 30%, with trisomies 21, 13, and 18 accounting for the majority of cases.[47] The rate of microdeletion 22q11 is found in 10% to 15% of fetuses and neonates with TOF,[48] and this risk increases in the presence of thymic hypoplasia,[10,49] right-sided aortic arch, extracardiac anomalies, or polyhydramnios in the second trimester of pregnancy.

### Pulmonary Atresia with Ventricular Septal Defect

#### Definition

Pulmonary atresia with ventricular septal defect (PA-VSD) is characterized by atresia of the pulmonary valve, hypoplasia of the pulmonary tract, membranous or infundibular VSD, and an overriding aorta (Fig. 11.36). Sources of pulmonary blood

flow include the ductus arteriosus and/or systemic–pulmonary collateral circulation. Systemic–pulmonary collateral circulation typically includes collateral arteries from the descending aorta to the lungs, called major aortopulmonary collateral arteries (MAPCAs).[50] PA-VSD has a prevalence of 0.07 per 1,000 live births.[6] A 10-fold increased risk of PA-VSD is seen in infants of diabetic mothers.[6]

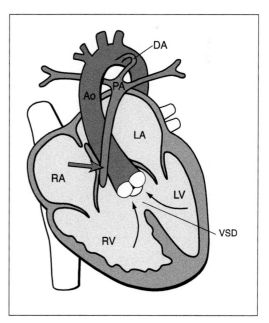

**Figure 11.36:** Schematic drawing of pulmonary atresia with ventricular septal defect (PA-VSD). See text for details. LA, left atrium; RA, right atrium; LV, left ventricle; RV, right ventricle; PA, pulmonary artery; Ao, aorta; DA, ductus arteriosus.

## Ultrasound Findings

The presence of an abnormal cardiac axis can be the first clue for the presence of PA-VSD (Fig. 11.37A). The 4CV is commonly normal in PA-VSD and the five-chamber view shows a dilated overriding aortic root (Fig. 11.37A) with an absence of a normal-sized pulmonary artery in the right ventricular outflow tract view. Color Doppler at the 3VT view shows a dilated transverse aortic arch with absence of antegrade flow across the pulmonary artery (Fig. 11.37B). Typically color Doppler demonstrates reverse flow in a tortuous ductus arteriosus and pulmonary artery in an oblique view of the chest, inferior to the aortic arch. The presence of MAPCAs is not detected in the first trimester of pregnancy.

## Associated Malformations

A right-sided aortic arch can be present in 20% to 50% of all cases.[51] Absence of the ductus arteriosus is also reported in about half of the cases. MAPCAs are associated in about 44% of cases[50] and are typically diagnosed in the second trimester of pregnancy. Associated extracardiac findings include a high incidence of chromosomal aberrations. In the Baltimore–Washington Infant Study, 8.3% of children with PA-VSD had chromosomal anomalies.[6] The incidence of 22q11 microdeletion is high and is found in 18% to 25% of fetuses with PA-VSD,[50] with an increased association in the presence of MAPCAs and/or a right aortic arch or hypoplastic thymus.

## Common Arterial Trunk

### Definition

CAT is characterized by a single arterial trunk that arises from the base of the heart and gives origin to the systemic, coronary, and pulmonary circulations (Fig. 11.38). A large VSD is almost always present in this anomaly, resulting from the near absence of the infundibular septum.[52] The spectrum of the disease is wide and is mainly related to the anatomic origin of the right and left pulmonary arteries, which may arise from a pulmonary trunk or as direct branches from the CAT or the descending aorta. The root of the CAT is large and has a biventricular origin in most cases (overrides the septal defect). In up to a third of CAT cases, however, the root appears to arise entirely from the right ventricle and, in rare cases, entirely from the left ventricle. The CAT valve has three leaflets (tricuspid) in about 69% of cases, four leaflets (quadricuspid) in 22% of cases, two leaflets (bicuspid) in 9% of cases, and, on very rare occasions, one, five, or more leaflets.[53] CAT is reported to occur in about 1.07 of 10,000 births.[30]

## Ultrasound Findings

Demonstrating the direct origin of the pulmonary arteries from the CAT is difficult in the first trimester and is facilitated by the application of color Doppler (Fig. 11.39). A typical feature of CAT is the presence of truncal valve regurgitation, which can help to differentiate CAT from other cardiac malformations involving an overriding aorta. A differentiating feature of CAT from PA-VSD is that the pulmonary arteries arise directly from the CAT rather than the right ventricle.

## Associated Malformations

Associated cardiac malformations are common with CAT. The ductus arteriosus is absent in 50% of the cases, and when present it remains patent postnatally in about two-thirds of patients.[54] Aortic arch abnormalities are common with

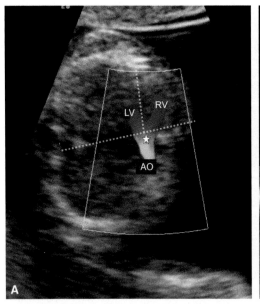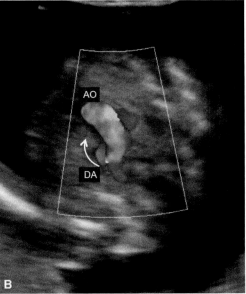

Figure 11.37: Transvaginal ultrasound at the level of the five-chamber view (A) and the transverse ductal arch view (B) in a fetus at 12 weeks of gestation with pulmonary atresia and ventricular septal defect. The five-chamber view (A) shows a large overriding aorta (AO) (*star*) and an abnormal cardiac axis (*dashed lines*). In the three-vessel-trachea view (B), reverse flow in the ductus arteriosus (DA) is demonstrated on color Doppler (*curved arrow*). RV, right ventricle; LV, left ventricle.

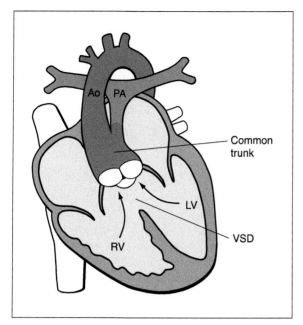

**Figure 11.38:** Schematic drawing of common arterial trunk. See text for details. LV, left ventricle; RV, right ventricle; VSD, ventricular septal defect; PA, pulmonary artery; Ao, aorta.

CAT, with right-sided arch noted in 21% to 36% of cases[54] (Fig. 11.39). Truncal valve dysplasia with incompetence is a common association. Extracardiac structural malformations are seen in up to 40% of CAT cases and are typically nonspecific (10). Numerical chromosomal anomalies are found in about 4.5% of the cases and include trisomies 21, 18, and 13. Microdeletion 22q11 is reported in 30% to 40% of cases.[55]

## Transposition of the Great Arteries

### Definition

Complete transposition of the great arteries (TGA) is a common cardiac malformation with AV concordance and ventriculoarterial discordance. This implies a normal connection between the atria and ventricles; the right atrium is connected to the right ventricle through the tricuspid valve and the left atrium is connected to the left ventricle through the mitral valve, but there is a switched connection of the great vessels, the pulmonary artery arising from the left ventricle, and the aorta arising from the right ventricle. Both great arteries display a parallel course, with the aorta anterior and to the right of the pulmonary artery (Fig. 11.40), hence the term D-TGA (D = "dexter"). D-TGA is a relatively frequent cardiac anomaly with an incidence of 0.315 cases per 1,000 live births.[56]

### Ultrasound Findings

In TGA, the great vessels assume a parallel course, which can be demonstrated in an oblique axial view of the fetal chest (Fig. 11.41B). This oblique view of the fetal chest is not a standard plane of the obstetric ultrasound examination and thus is not displayed on routine ultrasound scanning. The demonstration on color Doppler of a single great vessel in the 3VT is often the first clue for the presence of TGA (Fig. 11.41A) in the first trimester. Once TGA is suspected on the 3VT view, the diagnosis can then be confirmed in the first trimester by demonstrating the parallel orientation of the great vessels in the oblique view of the fetal chest (Fig. 11.41B). The 4CV is commonly normal in TGA with the exception of an abnormal cardiac axis in some cases with mesocardia.

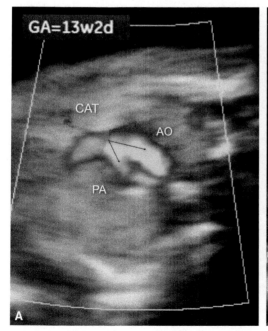
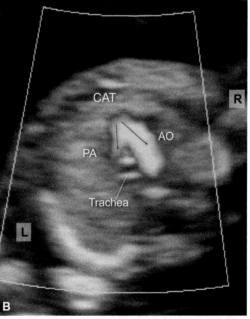

**Figure 11.39:** Common arterial trunk (CAT) in a fetus at 13 weeks of gestation. Note in planes **A** and **B** the bifurcation of the CAT into the aorta (AO) and the pulmonary artery (PA). Also note that the aortic arch courses to the right of the trachea, as a right-sided aortic arch. R, right; L, left.

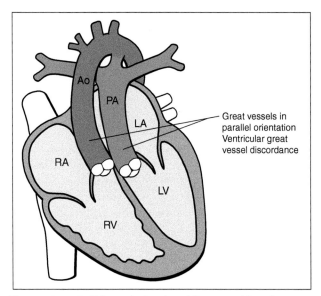

**Figure 11.40:** Schematic drawing of D-transposition of great arteries (D-TGA). See text for details. LA, left atrium; RA, right atrium; LV, left ventricle; RV, right ventricle; PA, pulmonary artery; Ao, aorta.

### Associated Malformations

VSDs and pulmonary stenosis (left ventricular outflow obstruction) are the two most common associated cardiac findings in D-TGA. VSDs are common and occur in about 40% of cases and are typically perimembranous but can be located anywhere in the septum.[56] Pulmonary stenosis coexists with a VSD in D-TGA patients in about 30% of cases, and the stenosis is usually more severe and complex than in D-TGA with intact ventricular septum.[56] Extracardiac anomalies may be present but rare, and numerical chromosomal aberrations are practically absent in D-TGA. Microdeletion of 22q11 could be present and should be ruled out, especially when extracardiac malformations or a complex D-TGA is present.

## Double Outlet Right Ventricle

### Definition

DORV encompasses a family of complex cardiac malformations where both great arteries arise primarily from the morphologic right ventricle (Fig. 11.42) but differ with regard to the variable spatial relationship of the great arteries, the location of the VSD that is commonly seen with DORV, and the presence or absence of pulmonary and less commonly aortic outflow obstruction. In DORV, four types of anatomic relationships of the aorta to the pulmonary artery at the level of the semilunar valves and four anatomic locations for the VSD have been described.[57] The exact subtype of DORV may be hard to characterize prenatally as the position of the VSD is difficult to establish with accuracy in fetal echocardiography. DORV has an incidence of approximately 0.09 per 1,000 live births.[5]

### Ultrasound Findings

DORV can occasionally be diagnosed in the first trimester due to the presence of an abnormal 4CV or 3VT view. An abnormal cardiac axis is commonly found in DORV and can be noted in the first trimester (Fig. 11.43A and B). The 3VT

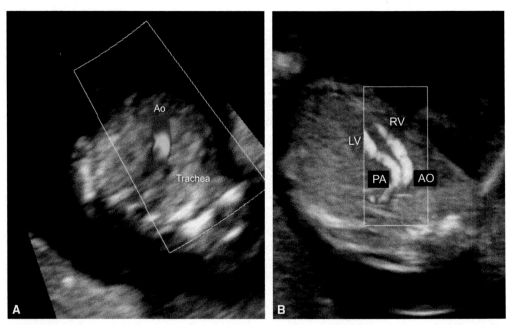

**Figure 11.41:** Color Doppler ultrasound at the three-vessel-trachea view **(A)** and an oblique view of the chest **(B)** at 12 weeks of gestation in a fetus with complete transposition of the great arteries (D-TGA). The three-vessel-trachea view **(A)** demonstrates the presence of a single great artery of normal size, representing the superiorly located aorta (Ao). The oblique view of the chest **(B)** shows the parallel course of the great vessels arising in discordance with the aorta (AO) from the right (RV) and the pulmonary artery (PA) from the left ventricle (LV).

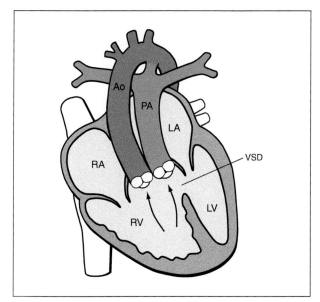

**Figure 11.42:** Schematic drawing of double outlet right ventricle. See text for details. LA, left atrium; RA, right atrium; LV, left ventricle; RV, right ventricle; Ao, aorta; PA, pulmonary artery; VSD, ventricular septal defect.

view typically shows discrepant size of the great arteries, a single large vessel (Fig. 11.43C), or parallel orientation of the great vessels (Fig. 11.44). When the 4CV is normal, DORV is difficult to diagnose in the first trimester.

## Associated Malformations

Associated cardiac findings are common and include a full spectrum of cardiac lesions. Pulmonary stenosis is the most common associated malformation and occurs in about 70% of cases.[58] Extracardiac anomalies are very common in fetuses with DORV and are nonspecific for organ systems.[59] Chromosomal abnormalities are frequently found in the range of 12% to 40% in fetuses with DORV and primarily include trisomies 18 and 13 and 22q11 microdeletion.[60]

## Right and Double Aortic Arch

### Definition

Right aortic arch is diagnosed when the transverse aortic arch is located to the right of the trachea on transverse imaging of the chest. A right aortic arch is associated with three main subgroups of arch abnormalities: right aortic arch with a right ductus arteriosus, right aortic arch with left ductus arteriosus, and double aortic arch (Fig. 11.45). Right aortic arch can be part of a complex cardiac malformation, but can often also be an isolated finding.[61] A right aortic arch occurs in about 1 in 1,000 of the general population,[62] but the prevalence of right aortic arch is probably higher in the presence of other cardiac anomalies.

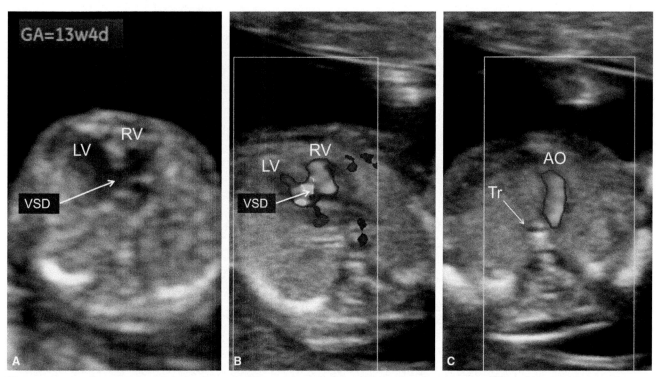

**Figure 11.43:** Four-chamber views in gray scale **(A)**, color Doppler **(B)**, and three-vessel-trachea view **(C)** in a fetus at 13 weeks of gestation with double outlet right ventricle. In **A** and **B**, the ventricular septal defect (VSD) is visualized in gray scale **(A)** and color Doppler **(B)**. Note the abnormal location of the heart in the chest with mesocardia in **A** and **B**. The three-vessel-trachea view **(C)** shows the aorta (AO) as a single vessel (superior to the pulmonary artery). In this case, the AO has a course to the right of the trachea (Tr), representing a right aortic arch. RV, right ventricle; LV, left ventricle.

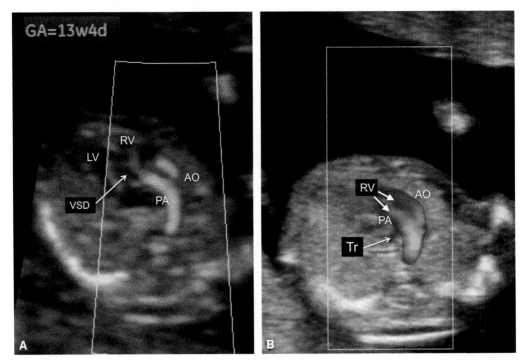

**Figure 11.44:** Oblique views **(A and B)** of the fetal thorax with color Doppler in a fetus at 13 weeks of gestation with double outlet right ventricle (same fetus as in Fig. 11.43). Note the presence of the ventricular septal defect (VSD) in **A**, and the origin of the aorta (AO) and pulmonary artery (PA) from the right ventricle (RV) in **A** and **B**. Aortic and ductal arches are seen to the right of the trachea (Tr) in **A** and **B**. LV, left ventricle.

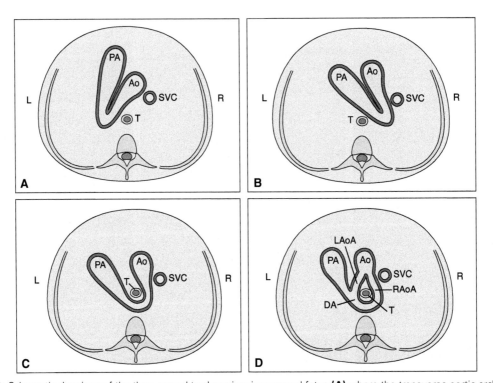

**Figure 11.45:** Schematic drawings of the three-vessel-trachea view in a normal fetus **(A)** where the transverse aortic arch (Ao) and isthmus merge with the pulmonary artery (PA) and ductus arteriosus (DA) into the descending aorta in a "V-shape" configuration to the left of the trachea (T). **B:** A right-sided aortic arch with a right-sided DA in a "V-shape" configuration to the right side of the trachea. **C:** A right aortic arch with the transverse aortic arch to the right side of the trachea; the DA is left-sided and the connection of aortic and ductal arches constitutes a vascular ring around the trachea in a "U-shape" configuration. **D:** A rare sub-form of right aortic arch with a left DA forming a double aortic arch with the transverse aortic arch bifurcating into a right and a left aortic arch (LAoA) surrounding the trachea and esophagus. L, left; R, right; SVC, superior vena cava; RAoA, right aortic arch.

## Ultrasound Findings

The diagnosis of a right aortic arch is possible in the first trimester and is enabled by the use of color Doppler at the 3VT view (Figs. 11.46 and 11.47). It is commonly suspected on transabdominal scanning when the relationship of the transverse aortic and ductal arches is evaluated. Transvaginal scanning can help in confirming the diagnosis. In recent years, we were able to diagnose right aortic arch with its three subgroups in the first trimester. Differentiating between the U-sign right aortic arch and the double aortic arch (lambda sign) may be difficult in the first trimester (Figs. 11.46 and 11.47). When suspected in the first trimester of pregnancy, the identification of the actual subtype of right aortic arch can be confirmed on follow-up ultrasound examination in the second trimester of pregnancy.

## Associated Malformations

Even if the right aortic arch appears as an isolated finding on ultrasound, fetal chromosomal karyotyping should be offered to rule out chromosomal aberrations, primarily 22q11 microdeletion[12] and occasionally trisomy 21 and other aneuploidies. Associated intracardiac anomalies are more common when the aorta and ductus arteriosus are on the right (V-sign) than with double aortic arch or with the U-sign right aortic arch.[1] Typical cardiac anomalies observed with a right aortic arch are TOF, pulmonary atresia with VSD, CAT, absent pulmonary valve, tricuspid atresia, and DORV.[61,63] The presence of a right aortic arch in association with a conotruncal anomaly increases the risk of 22q11 microdeletion.[61,63]

## Anomalies of the Systemic and Pulmonary Veins

The systemic and pulmonary veins in the first trimester are generally too small in size to be clearly evident on gray-scale ultrasound, making detection of venous malformations extremely difficult. Anomalies of the abdominal venous vasculature are discussed in Chapter 12. The presence of a left persistent superior vena cava may be rarely detected in the first trimester. Anomalies of the pulmonary venous system are still considered not diagnosable in the first trimester, unless in combination with isomerism, which provides a clue to the presence of anomalous pulmonary venous return. A follow-up in the second trimester of pregnancy is recommended when pulmonary venous malformations are suspected in the first trimester.

## Aberrant Right Subclavian Artery

ARSA can be demonstrated in the first trimester in the 3VT view in color Doppler by reducing the velocity of flow in order to demonstrate the small subclavian artery. The ability to image the ARSA is significantly enhanced when transvaginal fetal ultrasound is performed (Fig. 11.48). ARSA has been associated with trisomy 21 and other aneuploidies. The patient's prior risk for aneuploidy should be taken into consideration when counseling is performed for the diagnosis of an isolated ARSA.

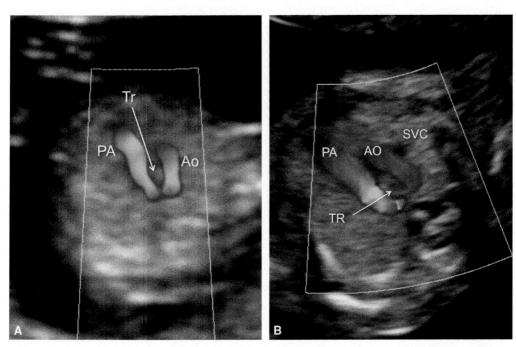

**Figure 11.46:** Three-vessel-trachea views in two fetuses at 13 weeks of gestation with a right aortic arch with a left ductus arteriosus (U-sign) demonstrated on transabdominal **(A)** and transvaginal **(B)** color Doppler. PA, pulmonary artery; Ao/AO, aorta; SVC, superior vena cava; TR, trachea; L, left.

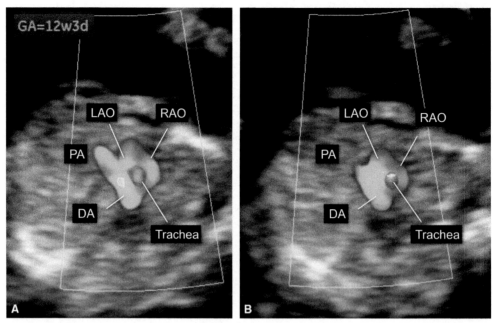

**Figure 11.47:** Transvaginal ultrasound in color Doppler in a fetus at 12 weeks of gestation with double aortic arch (A,B). Note the left (LAO) and right (RAO) aortic arches surrounding the trachea. Differentiating a RAO (see Fig. 11.46) from a double arch is more commonly performed in the second trimester of pregnancy. PA, pulmonary artery; DA, ductus arteriosus.

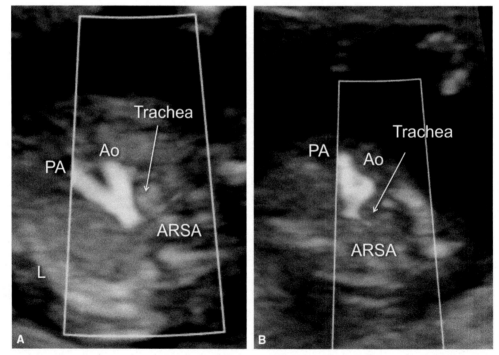

**Figure 11.48:** Transvaginal ultrasound of an axial view of the fetal chest at the three-vessel-trachea view showing an aberrant right subclavian artery (ARSA) in two fetuses (A and B), both at 13 weeks of gestation noted during the nuchal translucency measurement. Ao, aorta; PA, pulmonary artery; L, left.

# REFERENCES

1. Abuhamad A, Chaoui R. *A Practical Guide to Fetal Echocardiography: Normal and Abnormal Hearts.* 3rd ed. Philadelphia, PA: Wolters Kluwer Health/Lippincott Williams & Wilkins; 2015

2. Gittenberger-de Groot AC, Bartelings MM, DeRuiter MC, et al. Basics of cardiac development for the understanding of congenital heart malformations. *Pediatr Res.* 2005;57:169–176.

3. Groot ACG-D, Bartelings MM, Poelmann RE, et al. Embryology of the heart and its impact on understanding fetal and neonatal heart disease. *Semin Fetal Neonatal Med.* 2013;18:237–244.

4. Srivastava D. Making or breaking the heart: from lineage determination to morphogenesis. *Cell.* 2006;126:1037–1048.

5. Hoffman JI, Christianson R. Congenital heart disease in a cohort of 19,502 births with long-term follow-up. *Am J Cardiol.* 1978;42:641–647.

6. Ferencz C. *Epidemiology of Congenital Heart Disease: The Baltimore-Washington Infant Study, 1981–1989.* 1st ed. Philadelphia, PA: WB Saunders; 1993.

7. Yoon PW, Olney RS, Khoury MJ, et al. Contribution of birth defects and genetic diseases to pediatric hospitalizations. A population-based study. *Arch Pediatr Adolesc Med.* 1997;151:1096–1103.

8. Jones KL, Jones MC, del Campo M. *Smith's Recognizable Patterns of Human Malformation.* 7th ed. Philadelphia, PA: Saunders; 2013.

9. Perez E, Sullivan KE. Chromosome 22q11.2 deletion syndrome (DiGeorge and velocardiofacial syndromes). *Curr Opin Pediatr.* 2002;14:678–683.

10. Chaoui R, Heling KS, Sarut Lopez A, et al. The thymic-thoracic ratio in fetal heart defects: a simple way to identify fetuses at high risk for microdeletion 22q11. *Ultrasound Obstet Gynecol.* 2011;37:397–403.

11. Besseau-Ayasse J, Violle-Poirsier C, Bazin A, et al. A French collaborative survey of 272 fetuses with 22q11.2 deletion: ultrasound findings, fetal autopsies and pregnancy outcomes. *Prenat Diagn.* 2014;34:424–430.

12. Perolo A, De Robertis V, Cataneo I, et al. Risk of 22q11.2 deletion in fetuses with right aortic arch and without intracardiac anomalies. *Ultrasound Obstet Gynecol.* 2016;48:200–203.

13. Chaoui R, Heling K-S, Zhao Y, et al. Dilated cavum septi pellucidi in fetuses with microdeletion 22q11. *Prenat Diagn.* 2016;36:911–915.

14. Lamouroux A, Mousty E, Prodhomme O, et al. La dysgénésie thymique: marqueur de microdélétion 22q11.2 dans le bilan d'un hydramnios. *J Gynécol Obstét Biol Reprod.* 2016;45:388–396.

15. Clur SA, Ottenkamp J, Bilardo CM. The nuchal translucency and the fetal heart: a literature review. *Prenat Diagn.* 2009;29:739–748.

16. Khalil A, Nicolaides KH. Fetal heart defects: potential and pitfalls of first-trimester detection. *Semin Fetal Neonatal Med.* 2013;18:251–260.

17. Maiz N, Nicolaides KH. Ductus venosus in the first trimester: contribution to screening of chromosomal, cardiac defects and monochorionic twin complications. *Fetal Diagn Ther.* 2010;28:65–71.

18. Huggon IC, DeFigueiredo DB, Allan LD. Tricuspid regurgitation in the diagnosis of chromosomal anomalies in the fetus at 11-14 weeks of gestation. *Heart.* 2003;89:1071–1073.

19. Sinkovskaya ES, Chaoui R, Karl K, et al. Fetal cardiac axis and congenital heart defects in early gestation. *Obstet Gynecol.* 2015;125:453–460.

20. Raymond FL, Simpson JM, Sharland GK, et al. Fetal echocardiography as a predictor of chromosomal abnormality. *Lancet.* 1997;350:930.

21. Natowicz M, Chatten J, Clancy R, et al. Genetic disorders and major extracardiac anomalies associated with the hypoplastic left heart syndrome. *Pediatrics.* 1988;82:698–706.

22. Rosenthal GL. Patterns of prenatal growth among infants with cardiovascular malformations: possible fetal hemodynamic effects. *Am J Epidemiol.* 1996;143:505–513.

23. Beekman RH. Aortic coarctation. In: Allen HD, Driscoll DJ, Shaddy RE, eds. *Moss and Adams' Heart Disease in Infants, Children, and Adolescents.* Baltimore, MD: Williams & Wilkins, 2012: 1044–1054.

24. Moene RJ, Gittenberger-de Groot AC, Oppenheimer-Dekker A, et al. Anatomic characteristics of ventricular septal defect associated with coarctation of the aorta. *Am J Cardiol.* 1987;59:952–955.

25. Rosenquist GC. Congenital mitral valve disease associated with coarctation of the aorta: a spectrum that includes parachute deformity of the mitral valve. *Circulation.* 1974;49:985–993.

26. Paladini D, Volpe P, Russo MG, et al. Aortic coarctation: prognostic indicators of survival in the fetus. *Heart.* 2004;90:1348–1349.

27. Todros T, Paladini D, Chiappa E, et al. Pulmonary stenosis and atresia with intact ventricular septum during prenatal life. *Ultrasound Obstet Gynecol.* 2003;21:228–233.

28. Shinebourne EA, Rigby ML, Carvalho JS. Pulmonary atresia with intact ventricular septum: from fetus to adult: congenital heart disease. *Heart.* 2008;94:1350–1357.

29. Tandon R, Edwards JE. Tricuspid atresia. A re-evaluation and classification. *J Thorac Cardiovasc Surg.* 1974;67:530–542.

30. Hoffman JIE, Kaplan S. The incidence of congenital heart disease. *J Am Coll Cardiol.* 2002;39:1890–1900.

31. Galindo A, Comas C, Martínez JM, et al. Cardiac defects in chromosomally normal fetuses with increased nuchal translucency at 10–14 weeks of gestation. *J Matern Fetal Neonatal Med.* 2003;13:163–170.

32. Berg C, Kremer C, Geipel A, et al. Ductus venosus blood flow alterations in fetuses with obstructive lesions of the right heart. *Ultrasound Obstet Gynecol.* 2006;28:137–142.

33. Wald RM, Tham EB, McCrindle BW, et al. Outcome after prenatal diagnosis of tricuspid atresia: a multicenter experience. *Am Heart J.* 2007;153:772–778.

34. Cetta F, Minich LL, Maleszewski JJ. Atrioventricular septal defects. In: Allen HD, Driscoll DJ, Shaddy RE, eds. *Moss and Adams' Heart Disease in Infants, Children, and Adolescents.* Baltimore, MD: Williams & Wilkins, 2012:691–712.

35. Delisle MF, Sandor GG, Tessier F, et al. Outcome of fetuses diagnosed with atrioventricular septal defect. *Obstet Gynecol.* 1999;94:763–767.

36. Rubio AE, Lewin MB. Ventricular septal defects. In: Allen HD, Driscoll DJ, Shaddy RE, eds. *Moss and Adams' Heart Disease in Infants, Children, and Adolescents.* Baltimore, MD: Williams & Wilkins; 2012: 713–721.

37. Gómez O, Martínez JM, Olivella A, et al. Isolated ventricular septal defects in the era of advanced fetal echocardiography: risk of chromosomal anomalies and spontaneous closure rate from diagnosis to age of 1 year. *Ultrasound Obstet Gynecol.* 2014;43:65–71.

38. Sharland GK, Chita SK, Allan LD. Tricuspid valve dysplasia or displacement in intrauterine life. *J Am Coll Cardiol.* 1991;17:944–949.

39. Earing MG, Hagler DJ, Edwards WD. Univentricular Atrioventricular Connection. In: Allen HD, Driscoll DJ, Shaddy RE, eds. *Moss and Adams' Heart Disease in Infants, Children, and Adolescents.* Baltimore, MD: Williams & Wilkins; 2012:1175–1194.

40. Van Praagh R, Ongley PA, Swan HJ. Anatomic types of single or common ventricle in man: morphologic and geometric aspects of sixty necropsied cases. *Am J Cardiol.* 1964;13:367–386.

41. O'Leary PM, Hagler DJ. Cardiac malpositions and abnormalities of atrial and visceral situs. In: Allen HD, Driscoll DJ, Shaddy RE, eds. *Moss and Adams' Heart Disease in Infants, Children, and Adolescents.* Baltimore, MD: Williams & Wilkins; 2012.

42. Sapire DW, Ho SY, Anderson RH, et al. Diagnosis and significance of atrial isomerism. *Am J Cardiol.* 1986;58:342–346.

43. Sharland GK, Cook AC. Heterotaxy syndromes/isomerism of the atrial appendages. In: Allan L, Hornberger L, Sharland G, eds. *Textbook of Fetal Cardiology.* London: Greenwich Medical Media; 2000:333–346.

44. Berg C, Geipel A, Kamil D, et al. The syndrome of right isomerism—prenatal diagnosis and outcome. *Ultraschall Med.* 2006;27:225–233.

45. Ticho BS, Goldstein AM, Van Praagh R. Extracardiac anomalies in the heterotaxy syndromes with focus on anomalies of midline-associated structures. *Am J Cardiol.* 2000;85:729–734.

46. Nakhleh N, Francis R, Giese RA, et al. High prevalence of respiratory ciliary dysfunction in congenital heart disease patients with heterotaxy. *Circulation.* 2012;125:2232–2242.

47. Poon LCY, Huggon IC, Zidere V, et al. Tetralogy of Fallot in the fetus in the current era. *Ultrasound Obstet Gynecol.* 2007;29:625–627.

48. Boudjemline Y, Fermont L, Le Bidois J, et al. Prevalence of 22q11 deletion in fetuses with conotruncal cardiac defects: a 6-year prospective study. *J Pediatr.* 2001;138:520–524.

49. Chaoui R, Kalache KD, Heling KS, et al. Absent or hypoplastic thymus on ultrasound: a marker for deletion 22q11.2 in fetal cardiac defects. *Ultrasound Obstet Gynecol.* 2002;20:546–552.

50. Vesel S, Rollings S, Jones A, et al. Prenatally diagnosed pulmonary atresia with ventricular septal defect: echocardiography, genetics, associated anomalies and outcome. *Heart.* 2006;92:1501–1505.

51. Bharati S, Paul MH, Idriss FS, et al. The surgical anatomy of pulmonary atresia with ventricular septal defect: pseudotruncus. *J Thorac Cardiovasc Surg.* 1975;69:713–721.

52. Cabalka AK, Edwards WD, Dearani JA. Truncus arteriosus. In: Allen HD, Driscoll DJ, Shaddy RE eds. *Moss and Adams' Heart Disease in Infants, Children, and Adolescents.* Baltimore, MD: Williams & Wilkins; 2012:990–1002.

53. Fuglestad SJ, Puga FJ, Danielson GK, et al. Surgical pathology of the truncal valve: a study of 12 cases. *Am J Cardiovasc Pathol.* 1988;2:39–47.

54. Butto F, Lucas RVJ, Edwards JE. Persistent truncus arteriosus: pathologic anatomy in 54 cases. *Pediatr Cardiol.* 1986;7:95–101.

55. Volpe P, Paladini D, Marasini M, et al. Common arterial trunk in the fetus: characteristics, associations, and outcome in a multicentre series of 23 cases. *Heart*. 2003;89:1437–1441.

56. Wernovsky G. Transposition of the great arteries. In: Allen HD, Driscoll DA, Shaddy RE, eds. *Moss and Adams' Heart Disease in Infants, Children, and Adolescents*. Baltimore, MD: Williams & Wilkins; 2012:1097–1146.

57. Sridaromont S, Feldt RH, Ritter DG, et al. Double outlet right ventricle: hemodynamic and anatomic correlations. *Am J Cardiol*. 1976;38:85–94.

58. Bradley TJ, Karamlou T, Kulik A, et al. Determinants of repair type, reintervention, and mortality in 393 children with double-outlet right ventricle. *J Thorac Cardiovasc Surg*. 2007;134:967–973.e6.

59. Gedikbasi A, Oztarhan K, Gul A, et al. Diagnosis and prognosis in double-outlet right ventricle. *Am J Perinatol*. 2008;25:427–434.

60. Obler D, Juraszek AL, Smoot LB, et al. Double outlet right ventricle: aetiologies and associations. *J Med Genet*. 2008;45:481–497.

61. Berg C, Bender F, Soukup M, et al. Right aortic arch detected in fetal life. *Ultrasound Obstet Gynecol*. 2006;28:882–889.

62. Achiron R, Rotstein Z, Heggesh J, et al. Anomalies of the fetal aortic arch: a novel sonographic approach to in-utero diagnosis. *Ultrasound Obstet Gynecol*. 2002;20:553–557.

63. Zidere V, Tsapakis EG, Huggon IC, et al. Right aortic arch in the fetus. *Ultrasound Obstet Gynecol*. 2006;28:876–881.

# CHAPTER 12

# The Fetal Gastrointestinal System

## INTRODUCTION

Ultrasound examination of the fetal abdomen in the first trimester includes the assessment of abdominal organs from the diaphragm superiorly to the genitalia inferiorly. This ultrasound examination allows for the determination of fetal abdominal situs and for the anatomic evaluation of major organs in the gastrointestinal and genitourinary systems. This chapter focuses on the gastrointestinal tract, whereas the genitourinary system is discussed in the following chapter.

## EMBRYOLOGY

The primitive gut is formed during the sixth menstrual week when the flat embryonic disc folds to form a tubular structure that incorporates the dorsal part of the yolk sac into the embryo (Fig. 12.1A–C). Ventral folding of the cranial, lateral, and caudal sections of the primitive gut forms the foregut, midgut, and hindgut, respectively (Fig. 12.2). In this process, the yolk sac remains connected to the midgut by the vitelline vessels (Fig 12.2). Three germ layers contribute to the formation of the gut, with the endoderm giving rise to the mucosal and submucosal surfaces; the mesoderm to the muscular, connective tissue and serosal surfaces; and the neural crest to the neurons and nerves of the submucosal and myenteric plexuses. The primitive gut is initially formed as a hollow tube, which is blocked by proliferating endoderm shortly after its formation. Recanalization occurs over the next 2 weeks by degeneration of tissue, and a hollow tube is formed again by the eighth menstrual week. Abnormalities of the recanalization process result in atresia, stenosis, or duplication of the gastrointestinal tract.

The foregut, supplied by the celiac axis, gives rise to the trachea and respiratory tract (see Chapter 10), esophagus, stomach, liver, pancreas, upper duodenum, gall bladder, and bile ducts. The midgut, supplied by the superior mesenteric artery, gives rise to the lower duodenum, jejunum,

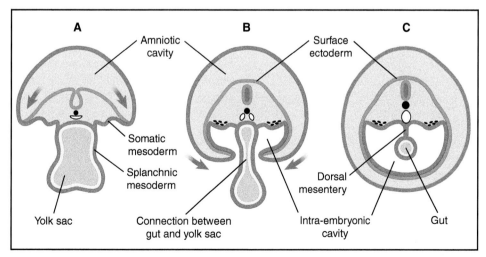

**Figure 12.1:** Axial views **(A–C)** of the developing embryo from the fourth week of gestation showing the formation of the primitive gut tube. Note the incorporation of part of the yolk sac into the embryo, shown in **A** and **B** and the primitive gut tube "gut" shown in **C**. See text for details.

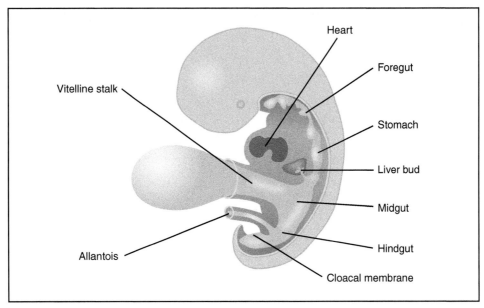

**Figure 12.2:** Schematic drawing of a sagittal view of the embryo at approximately 5 to 6 menstrual weeks showing the formation of the primitive gastrointestinal tract (foregut, midgut, and hindgut) and the liver bud. Note the connection of the midgut to the vitelline duct. See text for details.

ileum, cecum, ascending colon, and proximal two-thirds of transverse colon. The hindgut, supplied by the inferior mesenteric artery, gives rise to the distal one-third of transverse colon, descending colon, sigmoid, rectum, and urogenital sinus. Because of lengthening of the gut and enlargement of upper abdominal organs, an intestinal loop from the midgut protrudes through the umbilical cord insertion into the abdomen at about the sixth week of embryogenesis (from fertilization). This intestinal loop returns to the intraabdominal cavity by about the 10th week of embryogenesis (from fertilization). Through the embryologic process, the midgut loop undergoes a series of three 90-degree counterclockwise rotations around the superior mesenteric artery.

## NORMAL SONOGRAPHIC ANATOMY

Sonographic visualization of the anatomy of the fetal abdomen is easily achieved in early gestation by the axial, sagittal, and coronal views of the fetus. We recommend a review of Chapter 5 on the systematic approach using the detailed first trimester ultrasound examination.

### Axial Planes

The authors recommend the systematic evaluation of abdominal organs through three axial planes at the level of the upper abdomen (subdiaphragmatic—stomach) (Fig. 12.3), mid-abdomen (cord insertion) (Figs. 12.4 and 12.5), and the pelvis (bladder) (Fig. 12.6). In the upper abdominal

axial plane, the fluid-filled anechoic stomach is imaged in the left upper abdomen and the slightly hypoechoic liver, as compared to the lungs, is seen to occupy the majority of the right abdomen (Fig. 12.3). The stomach is consistently seen at 12 weeks of gestation and beyond. This axial plane in the upper abdomen (Fig. 12.3) is important for the assessment of the abdominal situs (see later). In normal situs, the stomach occupies the left side of the abdomen, the liver and gall bladder occupy the right side of the abdomen, and the inferior vena cava (IVC) is seen anterior and to the right side of the descending aorta (Fig. 12.3B). The gall bladder is usually seen in about 50% of fetuses by the 13th week of gestation and practically in all fetuses by the 14th week of gestation.[1] The mid-abdominal axial plane is important for the assessment of the cord insertion into the abdomen and the anterior abdominal wall (Fig. 12.4). In the mid-abdominal axial plane, the bowel is seen with a slightly hyperechoic sonographic appearance when compared to the liver (Fig. 12.4). Both kidneys can be seen in cross-section in the posterior aspect of the abdomen (Fig. 12.4A). It is important to note that physiologic bowel herniation is noted up until the 12th week of gestation (Fig. 12.5). Studies have shown that the midgut herniation should not exceed 7 mm in transverse measurements at any gestation and that the physiologic herniation is almost never seen at crown-rump length measurements exceeding 45 mm.[2,3] The axial plane at the level of the pelvis reveals the bowel surrounding a small urinary bladder (Fig. 12.6). The two iliac crests can be seen in this plane in the posterior aspect of the pelvis (Fig. 12.6B). A slightly oblique plane of the pelvis in color Doppler demonstrates the two umbilical arteries surrounding the urinary bladder with an intact abdominal wall (Fig. 12.6B).

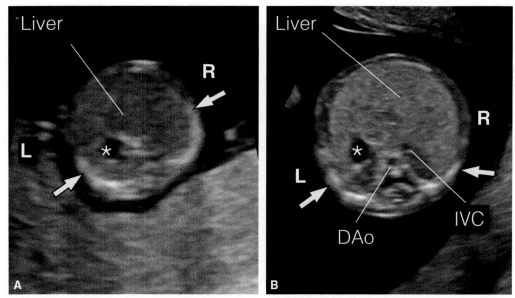

**Figure 12.3:** Axial planes at the level of the upper abdomen in two fetuses at 13 weeks of gestation. The fetus in **A** was examined transabdominally and the fetus in **B** transvaginally. Note the presence of fluid-filled stomachs (*asterisks*) in the upper left abdomen in **A** and **B**. Ribs (*arrows*) are visualized bilaterally along with the liver and inferior vena cava (IVC) in the right (R) abdomen. The descending aorta (DAo) is seen posterior and to the left of the IVC. Improved resolution is noted in fetus in **B** because of the transvaginal approach, thus allowing clear depiction of the IVC and DAo. L, left.

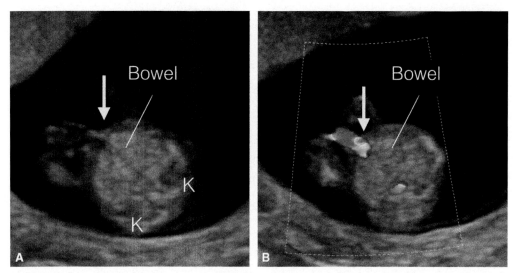

**Figure 12.4:** Axial plane of the middle abdomen in gray scale **(A)** and color Doppler **(B)** at the level of the umbilical cord attachment (*arrow*) in a fetus at 12 weeks of gestation. Note the presence of an intact anterior abdominal wall (*arrow*) and the fetal bowel appearing slightly more hyperechoic than surrounding tissue. Both kidneys (K) are seen in the posterior abdomen in **A**.

## Sagittal Planes

In the sagittal and coronal planes of the fetus, the chest, abdomen, and pelvic organs are seen and are differentiated by their echogenicity. The lung and bowel are hyperechoic, the liver is hypoechoic, and the stomach and bladder are anechoic (Fig. 12.7). Lungs and liver are well separated by the concave-shaped diaphragm (Fig. 12.7). As in the second trimester, the parasagittal views do not exclude a diaphragmatic

hernia. In the midsagittal view of the abdomen, the anterior abdominal wall with the umbilical cord insertion can be demonstrated (Fig. 12.7B) either on two-dimensional (2D) color Doppler or on three-dimensional (3D) ultrasound. This plane is ideally used in combination with color Doppler to visualize the course of the umbilical artery, vein, and ductus venosus (DV) (Fig. 12.8). The midsagittal plane of the abdomen is the most optimal plane for Doppler interrogation of the DV in early gestation (see Fig. 1.4).

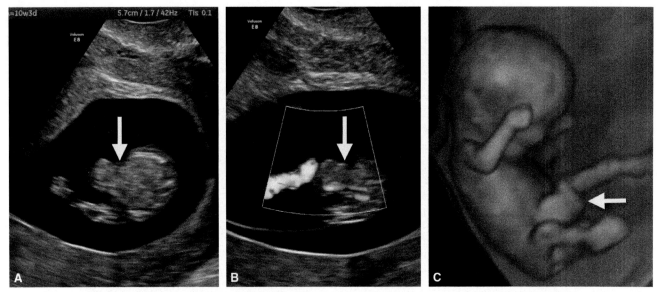

**Figure 12.5:** Axial views of the fetal abdomen in gray scale **(A)** and color Doppler **(B)** of a fetus at 10 weeks of gestation demonstrating the presence of a physiologic midgut herniation (*arrow*). In the corresponding 3D ultrasound in surface mode **(C)**, the midgut herniation is shown as a bulge at the site of cord insertion into the abdomen (*arrow*).

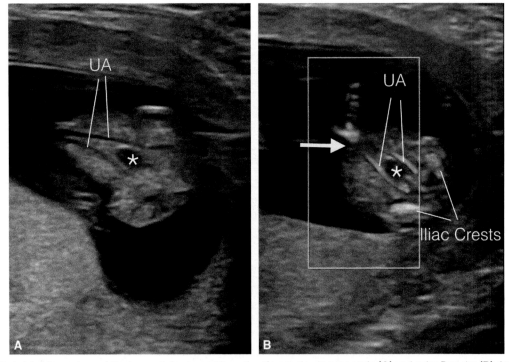

**Figure 12.6:** Axial oblique plane of the lower abdomen at 13 weeks of gestation in gray scale **(A)** and color Doppler **(B)** demonstrating the fluid-filled urinary bladder (*asterisk*), surrounded by the left and right umbilical arteries (UA). This view is best visualized with color Doppler **(B)**, which can also confirm the intact abdominal wall (*arrow*). Note the posterior location of the iliac crests in **B**.

## Coronal Planes

A coronal view is rarely necessary in the first trimester, but it has been our experience that the coronal view is best suited to evaluate the position of the stomach when the diagnosis of diaphragmatic hernia is suspected (see Chapter 10). Transvaginal ultrasound examination of the abdomen in the first trimester provides high-resolution display of organs, which is helpful when abnormalities are suspected. It is important to note, however, that the fetal bowel appears more echogenic on transvaginal imaging, and differentiating normal bowel from hyperechogenic bowel because of pathologic conditions is difficult in early gestation. This is discussed later in this chapter.

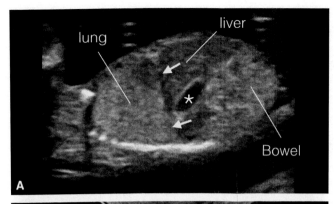

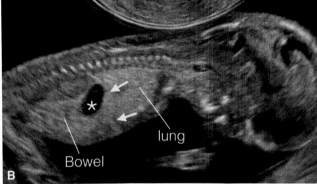

**Figure 12.7:** Parasagittal plane in two fetuses at 13 **(A)** and 12 **(B)** weeks of gestation demonstrating the thorax and abdomen. The filled stomach (*asterisk*) is seen under the diaphragm (*arrows*). Fetus **A** is presenting in a dorso-posterior position and fetus **B** in a dorso-anterior position. Note the hyperechoic lungs and bowel, the hypoechoic liver, and anechoic stomach and bladder (not shown).

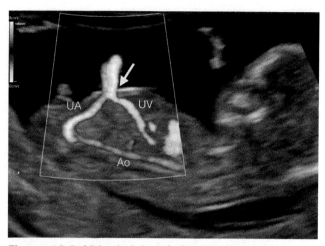

**Figure 12.8:** Midsagittal view of a fetus at 13 weeks of gestation in color Doppler demonstrating the cord arising from the abdomen (*arrow*) with the umbilical artery (UA) and vein (UV). Ao, descending aorta.

## Three-Dimensional Ultrasound of the Fetal Abdomen

Similar to the use of 3D ultrasound in surface mode in the second and third trimester of pregnancy, 3D ultrasound in the first trimester provides additional information to the 2D ultrasound views.[4] Surface mode is especially helpful for the demonstration of a normal and abnormal abdominal wall (Fig. 12.9), as illustrated in this chapter. For the assessment of the intraabdominal organs, 3D ultrasound can also be used in

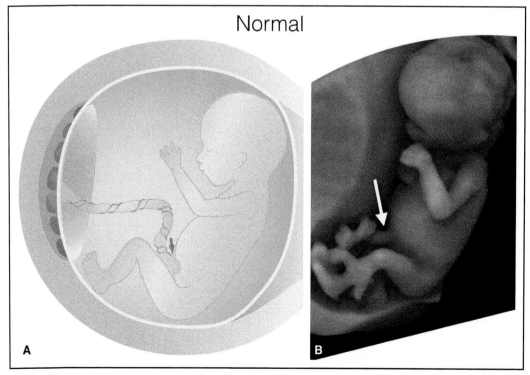

**Figure 12.9:** Schematic drawing **(A)** and corresponding 3D ultrasound image in surface mode of a fetus at 12 weeks of gestation. Note the normal insertion of the umbilical cord in the abdomen in **A** and **B** (*arrows*).

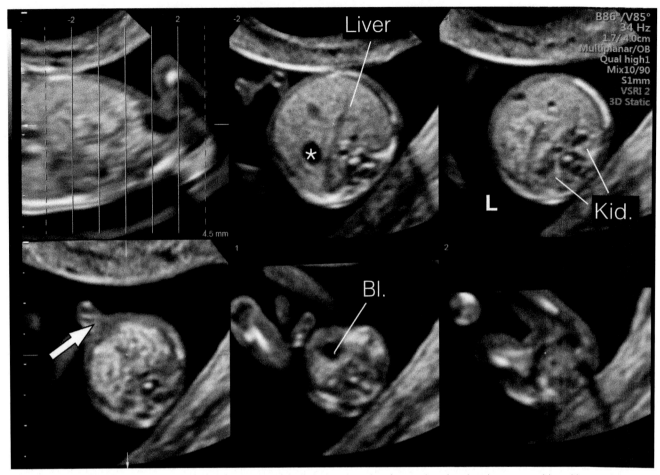

**Figure 12.10:** Tomographic axial views of the abdomen in a fetus at 12 weeks of gestation showing the upper, mid, and lower abdomen. Note the presence of the stomach (*asterisk*) and liver in the upper abdomen, kidneys (Kid.) and abdominal cord insertion (*arrow*) in the mid-abdomen, and the urinary bladder (Bl.) in the lower abdomen. L, left.

multiplanar display, with reconstruction of planes for the specific evaluation of target anatomic regions displayed in tomographic view of axial (Fig. 12.10) or coronal (Fig. 12.11) planes. For more details on the use of 3D ultrasound in the first trimester, refer to Chapter 3 in this book and a recent book on the clinical use of 3D in prenatal medicine.[4] Figures 12.5C and 12.9 show surface mode of the fetal anterior abdominal wall and Figures 12.10 and 12.11 show the use of multiplanar mode with plane reconstruction of axial and coronal views. In our experience, multiplanar mode can be of help especially in the transvaginal approach where transducer manipulation is limited (Figs. 12.10 and 12.11).

## VENTRAL WALL DEFECTS

Defects of the abdominal wall are common anomalies in the fetus, and large defects are often detected in the first trimester.[5] These anomalies include omphalocele, gastroschisis, Pentalogy of Cantrell, and body stalk anomaly (Table 12.1). Bladder exstrophy and cloacal exstrophy are often listed as abdominal wall defects, but are discussed in Chapter 13 as part of the urogenital anomalies.

## Omphalocele

### Definition

Omphalocele, also known as exomphalos, is a congenital defect of the anterior midline abdominal wall with herniation of abdominal viscera, such as bowel and/or liver into the base of the umbilical cord. Embryologically, omphalocele results from failure of fusion of the lateral folds of the primitive gut. Omphalocele has a covering sac made of peritoneum on the inner surface, Wharton's jelly in the middle, and amnion on the outer surface. The typical location of an omphalocele is in the middle of the abdominal wall at the level of the umbilical cord attachment, and the umbilical cord typically inserts on the dome of the herniated sac. On rare occasions, the covering membrane can rupture prenatally. When this occurs, differentiating an omphalocele from gastroschisis on prenatal ultrasound is difficult. The size of the omphalocele differs based upon its content, which may include bowel alone or bowel with liver and other organs. Omphaloceles are commonly associated with fetal genetic and structural abnormalities. Birth prevalence of omphalocele is reported around 1.92 per 10,000 live births.[6]

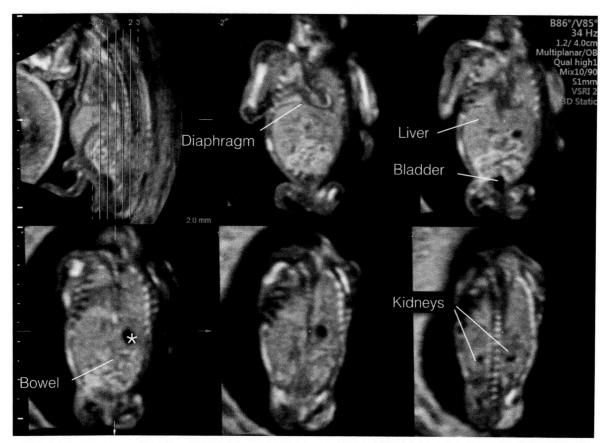

**Figure 12.11:** Tomographic coronal views of the fetal chest and abdomen at 13 weeks of gestation. In this view, the diaphragm, liver, stomach (*asterisk*), bowel, kidneys, and urinary bladder can be seen. Note that the bowel appears echogenic because of the transvaginal approach.

## Table 12.1 • First Trimester Ultrasound and Ventral Wall Defects

| | |
|---|---|
| Physiologic midgut herniation | Herniation of small bowel in a small midline sac, measuring less than 7 mm and physiologically seen until the 12th week of gestation |
| Omphalocele | Midline defect with viscera covered by a membrane. Umbilical cord arises from the dome of the sac. Content can be small with bowel, but can also be large including bowel, liver, stomach, and other organs |
| Gastroschisis | Paraumbilical defect typically to the right of the umbilical cord insertion with evisceration of bowel. No covering membrane |
| Pentalogy of Cantrell | Five features: Abdominal defect similar to omphalocele but higher on abdomen (1), anterior defect of diaphragm (2), distal sternal defect (3), pericardial defect (4), cardiac abnormalities with partial or complete ectopia cordis (5) |
| Ectopia cordis | Sternal defect with the heart partly or completely exteriorized, with or without cardiac abnormalities |
| Body stalk anomaly (limb-body wall complex) | Complex large anterior wall defect with the fetus fixed to the placenta because of a short or absent umbilical cord. Deformities of body, spine, and limbs. Body stalk anomaly can also result from an amniotic band syndrome with a normal umbilical cord. See also in OEIS |
| Bladder exstrophy | Defect in the abdominal wall below the attachment of the umbilical cord. The insertion of the cord is low and below it bladder tissue is exteriorized. Urinary bladder is not visible. Female and male genitalia malformed. Can be part of cloacal exstrophy |
| Cloacal exstrophy, (OEIS complex) | In addition to bladder exstrophy, a low omphalocele is present in association with rectal and anorectal malformations and distal spine anomaly. Anomaly of genitalia is part of complex. OEIS complex is rare and stands for omphalocele, exstrophy of bladder, imperforate anus, and spinal defect. A body stalk anomaly of the lower body can present as OEIS complex, usually legs are completely or partly absent. |

### Ultrasound Findings

The physiologic midgut herniation (Fig. 12.5) is present between the 6th and 11th week of gestation and at crown-rump length of less than 45 mm.[2] Therefore, the diagnosis of a *small* omphalocele cannot be performed reliably before the 12th week of gestation. The omphalocele is seen as a protrusion at the level of the cord insertion into the abdomen. The omphalocele-covering sac is seen as clear borders on ultrasound. Omphaloceles can be easily demonstrated on sagittal or axial views obtained at mid-abdomen (Figs. 12.12 to 12.16). Figure 12.12 shows a schematic drawing of an omphalocele along with its corresponding 3D ultrasound in surface mode. In the first trimester, the omphalocele sac is either relatively small containing bowel loops (Fig. 12.13A) or large containing liver and bowel (Fig. 12.13B). Figure 12.14 shows parasagittal and axial views of a fetus with a large omphalocele, containing liver at 12 weeks of gestation, and Figure 12.15 shows a large omphalocele in two fetuses at 12 and 13 weeks of gestation containing bowel, liver, and stomach. The size of the omphalocele sac has an inverse relationship with chromosomal abnormalities. The presence of a small omphalocele in the first trimester with a thickened nuchal translucency should raise suspicion for the presence of associated fetal malformations and chromosomal aneuploidy (Figs. 12.13A and 12.16). Color Doppler helps in the demonstration of the umbilical cord attachment at the dome of the omphalocele, which can differentiate it from gastroschisis (Fig. 12.17). 3D ultrasound helps in the demonstration and documentation of the size of the omphalocele (Fig. 12.12). Transvaginal ultrasound provides detailed information of the omphalocele content and

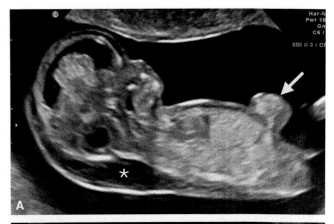

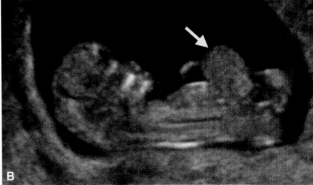

**Figure 12.13:** Midline sagittal plane in two fetuses with small **(A)** and large **(B)** omphalocele (*arrows*) at 12 weeks of gestation. In fetus **A**, the omphalocele is small and contains bowel only, whereas in fetus **B**, the omphalocele is relatively large and contains liver and bowel. Note the presence of an enlarged nuchal translucency (*asterisk*) in fetus **A** and workup revealed trisomy 18 in this fetus.

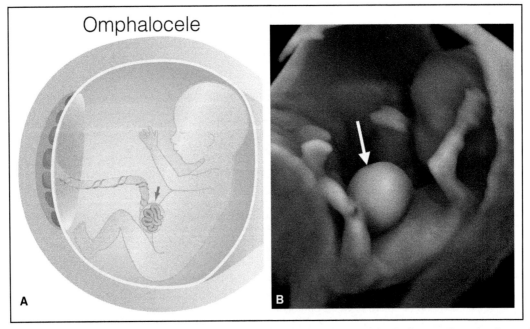

**Figure 12.12:** Schematic drawing **(A)** and corresponding 3D ultrasound image in surface mode of a fetus at 12 weeks of gestation with an omphalocele (*arrows*). Note in **A** the presence of an omphalocele sac covering the protruding intraabdominal organs (bowel, with or without liver), with the umbilical cord attached to the top of the omphalocele. The umbilical cord is not seen in **B**, as the lower extremities obscure it.

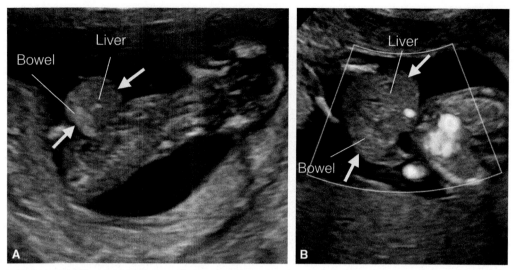

**Figure 12.14:** Parasagittal **(A)** and axial **(B)** view of a fetus at 12 weeks of gestation with a large omphalocele (*arrows*). Note the presence of liver and bowel within the omphalocele.

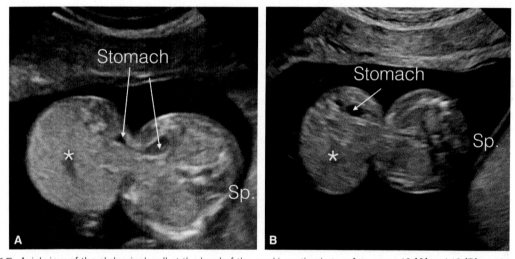

**Figure 12.15:** Axial view of the abdominal wall at the level of the cord insertion in two fetuses at 12 **(A)** and 13 **(B)** weeks of gestation. Note the presence of a large omphalocele (*asterisks*) with liver and bowel content in both fetuses. In fetus **A** the stomach is partly in the omphalocele, whereas in fetus **B** the stomach has completely protruded into the omphalocele. Sp, spine.

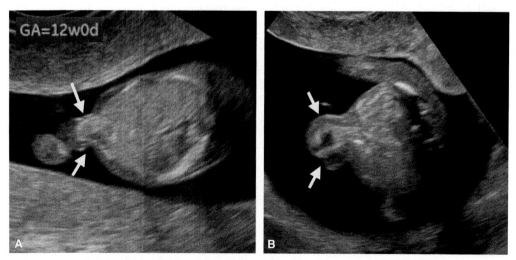

**Figure 12.16:** Axial view of the abdominal wall at the level of the cord insertion in two fetuses at 12 **(A)** and 13 **(B)** weeks of gestation. Note the presence of a small omphalocele (*arrows*) in fetus **A** and **B**, with only bowel content. Trisomy 18 was diagnosed in both fetuses.

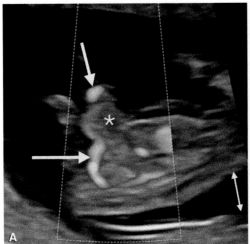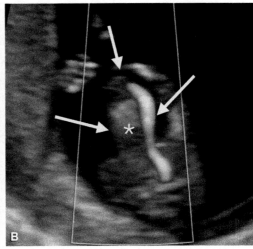

**Figure 12.17:** Sagittal **(A)** and axial **(B)** planes of the mid-abdomen in color Doppler in a fetus at 12 weeks of gestation with trisomy 18. Note the presence of a small omphalocele (*asterisk*) in **A** and **B** and a thickened nuchal translucency (*double headed arrow*) in **A**. The use of color Doppler is helpful because it shows the umbilical cord arising from the top of the omphalocele in **A** (*arrow*) (compare with Fig. 12.12A) and a single umbilical artery in **B** (*arrow*).

additional anomalies of the heart, brain, kidneys, and spine. On occasion, the omphalocele can be as large or even larger than the abdominal circumference (Fig. 12.15). Follow-up of a first trimester isolated small omphalocele with a normal karyotype and nuchal translucency into the late second trimester is important because resolution of such cases has been documented in about 58% of fetuses.[7] The presence of the liver in the omphalocele precludes resolution.

### Associated Malformations

Associated anomalies are common and are present in the majority of omphaloceles.[6] Cardiac malformations are the most common associated structural abnormalities, and detailed cardiac imaging is thus recommended when an omphalocele is diagnosed in the first trimester[6,8] (see Chapter 11). Chromosomal abnormalities, commonly trisomies 18, 13, and 21, are seen in about 50% of cases diagnosed in the first trimester.[8] Omphaloceles associated with chromosomal abnormalities are typically small, with thickened nuchal translucency and other fetal structural abnormalities. Trisomy 18 represents the most common chromosomal abnormality in fetuses with omphaloceles. Large omphaloceles containing liver were assumed not to be commonly associated with aneuploidy,[9] but recent studies do not support this observation. In a recently published large study on 108,982 fetuses including 870 fetuses with abnormal karyotypes, omphalocele was found in 260 fetuses for a prevalence of 1:419.[10] The majority of omphaloceles (227/260 [87.3%]) had bowel as the only content, with only 33/260 (12.7%) containing liver. In this study, the rate of aneuploidy in association with an omphalocele was 40% (106/260), and this rate was independent from the omphalocele content. The most common aneuploidy was trisomy 18 (55%), followed by trisomy 13 (24%), whereas trisomy 21, triploidy, and others were found in 6%, 5%, and 7%, respectively.[10] The presence of a genetic

syndrome should be considered in the presence of an isolated omphalocele with a normal karyotype. Beckwith–Wiedemann syndrome, reported to be present in about 20% of isolated omphaloceles, should be considered especially if first trimester biochemical markers of aneuploidy, such as β-human chorionic gonadotropin and pregnancy-associated plasma protein-A values, are elevated[11] (Fig. 12.18). The diagnosis of Beckwith–Wiedemann syndrome is typically suspected in the second and third trimester when an omphalocele is seen in association with macroglossia, polyhydramnios, renal and liver enlargements, and a thickened placenta called mesenchymal dysplasia of the placenta. Associated ultrasound findings that suggest the presence of a genetic syndrome in omphaloceles are rarely seen in the first trimester. Differential diagnosis of ventral wall defects is summarized in Table 12.1.

## Gastroschisis

### Definition

Gastroschisis is a full-thickness, paraumbilical defect of the anterior abdominal wall with herniation of the fetal bowel into the amniotic cavity (Figs. 12.19 and 12.20). The defect is typically located to the right side of the umbilical cord insertion (Fig. 12.21). The herniated bowel is without a covering membrane and is freely exposed to the amniotic fluid. Gastroschisis has traditionally been regarded as a vascular lesion resulting from compromise of the right umbilical vein (UV) or the omphalomesenteric artery, with resultant ischemic injury of the abdominal wall. Recent theories challenge this pathogenesis and propose that gastroschisis results from faulty embryogenesis with failure of incorporation of the yolk sac and vitelline structures into the umbilical stalk, resulting in an abdominal wall defect, through which the midgut egresses into the amniotic cavity.[12] Gastroschisis is more common in pregnant women of young age.[13] Unlike omphalocele,

## Beckwith-Wiedemann Syndrome

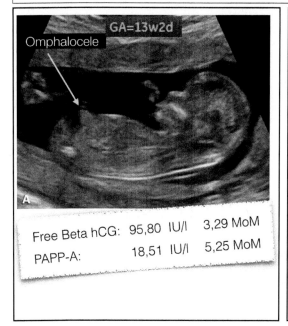

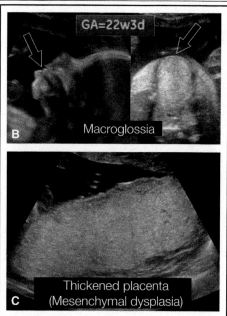

**Figure 12.18:** Fetus with Beckwith–Wiedemann syndrome. At 13 weeks of gestation a small omphalocele with bowel content was detected, as shown in a midsagittal plane of the fetus in **A**. In addition, free β human chorionic gonadotropin (hCG) and pregnancy-associated plasma protein-A were elevated. Chorionic villous sampling revealed a normal karyotype. At 22 weeks of gestation, no omphalocele was found but macroglossia was noted as shown in a midsagittal and coronal planes of the face in **B** (*arrows*). The placenta also appeared thickened at 22 weeks of gestation, suggesting mesenchymal dysplasia **(C)**. Sonographic signs were suggestive of Beckwith–Wiedemann syndrome, which was confirmed postnatally with molecular genetics.

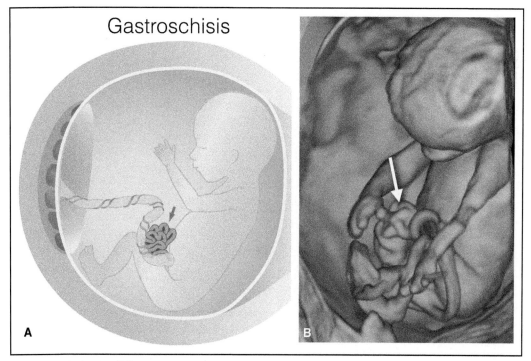

**Figure 12.19:** Schematic drawing **(A)** and corresponding 3D ultrasound image in surface mode of a fetus at 13 weeks of gestation with gastroschisis. Note in **A** and **B** the presence of bowel loops anterior to the abdominal wall (*arrows*). There is no covering sac around the bowel and the surface of herniated bowel appears irregular.

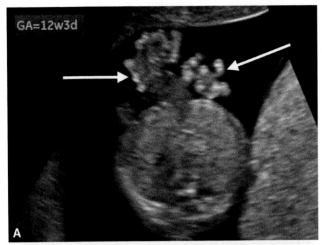

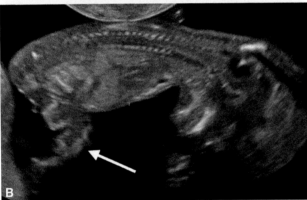

**Figure 12.20:** Axial **(A)** and sagittal **(B)** views of a fetus with a gastroschisis at 12 weeks of gestation. Note in **A** and **B** the presence of fetal bowel outside of the abdominal cavity (*arrows*). Also note that the herniated bowel loops appear irregular (*arrow*).

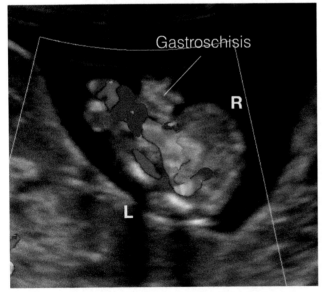

**Figure 12.21:** Axial view in color Doppler of the fetal abdomen in a fetus at 12 weeks of gestation with gastroschisis. Note the normally inserted umbilical cord into the abdomen to the left of the gastroschisis defect. L, left; R, right.

gastroschisis is rarely associated with chromosomal or structural abnormalities. There has been an increase in the prevalence of gastroschisis worldwide.[13]

### Ultrasound Findings

Prenatal diagnosis on ultrasound can be achieved after 11 weeks of gestation and is based on the visualization of the herniated, free-floating, bowel loops in the amniotic cavity with no covering sac (Figs. 12.19 to 12.23). The superior surface (dome) of the herniated bowel in gastroschisis appears irregular on ultrasound examination (like a cauliflower), an important differentiating feature from omphalocele, which typically has a smooth surface (compare Fig. 12.12 with 12.19). Color Doppler helps in identifying the normally inserting umbilical cord into the fetal abdomen, commonly to the left of the herniated bowel (Fig. 12.21). 3D and transvaginal ultrasound are helpful in the demonstration and documentation of detailed anatomic findings in gastroschisis (Figs. 12.19, 12.22, 12.23).

### Associated Malformations

Large series of fetal gastroschisis have shown additional unrelated fetal malformations and chromosomal aneuploidy in 12% and 1.2%, respectively.[14] The presence of hyperechoic bowel loops in the first trimester may represent bowel underperfusion, and follow-up of such cases into the second and third trimester is recommended to assess for the presence of bowel atresia.[15] Follow-up ultrasound examination in later gestation is also recommended given the association of gastroschisis with fetal growth restriction and oligohydramnios.

## Pentalogy of Cantrell and Ectopia Cordis

### Definition

Pentalogy of Cantrell is a syndrome encompassing five anomalies: midline supraumbilical abdominal defect, defect of the lower sternum, defect in the diaphragmatic pericardium, deficiency of the anterior diaphragm, and intracardiac abnormalities. The presence of an omphalocele and displacement of the heart partially or completely outside the chest (ectopia cordis) are hallmarks of this syndrome (Fig. 12.24). The structural abnormalities in Pentalogy of Cantrell show a wide spectrum, but the outcome primarily depends on the size of the chest and abdominal wall defects and the type of cardiac malformations. The location of the omphalocele on the abdominal wall is important, and close attention should be given to that during the ultrasound examination. Typically, omphaloceles are located in the mid-abdominal wall region at the level of the umbilical cord insertions. A higher position of an omphalocele on the abdominal wall can be suggestive for the presence of a supraumbilical abdominal defect, which is likely to be part of Pentalogy of Cantrell even in the absence of ectopia cordis.

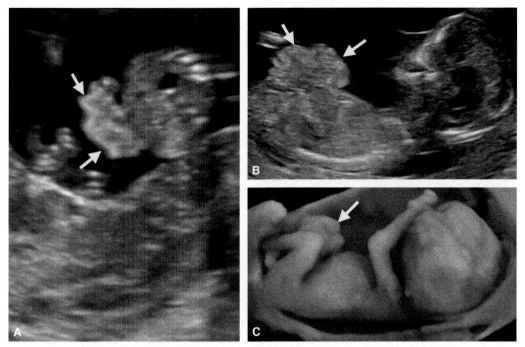

**Figure 12.22:** Axial **(A)**, sagittal **(B)** views in two-dimensional ultrasound and corresponding three-dimensional ultrasound surface mode **(C)** of a fetus at 13 weeks of gestation with gastroschisis. Note the irregular surface appearance of the herniated bowel loops (*arrows*), which is typical for gastroschisis.

Ectopia cordis is an anomaly where the heart is partially or completely located outside the thorax. It is often found together with a Pentalogy of Cantrell, with body stalk anomaly,[16] but can be isolated as well, in the presence of a split sternum with closed abdominal wall or in the presence of amniotic band syndrome.

## Ultrasound Findings

The prenatal diagnosis of Pentalogy of Cantrell is easily made in the first trimester by the demonstration of the omphalocele and ectopia cordis (**Figs. 12.24 and 12.25**). The midsagittal view of the chest and abdomen is optimal

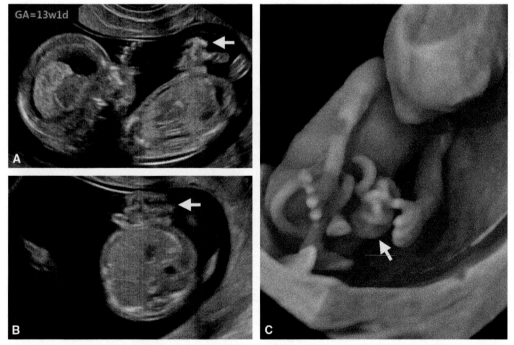

**Figure 12.23:** Parasagittal **(A)** and axial **(B)** views in two-dimensional ultrasound and corresponding three-dimensional (3D) ultrasound in surface mode **(C)** of a fetus at 13 weeks of gestation with gastroschisis. Note that the herniated bowel (*arrows*) is echogenic in **A** and **B**. **C:** Free bowel loops on 3D ultrasound. Bowel dilation in gastroschisis is first evident in the second trimester of pregnancy.

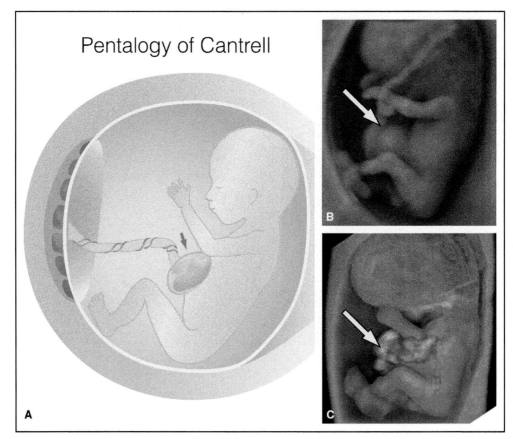

**Figure 12.24:** Schematic drawing **(A)** and corresponding 3D ultrasound image in surface mode **(B)** and glass-body mode **(C)** in a fetus at 11 weeks of gestation with Pentalogy of Cantrell. Note the presence of a high omphalocele with ectopia cordis (*arrows*). Ectopia cordis could be partial or complete (complete in this case). Pentalogy of Cantrell is often associated with a cardiac anomaly (see text for details).

because it demonstrates the abdominal wall defect and the ectopia cordis in one plane (Figs. 12.26 to 12.28). Typically, the omphalocele is large, is positioned high on the abdominal wall, and contains liver (Figs. 12.24 to 12.28). The lower part of the abdomen appears normal. In a sagittal or axial view, the heart appears to be partly or completely protruding toward the omphalocele (Figs. 12.24 and 12.25). 3D ultrasound in surface mode can show the high position of the omphalocele and demonstrate ectopia cordis (Fig. 12.24). Once the diagnosis of Pentalogy of Cantrell

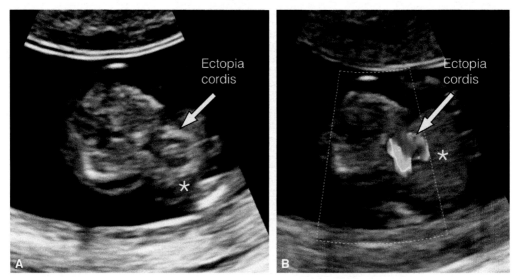

**Figure 12.25:** Axial views at the level of the thorax in gray scale **(A)** and color Doppler **(B)** in a fetus at 11 weeks of gestation with Pentalogy of Cantrell. Note the prisence of an omphalocele (*asterisks*) with ectopia cordis (*arrows*).

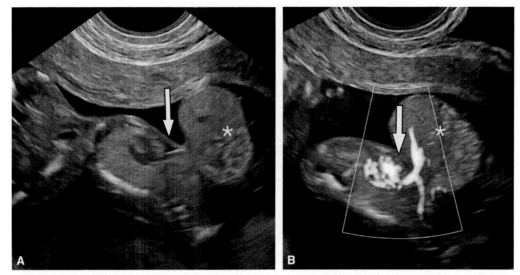

**Figure 12.26:** Sagittal views at the level of the thorax and abdomen in gray scale **(A)** and color Doppler **(B)** in a fetus at 13 weeks of gestation with a mild form of Pentalogy of Cantrell with partial ectopia cordis. Note the presence of a high omphalocele (*asterisks*), inferiorly displaced heart, pericardial defect, and an anterior defect in the chest (*arrow*).

is made, identifying the associated cardiac malformation is important for patient counseling. This can be challenging in the first trimester given the presence of ectopia cordis and cardiac malrotation. A follow-up ultrasound at around 14 to 15 weeks of gestation is helpful in confirming the associated type of cardiac abnormality. One study noted that the degree of cardiac protrusion tends to regress with advancing gestation (Fig. 12.28).[17]

The diagnosis of an isolated ectopia cordis has been reported in the first trimester as well. In general, it is rather rare, however. In a series of seven cases of ectopia cordis, Sepulveda et al. noted only one isolated case, whereas in the remaining cases Pentalogy of Cantrell and body stalk anomaly were associated findings.[16] The diagnosis of a heart outside of the thoracic cavity can be performed even earlier than 11

weeks of gestation. Associated intracardiac and extracardiac anomalies are common.[18]

## Associated Abnormalities

Enlarged nuchal translucency and cystic hygroma have been reported in association with Pentalogy of Cantrell.[16] Many associated fetal malformations have also been reported to include neural tube defects, encephalocele, craniofacial defects, and limb defects among others. Chromosomal anomalies can be present, and invasive procedure should be offered.[16] When the full spectrum of Pentalogy of Cantrell is present, the prognosis is typically poor, with neonatal mortality reported in the range of 60% to 90%. In fetuses with variants of the syndrome, prognosis is improved.

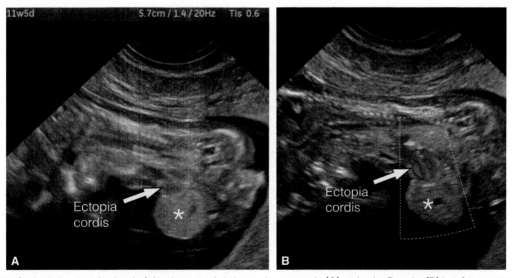

**Figure 12.27:** Sagittal views at the level of the thorax and abdomen in gray scale **(A)** and color Doppler **(B)** in a fetus at 11 weeks of gestation with Pentalogy of Cantrell. Note the presence of a high omphalocele (*asterisks*) with ectopia cordis (*arrows*).

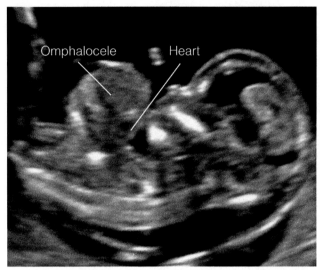

**Figure 12.28:** Sagittal view of the fetal chest and abdomen in a fetus at 12 weeks of gestation with a high omphalocele and ectopia cordis (heart) as part of Pentalogy of Cantrell. This fetus was also found to have tetralogy of Fallot. Upon follow-up ultrasound examinations in the late second and third trimesters, the fetal heart retracted into the chest. The newborn underwent corrective surgery and is currently alive and well.

## Body Stalk Anomaly

### Definition

Body stalk anomaly is a severe abnormality resulting from failure of formation of the body stalk and involves a combination of multiple malformations to include the thoracoabdominal wall (Figs. 12.29 and 12.30), craniofacial structures, spine, and extremities.[19] The umbilical cord is either very short or absent (Fig. 12.31). Typically, the abdominal organs lie in a sac outside the abdominal cavity and are covered by amnion and placental tissue (Figs. 12.29 and 12.30). In a study involving 17 cases of body stalk anomalies diagnosed at a median gestational age of 12 + 3 weeks, liver and bowel herniation into the coelomic cavity, along with an intact amniotic sac containing the rest of the fetus and normal amount of amniotic fluid, was noted in all fetuses.[20] Additionally, absent or short umbilical cord and severe kyphoscoliosis and positional abnormalities of the lower limbs were common associated findings.[20] The authors noted that examination of the amniotic membrane continuity, content of both the amniotic sac and coelomic cavity, and short or absent umbilical cord help in differentiating this condition from other abdominal wall defects.[20]

Although body stalk anomaly is not primarily related to the gastrointestinal anomalies, the associated abdominal/chest wall defect is quite large, which typically leads to the initial suspicion of the defect. The embryogenesis of this anomaly is primarily related to defective development of the germinal disc, probably because of a vascular insult, resulting in amnion rupture with amniotic band-type defects.[19,21] Three main types of malformations in body stalk anomaly include body wall defects, limb deformities/amputations, and craniofacial defects. The conditions affecting the spine such as sacral agenesis or interrupted spine are discussed separately in Chapter 14.

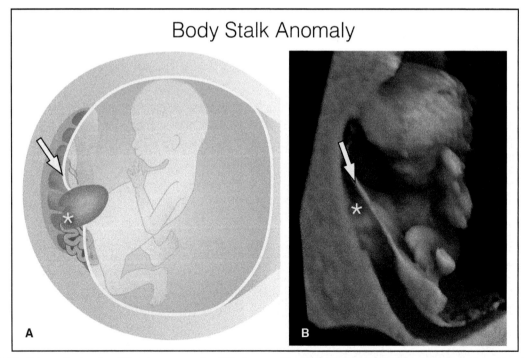

**Figure 12.29:** Schematic drawing **(A)** and corresponding 3D ultrasound image in surface mode **(B)** in a fetus at 11 weeks of gestation with a body stalk anomaly. Note the presence of a large anterior wall defect, with a nearly absent umbilical cord. The fetus is stuck to the placenta, and the whole body is severely deformed (see also Fig. 12.30). Also note that the fetal liver and bowel (*asterisks*) are outside of the amniotic cavity. *Arrows* point to the amniotic membrane.

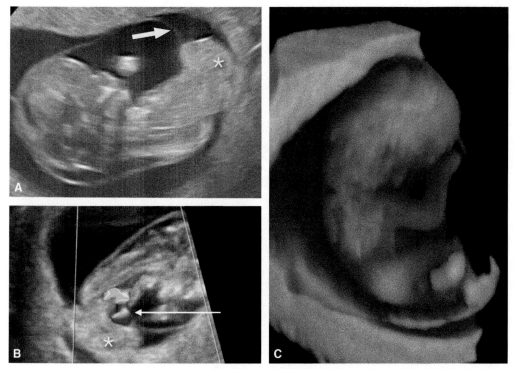

**Figure 12.30:** Two-dimensional ultrasound in gray scale **(A)** and color Doppler **(B)** along with the corresponding three-dimensional ultrasound in surface mode **(C)** in a fetus at 11 weeks of gestation with a body stalk anomaly. Note that the liver is outside the amniotic cavity (*asterisks* in **A** and **B**). The *yellow arrow* points to the amniotic membrane in **A**. There is also ectopia cordis noted in **B** on color Doppler (*long white arrow*). Body deformity is noted on the three-dimensional ultrasound in **C**.

## Ultrasound Findings

The ultrasound diagnosis of body stalk anomaly is generally straightforward, and the anomaly can be detected even before 11 weeks of gestation. A large chest and abdominal wall defect with massive evisceration of organs is seen on ultrasound along with spinal abnormalities such as kyphoscoliosis (**Figs. 12.29 and 12.30**). Because of severe anatomic distortion, a midsagittal plane of the fetus is typically not possible (**Fig. 12.30**). The presence of a

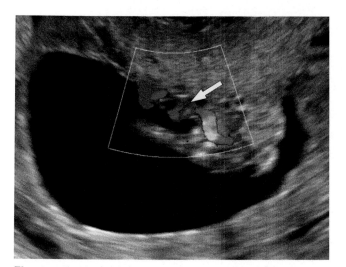

**Figure 12.31:** Axial view in color Doppler of the fetal abdomen in a fetus with body stalk anomaly at 12 weeks of gestation. Note the presence of a short cord (*arrow*). The fetus also had multiple complex malformations.

very short or absent cord and the proximity of the fetus to the placenta help to confirm the diagnosis (**Fig. 12.31**). 3D ultrasound in surface mode and in multiplanar display of the whole fetus is ideal in order to demonstrate the complete picture of this severe anomaly (**Figs. 12.29 and 12.30**). On many occasions, body stalk anomaly is easier to diagnose in the first trimester. In the second and third trimesters, the associated presence of oligohydramnios and fetal crowding makes the diagnosis of body stalk anomaly more challenging. Occasionally, a body stalk anomaly is associated with amniotic bands, which can be visualized on transvaginal ultrasound by the demonstration of reflective membranes connected to the wall defect.

## Associated Malformations

Associated malformations are many, include all organ systems, and are features of body stalk anomaly. Neural defects, facial deformities, and skeletal abnormalities are common. On occasion, a lower extremity is partly or completely absent. Anomalies of the chest and abdominal walls are nearly always present. In addition, a thickened nuchal translucency is found in most cases. Fetal karyotype is usually normal, and body stalk anomaly is uniformly fatal.

## Cloacal Exstrophy and OEIS Syndrome

Cloacal exstrophy is a spectrum of malformations with its severity related to the time of embryologic disruption in the development of the genitourinary system. Epispadia represents the milder

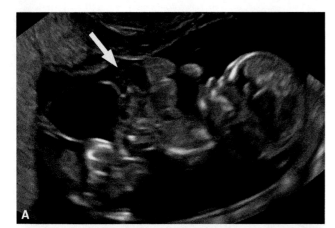

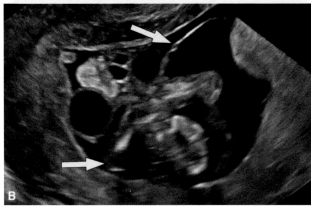

**Figure 12.32:** Ultrasound images of a fetus at 12 weeks of gestation with OEIS. OEIS includes the presence of an **O**mphalocele, **E**xstrophy of the bladder, **I**mperforate anus, and **S**pinal defect. OEIS is the most severe form of body stalk anomaly with parts of the body missing and others outside of the amniotic cavity. Note the presence of severe body deformity and a significant part of the embryo outside of the amniotic cavity in **A** and **B**. *Arrows* point to the amniotic membrane.

form and bladder/cloacal exstrophy represents the severe form of cloacal exstrophy spectrum. The association of cloacal exstrophy with imperforate anus, omphalocele, and vertebral defects has often been referred to as OEIS complex. OEIS therefore represents the combination of omphalocele, exstrophy of the bladder, imperforate anus, and spinal defects (Figs. 12.32 and 12.33). Often, the appearance can be suggestive of a body stalk anomaly, severe sacral agenesis with spinal defects or a cloaca, and the first trimester diagnosis can therefore be technically difficult.

In a series involving 12 cases of OEIS reported in the literature, all had exstrophy of the bladder.[22] Neural tube defects, omphalocele, and anal atresia were found in 10/12, 9/12, and 9/12 cases, respectively.[22] Vertebral defects, along with lower extremity abnormalities, were found in less than half of cases.[22] Additional malformations involved central nervous system, cardiac, and renal organs. All fetuses in this series had normal karyotype.[22] OEIS complex is rare, with an incidence ranging from 1/200,000 to 1/400,000.[23,24] Almost all cases of OEIS occur sporadically.[25]

## GASTROINTESTINAL OBSTRUCTIONS

The following gastrointestinal obstructions are commonly diagnosed in the second trimester of pregnancy, and their sonographic features are rarely identified before the 14th week of gestation. We are hereby listing them for completion sake. Despite reported cases of gastrointestinal obstruction diagnosed in the first trimester, the authors believe that these represent the exception rather than the rule because most cases of gastrointestinal obstruction are associated with normal first trimester ultrasound. Detailed presentation of ultrasound

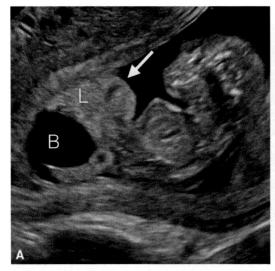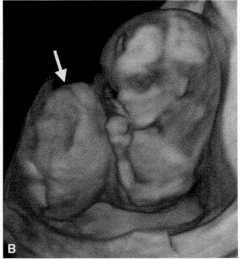

**Figure 12.33:** Sagittal views in gray scale **(A)** and the corresponding three-dimensional ultrasound in surface mode in **B** in a fetus with OEIS complex (see Fig. 12.32 for explanation) at 13 weeks of gestation. Note the presence of major body deformities with absence of the majority of the lower body. A large abdominal wall defect *(arrow)* is noted with liver (L) and bladder (B) stuck to the uterine wall.

findings, associated malformations, and outcome is beyond the scope of this chapter.

## Esophageal Atresia

The classic sonographic features of esophageal atresia in the second and third trimester of pregnancy, such as an empty stomach and polyhydramnios, are not seen in the first trimester. The stomach in the first trimester of pregnancy is primarily filled because of gastric secretions, and polyhydramnios is seen in the late second and third trimester of pregnancy. A normally filled stomach in the upper left abdomen therefore does not exclude esophageal atresia in the first trimester. Indeed, the authors have observed normal sonographic anatomy of the gastrointestinal tract in the first trimester in fetuses that were later diagnosed with esophageal atresia in the second trimester of pregnancy. In pregnancies at high risk for esophageal atresia because of a prior family history or in the presence of associated anomalies, we recommend direct visualization of the esophagus as a continuous hyperechogenic structure (Fig. 12.34), rather than looking for indirect signs such as stomach filling. The two reported cases of first trimester diagnosis of esophageal atresia were associated with duodenal atresia.[26,27]

## Duodenal Atresia

The prenatal diagnosis of duodenal atresia is occasionally possible in the first trimester, and few case reports have described the appearance of the classic double bubble sign (dilated stomach and proximal duodenum) in the first and early second trimester of pregnancy.[28] An associated esophageal atresia was present in few reported cases in the literature.[26,27] The authors are cautious about making the diagnosis of duodenal atresia in the first trimester given the scarcity of follow-up data on this subject. When duodenal atresia is suspected in the first trimester (Fig. 12.35), risk assessment for aneuploidy should be performed and follow-up ultrasound examinations into the second trimester are recommended before a final diagnosis is attained. In our experience, most cases of duodenal atresia are evident after the 23rd week of gestation.

## Anorectal Atresia

The prenatal diagnosis of anorectal atresia is a challenge in the second and third trimester of pregnancy because several cases escape prenatal identification. Interestingly, sonographic markers of anorectal atresia in the first trimester have been reported.[29–32] The detection of an anechoic sausage-shaped structure in the lower abdomen in the first trimester, representing a dilated colon or rectum (Fig. 12.36), can be a clue to the presence of anorectal atresia.[29–31,33] Commonly, this marker resolves in the second trimester and often reappears in the third trimester of pregnancy. The presence of other fetal abnormalities increases the risk for an associated anorectal atresia, especially when a VATER (Vertebral anomaly, Anorectal atresia, Trachea-Esophageal fistula, and Renal anomaly) association is suspected[33] (Fig. 12.36). The risk for associated

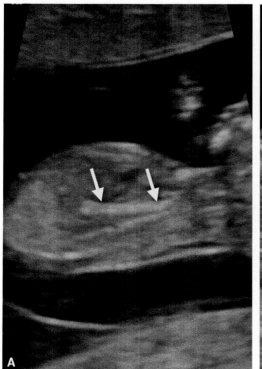
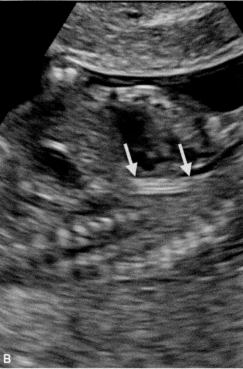

**Figure 12.34:** Transabdominal **(A)** and transvaginal **(B)** parasagittal ultrasound images of the chest and upper abdomen in two fetuses at 13 weeks of gestation demonstrating echogenic esophagus (*arrows*). High-resolution ultrasound transducers enable imaging of the esophagus in early gestation.

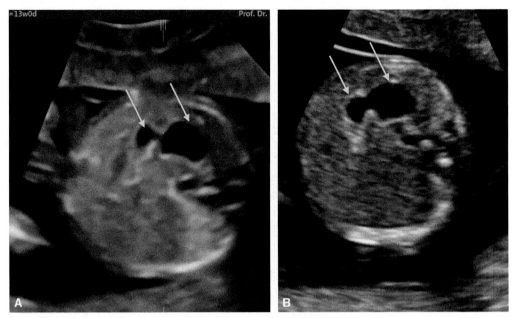

**Figure 12.35:** Axial views of the abdomen in a fetus at 13 weeks of gestation demonstrating a "double bubble" (*arrows*). **A and B:** Two phases of stomach peristalsis. Follow-up ultrasound examination at 17 weeks of gestation noted absence of the double bubble and workup revealed normal karyotypic analysis. Note in **A** and **B** that the "double bubble" does not cross the midline of the abdomen.

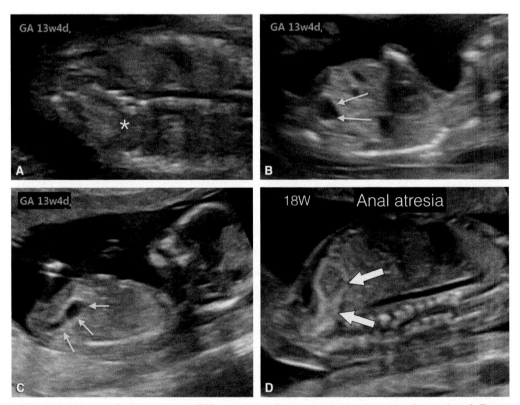

**Figure 12.36:** Ultrasound images of a fetus with a VATER association, first suspected at 13 weeks of gestation. **A:** The presence of hemivertebra (*asterisk*) at 13 weeks of gestation. **B:** A cystic structure in the lower abdomen (*arrows*) at 13 weeks of gestation. **C:** A sagittal view of the abdomen and pelvis showing the cystic structure as a dilated rectum with echogenic borders (*arrows*). **D:** A sagittal view of the pelvis at 18 weeks of gestation demonstrating the rectum and colon with increased echogenic borders (*arrows*), suggesting the presence of anal atresia. The bowel echogenicity disappeared on follow-up ultrasound with advancing gestation. Postnatally, VATER association and anal atresia were confirmed.

gastrointestinal obstruction is increased when single umbilical artery, absent kidney, hemivertebra, and/or other malformations are noted (Fig. 12.36). In a metaanalysis of 33 fetuses with intraabdominal cysts in the first trimester of pregnancy, four had anorectal malformations at birth.[33]

## OTHER GASTROINTESTINAL SYSTEM ABNORMALITIES

### Abnormal Abdominal Situs

An accurate comprehensive examination of the abdominal situs is recommended during the ultrasound examination in the first trimester (Fig. 12.37). The presence of abnormal abdominal situs is an important aspect of fetal anatomy survey because it can be a clue to the presence of heterotaxy and complex congenital heart disease (Fig. 12.38). Abdominal situs abnormality is first suspected when the stomach is not located in the left abdominal cavity (Fig. 12.38) or in the presence of abnormal venous connections (Fig. 12.39).

### Echogenic Bowel

The diagnosis of echogenic bowel in the first trimester is similar to that in the second trimester and is based on bowel echogenicity equal to bone (Fig. 12.40). This is a subjective assessment that is tricky in the first trimester, especially when transvaginal ultrasound is used, because enhanced tissue resolution provides for increased bowel echogenicity under normal conditions (Fig. 12.41). In order to avoid false-positive diagnosis, the authors recommend that the diagnosis of

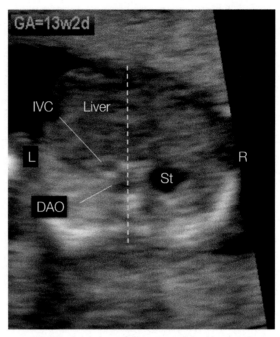

**Figure 12.38:** Axial view of the upper abdomen showing abnormal abdominal situs in a fetus with right isomerism suspected because of a complex cardiac anomaly at 13 weeks of gestation. Note the presence of a right-sided stomach (St), whereas the descending aorta (DAO), inferior vena cava (IVC), and liver are left sided. L, left; R, right.

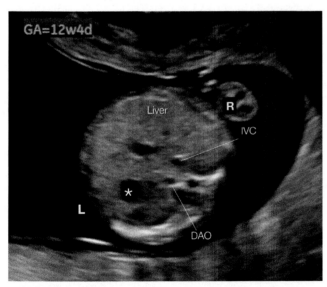

**Figure 12.37:** Axial view of the upper abdomen in a normal fetus at 12 weeks of gestation, imaged by high-resolution transvaginal ultrasound. The stomach (*asterisk*) and the descending aorta (DAO) are left sided, whereas the inferior vena cava (IVC) and liver are right sided. This plane is visualized routinely in order to exclude situs anomalies, especially if a cardiac defect has been suspected. L, left; R, right.

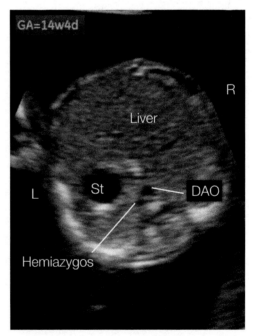

**Figure 12.39:** Axial view of the upper abdomen, obtained with high-resolution transvaginal scanning, showing abnormal abdominal situs in a fetus with left isomerism suspected because of a complex cardiac anomaly at 14 weeks of gestation. Note the presence of a left-sided stomach (St), an interrupted inferior vena cava, and a hemiazygos vein continuation shown to the left of the descending aorta (DAO). L, left; R, right.

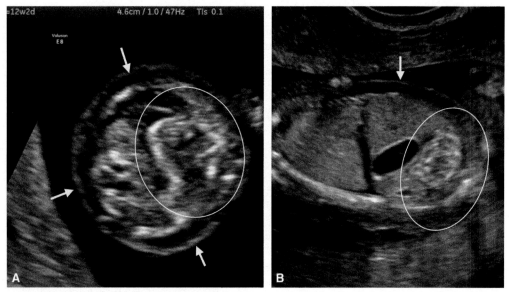

**Figure 12.40:** Axial view **(A)** at 12 weeks of gestation and parasagittal view **(B)** at 13 weeks of gestation in two fetuses with echogenic bowel (*circle*) and trisomy 21. Note that the bowel is as bright as bone and the presence of hydropic skin (*arrows*) in both fetuses. Echogenic bowel in trisomy 21 is rarely an isolated finding.

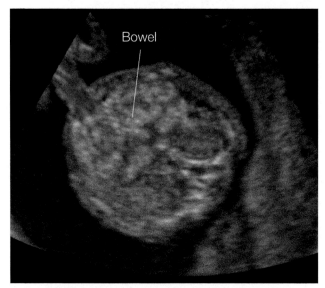

**Figure 12.41:** Axial view of the fetal abdomen at 13 weeks of gestation obtained with transvaginal ultrasound. Note that the bowel is echogenic because of the high resolution of the ultrasound transducer. Differentiating echogenic bowel from normal bright bowel in early gestation can be challenging, especially when high-resolution transducers are used in transvaginal scanning.

echogenic bowel in the first trimester be reserved for bowel that is unequivocally as bright as bone and a follow-up ultrasound examination is performed. Workup includes risk assessment and/or diagnostic testing for genetic abnormalities, screening for infectious etiologies, and detailed anatomic survey.

### Intraabdominal Cysts

The presence of intraabdominal cysts in the fetus can be detected by ultrasound in the first trimester[34–36] as anechoic structures in the fetal abdomen that are distinct from the stomach and bladder (Fig. 12.42). The shape, location, size, and content of the cyst(s)

reveal its possible etiology. Abdominal cysts that are present in the liver are typically circular and tend to resolve spontaneously by the second trimester (Fig. 12.43). Occasionally, a remnant echogenic intrahepatic focus can be seen following resolution (Fig. 12.43). Intraabdominal cysts in the lower abdomen, especially with abnormal shape and echogenic content, are commonly bowel in origin and may be related to an abnormal genitourinary system such as a cloaca (Figs. 12.44 to 12.46) or an anorectal atresia[33] (Fig. 12.36). Often, upon follow-up of lower abdominal cysts that are suspected to be related to abnormal genitourinary system, echogenic debris are found as evidence for enterolithiasis (Fig. 12.46). The presence of peristalsis in an intraabdominal cyst suggests a gastrointestinal origin. A large dilated cystic structure in the lower abdomen may represent a dilated bladder related to an obstructed urethra (see Chapter 13). Omphalomesenteric cysts can originate in the abdomen and migrate into the umbilical cord (see Chapter 15).[35] Fetal intraabdominal cysts are rare in the first trimester, and in the majority of cases they represent an isolated finding.[33] When isolated, intraabdominal cysts are usually associated with a good prognosis and tend to resolve on follow-up ultrasound in about 80% of cases[33] (Figs. 12.42 and 12.43). Follow-up ultrasound in the second and third trimester is recommended even when resolution of the cysts occurs, given a reported association with anorectal and other gastrointestinal malformations.[33,36]

## INTRAABDOMINAL ARTERIAL AND VENOUS ABNORMALITIES

### Normal Sonographic Anatomy

The fetal vascular anatomy of the umbilical, hepatic, and portal venous systems along with the IVC is complex, because of small vasculature, the presence of normal anatomic variations, and the close spatial relationship of the vessels.

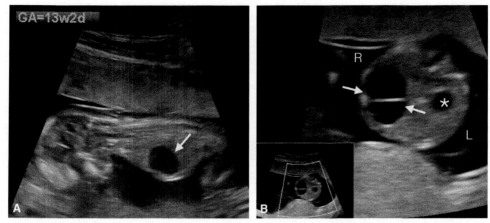

**Figure 12.42:** Sagittal **(A)** and axial **(B)** views of a fetus at 13 weeks of gestation with a large intrahepatic cyst (*arrows*). The stomach is seen in **B** (*asterisk*). Expectant management and follow-up ultrasound at 16 weeks of gestation (Fig. 12.43) showed resolution of cyst. L, left; R, right.

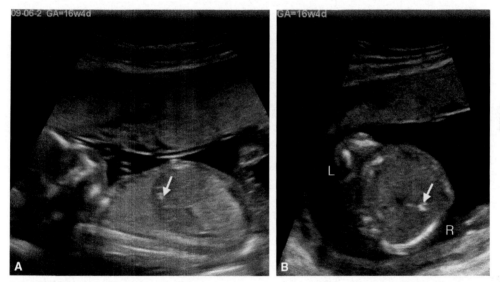

**Figure 12.43:** Sagittal **(A)** and axial **(B)** views of the same fetus in Figure 12.42, now at 16 weeks of gestation. Note the resolution of the large intrahepatic cyst within 3 weeks. An echogenic focus (*arrow*) is now present within the liver. L, left; R, right.

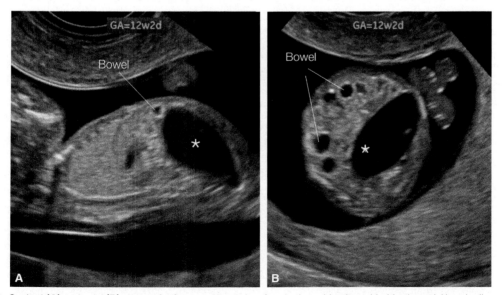

**Figure 12.44:** Sagittal **(A)** and axial **(B)** views of a fetus at 12 weeks of gestation with a large bladder (*asterisk*) and adjacent dilated bowel loops with echogenic walls. These findings are suspicious for bowel obstruction with a fistula into a cloaca. See Figures 12.45 and 12.46.

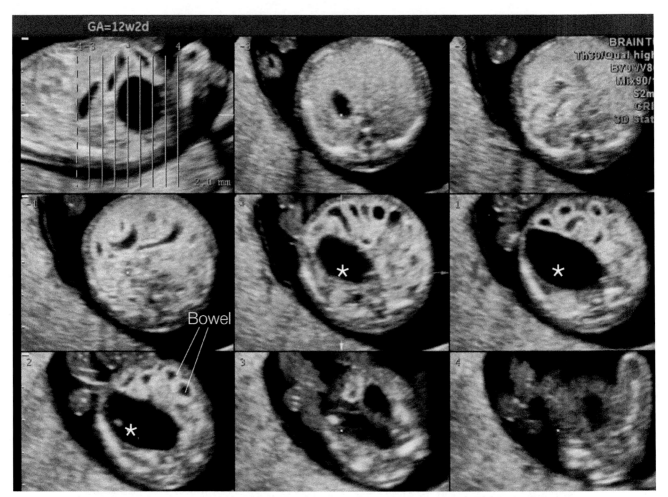

**Figure 12.45:** Three-dimensional ultrasound in tomographic display of a fetus at 12 weeks of gestation with a large bladder (*asterisk*) and dilated bowel loops (same fetus as in Fig. 12.44). Note the presence of multiple dilated bowel loops with echogenic borders.

The umbilical vein (UV) enters the fetal abdomen in the midline and has a short extrahepatic course before entering into the liver with a slight right tilt (Fig. 12.47). The UV drains into a confluence called the portal sinus. The ductus venosus (DV) is a thin hourglass-shaped fetal vessel that connects the UV to the heart. The DV arises from the region of the portal sinus and joins the IVC at the level of the subdiaphragmatic vestibulum (Fig. 12.47). The hepatic veins are the intrinsic

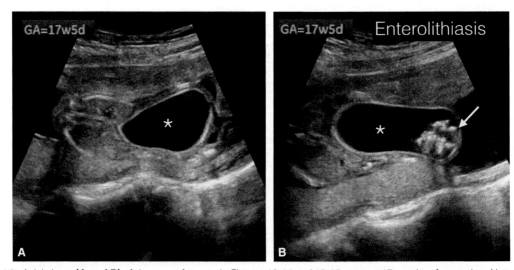

**Figure 12.46:** Axial views (**A and B**) of the same fetus as in Figures 12.44 and 12.45, now at 17 weeks of gestation. Note the presence of a dilated cloaca (*asterisks*) with echogenic wall. **B:** The presence of enterolithiasis with echogenic debris within the cyst (*arrow*).

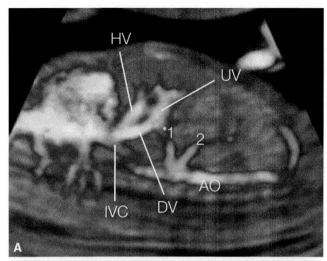

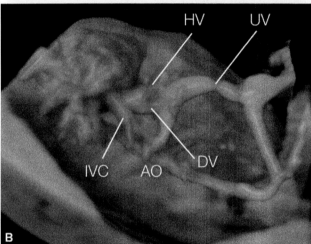

**Figure 12.47:** Sagittal view of the thorax and abdomen in color Doppler **(A)** and in 3D glass-body mode **(B)** in a normal fetus at 13 weeks of gestation, demonstrating the main intraabdominal vasculature. Note that the ductus venosus (DV), the inferior vena cava (IVC), and the left hepatic vein (HV) merge together to enter the heart. From the descending aorta (AO) arise the celiac trunk (*1*) and the superior mesenteric artery (*2*). UV, umbilical vein.

veins of the liver; they converge into three main hepatic veins and join the inferior vena cava (IVC) and DV at the subdiaphragmatic vestibulum, which drains into the right atrium. The IVC in the abdomen courses on the right side of the spine and assumes a more ventral position along the posterior liver surface as it enters the subdiaphragmatic vestibulum.

The descending aorta gives rise to several branches in the abdomen to include, among others, four main ones: the celiac trunk at level of T12 (Fig. 12.47), the superior mesenteric artery at level L1 (Fig. 12.47), the renal arteries at level L1 to L2, and the inferior mesenteric artery at level L3. Three branches arise from the celiac trunk including the common hepatic, splenic, and left gastric artery. The superior mesenteric artery provides several branches to the small bowel and part of large bowel.

Most reports in the literature on the sonographic imaging of the abdominal vasculature are from the second and third trimester of pregnancy. Because of the small size of abdominal

vasculature in early gestation, the sonographic imaging in the first trimester is quite difficult and is only achieved with color Doppler and in optimal imaging conditions. A slightly oblique plane of the abdomen at the level of the liver, pointing toward the left shoulder, is best for the visualization of the three hepatic veins. The DV can be visualized in an axial plane of the upper abdomen, but imaging of the DV in the first trimester is best seen in a midsagittal longitudinal view of the abdomen (Fig. 12.47). In this approach, the junction between the DV and the UV is seen, and the narrow size of the DV is appreciated (Fig. 12.47). Because of its narrow and short size, visualization of the DV is facilitated by the use of color Doppler, which reveals the presence of color aliasing, an important feature that helps in the identification of DV (Figs. 12.47 and 3.11). The IVC is visualized by an oblique insonation of the abdomen in a midsagittal view as shown in Figure 3.12. The celiac trunk with its hepatic artery branch along with the superior mesenteric artery is best seen when the fetus is in a dorsoposterior position and the aorta is in a horizontal orientation (Figs. 12.8 and 12.47). This fetal orientation allows for flow in the celiac trunk and mesenteric arteries to be parallel to the ultrasound beam, which optimizes visualization (Fig. 12.47). In our experience, the midsagittal plane of the abdomen in low-velocity color Doppler is the most optimal view for the visualization of the main abdominal vasculature to include the UV, DV, IVC, and hepatic artery. For a more detailed discussion on the sonographic anatomy of the intraabdominal venous system, we recommend our two review articles on this subject.[37,38]

## Intraabdominal Venous and Arterial Anomalies

Prenatal reports on anomalies of the abdominal venous system in the first trimester are scarce. In general, there are two groups of abnormalities, one related to anomalies affecting the DV, such as agenesis or the anomalous connections of the DV, and the other related to interruption of the IVC with azygos continuity. These conditions are briefly discussed in the following sections.

### Agenesis or Abnormal Connection of the Ductus Venosus

As known from reports in the second trimester, anomalies of the DV include its complete agenesis (Fig. 12.48) or its anomalous connection to the IVC, hepatic system, other abdominal vasculature, or directly to the right atrium and other sites.[37,38] In general, abnormalities of DV are suspected when the examiner is looking for the DV in a midsagittal plane in color Doppler in order to perform pulse Doppler sampling. There are no large series on the clinical relevance of DV anomalies in the first trimester, but such abnormalities are known to be associated with cardiac defects, aneuploidies such as trisomy 21, 13, 18, Turner syndrome, and syndromic conditions as in Noonan syndrome and others (Figs. 12.49 and 12.50). The risk for aneuploidy is higher when the DV connects at an abnormal level on the IVC (intrahepatic portion) rather than

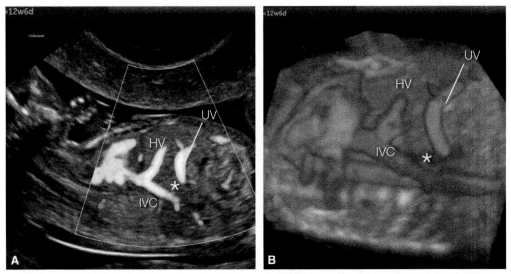

**Figure 12.48:** Sagittal view of the thorax and abdomen in color Doppler **(A)** and in 3D glass-body mode **(B)**, in a fetus at 12 weeks of gestation with agenesis of the ductus venosus (*asterisk*). Compare with the normal abdominal vasculature in Figure 12.47. IVC, inferior vena cava; HV, left hepatic vein; UV, umbilical vein.

in its normal location at the subdiaphragmatic vestibulum (Figs. 12.49 and 12.50).[39] Abnormal direct connection of the UV to the IVC is also associated with increased risk of aneuploidy.[39] In one study on 37 fetuses with trisomy 21, it was shown that 11% of cases had a direct connection of the DV to the intrahepatic portion of the IVC.[39] This observation has also mirrored our clinical experience as we have found similar associations with aneuploidies and Noonan syndrome (Figs. 12.49 and 12.50). Because anomalies of the DV can also be associated with cardiac anomalies, as well as other anomalies of the umbilicoportal system when seen in the first trimester (Fig. 12.51), a careful examination of these two anatomic regions should be performed and follow-up ultrasound in the second trimester is recommended. We propose

a workup of DV or UV abnormalities diagnosed in the first trimester in **Table 12.2**.

## Interruption of the Inferior Vena Cava

Interruption of the IVC with azygos continuation is an anomaly that is commonly seen in the presence of heterotaxy syndrome mainly in left atrial isomerism, but can also occur in isolation.[40] Its detection in the first trimester is very difficult because of the small size of the azygos vein. When suspected in the first trimester by the presence of complex cardiac defects or abnormal situs, color Doppler can reveal the absence of the IVC and the presence of a dilated azygos vein with a course side-by-side to the descending aorta, thus confirming the

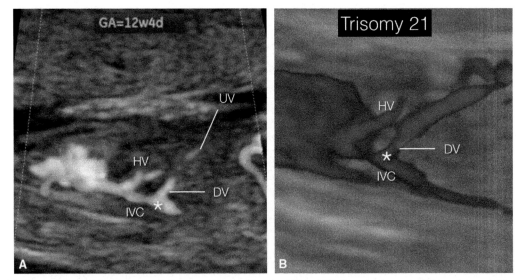

**Figure 12.49:** Sagittal view of the thorax and abdomen in color Doppler **(A)** and 3D glass-body mode **(B)** in a fetus at 12 weeks of gestation with trisomy 21. Note the direct connection (*asterisk*) of the ductus venosus (DV) with the inferior vena cava (IVC) and the separate attachment of the hepatic vein (HV) to the IVC. The fetus also had thickened nuchal translucency (not shown).

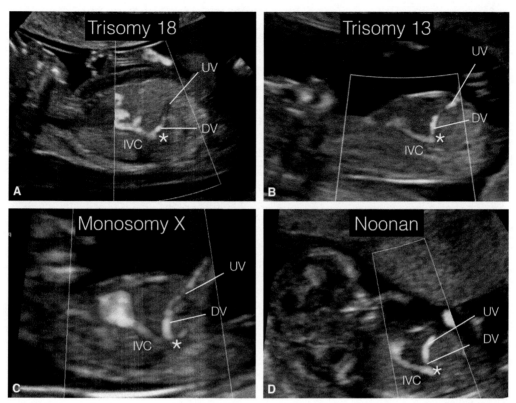

**Figure 12.50:** Sagittal views of the abdomen in color Doppler in four fetuses with trisomy 18 **(A)**, trisomy 13 **(B)**, monosomy X **(C)**, and Noonan syndrome **(D)**, respectively, obtained between 12 and 13 weeks of gestation. Note that all four fetuses **(A–D)** show the direct connection (*asterisks*) of the ductus venosus (DV) or umbilical vein (UV) to the inferior vena cava (IVC). Additional markers of aneuploidy were found in all fetuses.

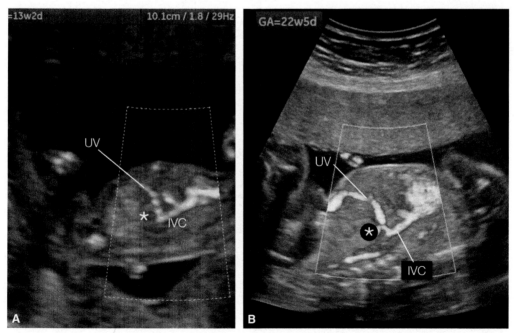

**Figure 12.51:** Sagittal views of the abdomen in color Doppler in the same fetus at 13 weeks of gestation **(A)** and at 22 weeks of gestation **(B)** demonstrating the direct connection (*asterisks*) of the umbilical vein (UV) to the inferior vena cava (IVC). No additional anomalies were found and fetal karyotype was normal. This finding was confirmed at 22 weeks of gestation **(B)**. The portal system was normally developed and abdominal ultrasound after birth showed a closure of the connection and no signs of portosystemic shunt.

## Table 12.2 • Workup of Ductus Venosus and/or Umbilical Vein Abnormalities

Assess the connecting site of the ductus venosus (if present) or umbilical vein (intrahepatic, extrahepatic, iliac, right atrium, etc.)

Check for aneuploidies such as trisomy 21, 13, 18, monosomy X, triploidy, and others

Check for the presence of syndromic sonographic markers (heterotaxy, Noonan syndrome, etc.)

Perform fetal echocardiography to rule out cardiac defects, including venous anomalies

Look for anomalies in other organs (renal, gastrointestinal, skeletal, central nervous system)

Check for the presence of early hydrops, and perform follow-up ultrasound for hydrops development

Assess in the second trimester for the presence of portal venous system abnormalities

Prognosis is good if none of the above additional conditions is present, but postnatal ultrasound of liver vasculature is recommended

Adapted from Chaoui, R, Heling, KS, Karl K. Ultrasound of the fetal veins. Part 1: The intrahepatic venous system. *Ultrasound in Med.* 2014;35:208–238, with permission, Copyright by Thieme Publishers.

diagnosis (Fig. 12.52). The authors have also noticed that in the presence of azygos continuation of an interrupted IVC in the first trimester, increased blood flow in the superior vena cava (SVC) or a persistent left SVC (possible site of drainage of azygos second to SVC) can be demonstrated on color Doppler in the three-vessel trachea view (Fig. 12.52).

### Intraabdominal Arterial Abnormalities

With the exception of the single umbilical artery, further information on anomalies of the other intraabdominal arteries in the first trimester is currently almost nonexistent in the literature. Abnormalities involving the hepatic artery and celiac trunk are probably the easiest to demonstrate in the first trimester. Doppler assessment of the hepatic artery in the first trimester has been described[41] (see Chapter 6). A fistula between the hepatic artery and the UV in a fetus with trisomy 21 presenting with hydrops in early gestation has been described by our group.[42] In addition, we observed three cases with the presence of an additional accessory hepatic artery arising from the aorta, superior to the celiac trunk, coursing along the diaphragm, and entering the liver cranially (Figs. 12.53 and 12.54). In one of the three fetuses, the diagnosis of trisomy 21 was made and in the other two, the finding disappeared likely because of spontaneous closure of the accessory artery. Conditions associated with a single umbilical artery are discussed in Chapter 15.

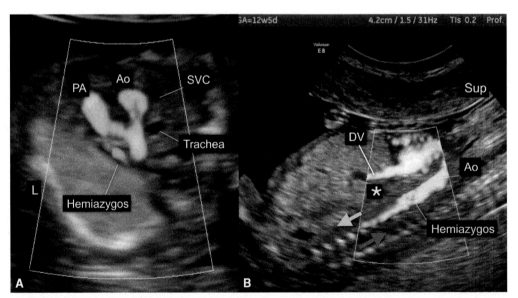

**Figure 12.52:** Three-vessel trachea view **(A)** and sagittal view **(B)** in color Doppler of a fetus at 12 weeks of gestation with a hemiazygos continuation. The fetal heart and stomach are left sided but the four-chamber view (not shown) revealed a cardiac anomaly. The three-vessel trachea view **(A)** shows an atypical vessel to the left of the pulmonary artery (PA), which was found to be the connection of a dilated hemiazygos vein into a persistent left superior vena cava. In the sagittal view **(B)**, the aorta (Ao) and hemiazygos vein are seen side-by-side and the IVC is absent (*asterisk*). The clue to the diagnosis of a hemiazygos (or azygos) is facilitated by color Doppler showing opposite direction of blood flow in the aorta and hemiazygos (*blue* and *red arrows*, respectively). This fetus had left atrial isomerism.

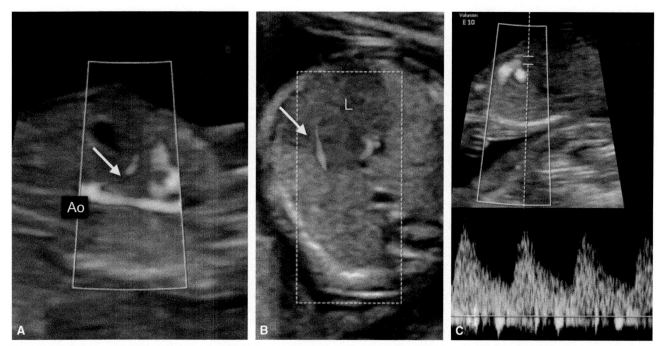

**Figure 12.53: A:** A sagittal view of the fetal abdomen in color Doppler in a fetus at 14 weeks of gestation with an aberrant liver artery (*arrow*) arising from the descending aorta (Ao) with a course toward the surface of the liver. **B:** A cross-section at the level of the diaphragm in the same fetus showing the course of the aberrant liver artery (*arrow*) on the top of the liver (L). **C:** The pulsed Doppler of the aberrant vessel with high arterial velocity. We have seen this condition in fetuses with trisomy 21. On occasions, the aberrant artery obliterates on follow-up ultrasound examination into the second trimester as in this case. See Figure 12.54.

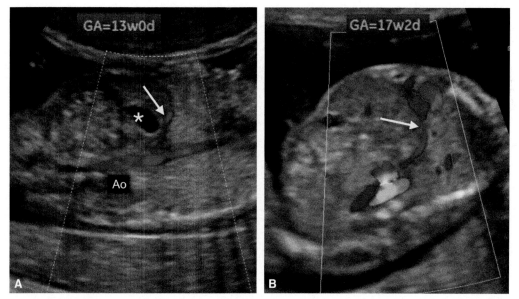

**Figure 12.54: A:** A sagittal view of the fetal abdomen in color Doppler in a fetus at 13 weeks of gestation with an aberrant liver artery (*arrow*) arising from the descending aorta (Ao) with a course toward the surface of the liver. The stomach is well seen (*asterisk*). **B:** A follow-up ultrasound examination at 17 weeks showing the aberrant liver artery (*arrow*). In this case, it persisted until the third trimester and had no postnatal impact on the outcome of the child.

# REFERENCES

1. Bronshtein M, Weiner Z, Abramovici H, et al. Prenatal diagnosis of gall bladder anomalies—report of 17 cases. *Prenat Diagn*. 1993;13:851–861.
2. Bowerman RA. Sonography of fetal midgut herniation: normal size criteria and correlation with crown-rump length. *J Ultrasound Med*. 1993;12:251–254.
3. Blaas HG, Eik-Nes SH, Kiserud T, et al. Early development of the abdominal wall, stomach and heart from 7 to 12 weeks of gestation: a longitudinal ultrasound study. *Ultrasound Obstet Gynecol*. 1995;6:240–249.
4. Chaoui R, Heling K-S. *3D-Ultrasound in Prenatal Diagnosis: A Practical Approach*. 1st ed. New York, NY: DeGruyter; 2016.
5. Syngelaki A, Chelemen T, Dagklis T, et al. Challenges in the diagnosis of fetal non-chromosomal abnormalities at 11–13 weeks. *Prenat Diagn*. 2011;31:90–102.
6. Marshall J, Salemi JL, Tanner JP, et al. Prevalence, correlates, and outcomes of omphalocele in the United States, 1995–2005. *Obstet Gynecol*. 2015;126:284–293.
7. Khalil A, Arnaoutoglou C, Pacilli M, et al. Outcome of fetal exomphalos diagnosed at 11–14 weeks of gestation. *Ultrasound Obstet Gynecol*. 2012;39:401–406.
8. Kagan KO, Staboulidou I, Syngelaki A, et al. The 11–13-week scan: diagnosis and outcome of holoprosencephaly, exomphalos and megacystis. *Ultrasound Obstet Gynecol*. 2010;36:10–14.
9. Groves R, Sunderajan L, Khan AR, et al. Congenital anomalies are commonly associated with exomphalos minor. *J Pediatr Surg*. 2006;41:358–361.
10. Syngelaki A, Guerra L, Ceccacci I, et al. Impact of holoprosencephaly, exomphalos, megacystis and high NT in first trimester screening for chromosomal abnormalities. *Ultrasound Obstet Gynecol*. 2016. doi:10.1002/uog.17286.
11. Wilkins-Haug L, Porter A, Hawley P, et al. Isolated fetal omphalocele, Beckwith-Wiedemann syndrome, and assisted reproductive technologies. *Birth Defects Res Part A Clin Mol Teratol*. 2009;85:58–62.
12. Stephenson JT, Pichakron KO, Vu L, et al. In utero repair of gastroschisis in the sheep (Ovis aries) model. *J Pediatr Surg*. 2010;45:65–69.
13. Fillingham A, Rankin J. Prevalence, prenatal diagnosis and survival of gastroschisis. *Prenat Diagn*. 2008;28:1232–1237.
14. Mastroiacovo P, Lisi A, Castilla EE, et al. Gastroschisis and associated defects: an international study. *Am J Med Genet A*. 2007;143A:660–671.
15. Fratelli N, Papageorghiou AT, Bhide A, et al. Outcome of antenatally diagnosed abdominal wall defects. *Ultrasound Obstet Gynecol*. 2007;30:266–270.
16. Sepulveda W, Wong AE, Simonetti L, et al. Ectopia cordis in a first-trimester sonographic screening program for aneuploidy. *J Ultrasound Med*. 2013;32:865–871.
17. Zidere V, Allan LD. Changing findings in pentalogy of Cantrell in fetal life. *Ultrasound Obstet Gynecol*. 2008;32:835–837.
18. Humpl T, Huggan P, Hornberger LK, et al. Presentation and outcomes of ectopia cordis. *Can J Cardiol*. 1999;15:1353–1357.
19. Sahinoglu Z, Uludogan M, Arik H, et al. Prenatal ultrasonographical features of limb body wall complex: a review of etiopathogenesis and a new classification. *Fetal Pediatr Pathol*. 2007;26:135–151.
20. Panaitescu AM, Ushakov F, Kalaskar A, et al. Ultrasound features and management of body stalk anomaly. *Fetal Diagn Ther*. 2016;40:285–290.
21. Daskalakis G, Sebire NJ, Jurkovic D, et al. Body stalk anomaly at 10–14 weeks of gestation. *Ultrasound Obstet Gynecol*. 1997;10:416–418.
22. Mallmann MR, Reutter H, Müller AM, et al. Omphalocele-exstrophy-imperforate anus-spinal defects complex: associated malformations in 12 new cases. *Fetal Diagn Ther*. 2016;41(1):66–70.
23. Ebert A-K, Reutter H, Ludwig M, et al. The exstrophy-epispadias complex. *Orphanet J Rare Dis*. 2009;4:23.
24. Carey JC. Exstrophy of the cloaca and the OEIS complex: one and the same. *Am J Med Genet*. 2001;99:270.
25. Boyadjiev SA, Dodson JL, Radford CL, et al. Clinical and molecular characterization of the bladder exstrophy-epispadias complex: analysis of 232 families. *BJU Int*. 2004;94:1337–1343.
26. Tsukerman GL, Krapiva GA, Kirillova IA. First-trimester diagnosis of duodenal stenosis associated with oesophageal atresia. *Prenat Diagn*. 1993;13:371–376.
27. Marquette GP, Skoll MAL, Yong SL, et al. First-trimester imaging of combined esophageal and duodenal atresia without a tracheoesophageal fistula. *J Ultrasound Med*. 2004;23:1232.
28. Petrikovsky BM. First-trimester diagnosis of duodenal atresia. *Am J Obstet Gynecol*. 1994;171:569–570.
29. Lam YH, Shek T, Tang MHY. Sonographic features of anal atresia at 12 weeks. *Ultrasound Obstet Gynecol*. 2002;19:523–524.
30. Taipale P, Rovamo L, Hiilesmaa V. First-trimester diagnosis of imperforate anus. *Ultrasound Obstet Gynecol*. 2005;25:187–188.
31. Chen M, Meagher S, Simpson I, et al. Sonographic features of anorectal atresia at 12 weeks. *J Matern Fetal Neonatal Med*. 2009;22:931–933.
32. Dhombres F, Friszer S, Castaing O, et al. Images kystiques abdominales fœtales du premier trimestre. *Gynecol Obstet Fertil*. 2015;43:491–495.
33. Khalil A, Cooke PC, Mantovani E, et al. Outcome of first-trimester fetal abdominal cysts: cohort study and review of the literature. *Ultrasound Obstet Gynecol*. 2014;43:413–419.
34. Zimmer EZ, Bronshtein M. Fetal intra-abdominal cysts detected in the first and early second trimester by transvaginal sonography. *J Clin Ultrasound*. 1991;19:564–567.
35. McCalla CO, Lajinian S, DeSouza D, et al. Natural history of antenatal omphalomesenteric duct cyst. *J Ultrasound Med*. 1995;14:639–640.
36. Ghezzi F, Raio L, Di Naro E, et al. Single and multiple umbilical cord cysts in early gestation: two different entities. *Ultrasound Obstet Gynecol*. 2003;21:215–219.
37. Sinkovskaya E, Klassen A, Abuhamad A. A novel systematic approach to the evaluation of the fetal venous system. *Semin Fetal Neonatal Med*. 2013;18:269–278.
38. Chaoui R, Heling K, Karl K. Ultrasound of the fetal veins. Part 1: The intrahepatic venous system. *Ultraschall Med*. 2014;35:208–228.
39. Achiron R, Gindes L, Gilboa Y, et al. Umbilical vein anomaly in fetuses with Down syndrome. *Ultrasound Obstet Gynecol*. 2010;35:297–301.
40. Abuhamad A, Chaoui R. *A Practical Guide to Fetal Echocardiography: Normal and Abnormal Hearts*. 3rd ed. Philadelphia, PA: Wolters Kluwer Health/Lippincott Williams & Wilkins; 2015.
41. Zvanca M, Gielchinsky Y, Abdeljawad F, et al. Hepatic artery Doppler in trisomy 21 and euploid fetuses at 11–13 weeks. *Prenat Diagn*. 2011;31:22–27.
42. Hartung J, Chaoui R, Kalache K, et al. Prenatal diagnosis of intrahepatic communications of the umbilical vein with atypical arteries (A-V fistulae) in two cases of trisomy 21 using color Doppler ultrasound. *Ultrasound Obstet Gynecol*. 2000;16:271–274.

# CHAPTER 13

# The Fetal Urogenital System

## INTRODUCTION

The first trimester examination of the fetal urogenital system primarily focuses on the demonstration of a fluid-filled bladder. When technically feasible or in specific high-risk conditions, visualization of both kidneys and fetal gender is attempted. With optimal imaging, and after the 12th week of gestation, evaluation of the fetal urogenital system is possible, but a conclusive diagnosis of normality requires confirmation later on in pregnancy, because some malformations are not visible until the second trimester or beyond. Several major urogenital malformations can be detected or suspected in the first trimester, however, and are discussed in this chapter. In a large prospective screening study for aneuploidies, including basic examination of fetal anatomy performed in 45,191 pregnancies, the detection of anomalies of the urogenital system in the first trimester was reported among the lowest of fetal malformations.[1]

## EMBRYOLOGY

Understanding the embryogenesis of the urogenital system is important as it relates to the evaluation of normal and abnormal anatomy. The urogenital system develops from the intermediate mesoderm, which forms a urogenital ridge on each side of the aorta. The urogenital ridge develops cranially to caudally into the pronephros, mesonephros, and metanephros, respectively, representing three sets of tubular nephric structures. The pronephros, the most cranial set of tubules, develops in the third week of embryogenesis and regresses a week later. The mesonephros, located in the midsection of the embryo, gives rise to the mesonephric tubules and the mesonephric ducts (Wolffian duct). The mesonephric tubules regress, but the mesonephric ducts persist bilaterally and open into the cloaca. The mesonephric ducts give rise to the ureters, renal pelves, and bladder trigone. In the male, the mesonephric ducts also give rise to the vasa deferens, epididymis, and seminal vesicles. An outgrowth of the caudal portion of the mesonephric duct on each side forms the ureteric bud, which grows toward the metanephric blastema, a mesenchymal condensation of metanephros (Fig. 13.1). The definitive adult kidney is formed by the ureteric bud, which gives rise to the renal pelvis, infundibula, collecting ducts, and calyces, and the metanephric tubules, which form the nephrons with capillary invagination. With the growth of the embryo, the kidney ascends from the pelvis into the upper retroperitoneum, and failure of renal migration results in a pelvic kidney.

At about the seventh week of embryogenesis, a urogenital membrane grows caudally, dividing the cloaca into ventral (urogenital sinus) and dorsal (rectum) components. The urethra is derived from the endoderm at the ventral urogenital sinus. An invagination of ectoderm in the most distal part of the urethra in males joins with the endodermal epithelium of the proximal urethra to create a continuous channel. Differentiation of the external genitalia into male and female occurs between the 8th and 11th week of embryogenesis. Detailed

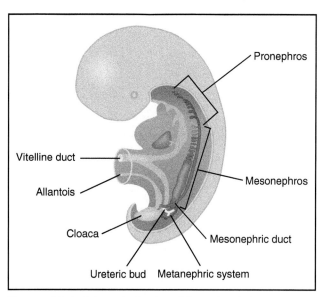

**Figure 13.1:** Schematic drawing of the embryologic development of the urogenital system at around the seventh menstrual week. See text for details.

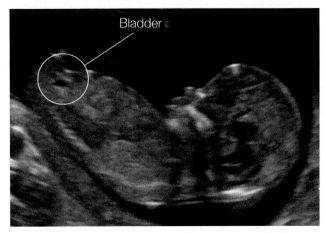

**Figure 13.2:** Midsagittal plane of the fetus at 13 weeks of gestation showing the bladder. This represents the same plane used for crown-length measurement in the first trimester.

development of the gonads and external genitalia is beyond the scope of this chapter.

## NORMAL SONOGRAPHIC ANATOMY

Visualization of the fetal urogenital system in the first trimester is performed by the identification of the bladder and when possible the kidneys, which can be seen on ultrasound as early as 10 weeks of gestation with high-resolution transvaginal transducers.

### Urinary Bladder

The fetal bladder appears as an anechoic structure in the anterior lower pelvis. The bladder is easily seen in the sagittal view of the fetus, in the same plane used for the crown-rump length (CRL) measurement (Fig. 13.2). The axial plane of the fetal pelvis also demonstrates the fetal bladder in a central–anterior location (Fig. 13.3). Visualization of the bladder in the first trimester is aided by color Doppler ultrasound, with the identification of the surrounding umbilical arteries (Fig. 13.4). Although the fetal stomach is almost always filled with fluid, the fetal bladder is occasionally empty in the first trimester and thus maybe difficult to image. When the fetal bladder is not clearly demonstrated in the first trimester, the ultrasound examiner should reassess for the presence of a bladder few minutes later to allow for bladder filling. The authors therefore recommend that visualization of the fetal bladder is performed at the beginning of the first trimester ultrasound examination in order to allow time for bladder filling if the bladder is not visible then. The longitudinal length of the normal bladder should be less than 7 mm in the first trimester (Fig. 13.5).[2,3] The fetal bladder is seen on ultrasound in about 88% of fetuses at 12 weeks of gestation and in 92% to 100% of fetuses at 13 weeks of gestation.[3,4]

### Kidneys and Adrenal Glands

With transabdominal ultrasound, the fetal kidneys are generally difficult to visualize and differentiate from the surrounding bowel in the first trimester. Visualization of the fetal kidneys by the transabdominal approach in the first trimester is improved

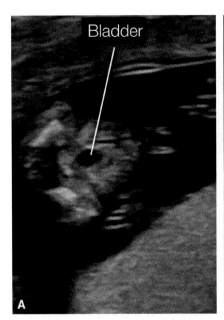
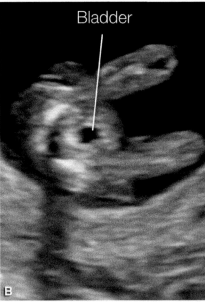
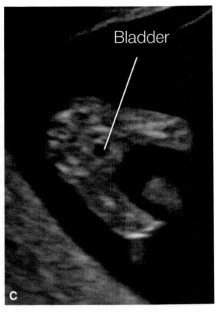

**Figure 13.3:** Axial views of the fetal lower pelvis in three fetuses (**A–C**) at 13, 13, and 12 weeks of gestation, respectively. Note that the bladder is seen in various stages of filing; with more filling in fetus **A** as compared to fetuses **B** and **C**. The bladder is best demonstrated in this axial view at the level of the pelvis. The addition of color Doppler, as shown in Figure 13.4, improves bladder visualization.

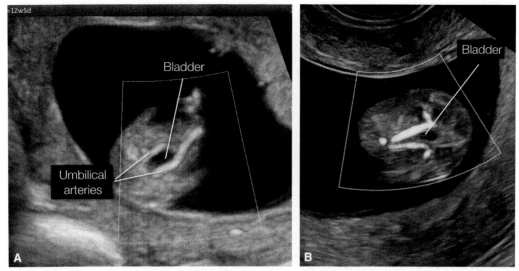

**Figure 13.4:** Axial views in color Doppler of the fetal lower pelvis in two fetuses **(A and B)** at 12 weeks of gestation. Note that the addition of color Doppler shows the umbilical arteries surrounding the bladder. This axial view is helpful for bladder imaging and also for confirming the presence of a three-vessel umbilical cord. Compare with Figures 3.10 ,13.33A and 13.34A..

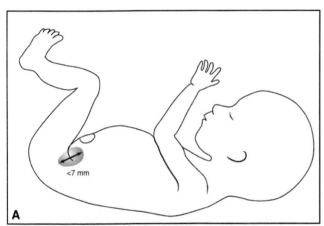

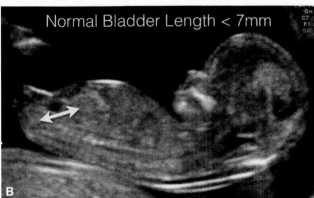

**Figure 13.5:** Schematic drawing **(A)** and corresponding ultrasound image **(B)** of the midsagittal plane of the fetus showing the bladder in the lower pelvis. The fetus in **B** is at 12 weeks of gestation. This midsagittal plane is used for measuring the longitudinal diameter of the bladder. A normal bladder in the first trimester should have a longitudinal diameter of less than 7 mm.

with the use of high-resolution transducers along with optimal scanning conditions (Figs. 3.2, 3.4, 13.6, and 13.7). The transvaginal approach substantially improves visualization of the fetal kidneys in the first trimester because of the proximity of the transducer to the fetal abdomen and increased resolution of the probe (Figs. 3.2 and 13.8).[4] The fetal kidneys appear in the first trimester as rounded, slightly bright structures in the posterior abdomen lateral to the spine, with the renal pelves noted as anechoic circles, centrally within the renal tissue (Figs. 13.7 and 13.8). Cranial to both kidneys, the slightly hypoechoic and large adrenal glands are seen (Fig. 13.7). The length of the adrenal gland is less than half the length of the kidney.[5] Visualization of the fetal kidneys in the first trimester can be achieved in the coronal, sagittal, or axial planes (Fig. 13.9) of the fetal abdomen. The coronal plane of the fetal abdomen is the optimal plane for first trimester imaging of the kidneys in our experience (Figs. 13.7, 13.8B, and 13.10). This coronal plane is also helpful for the demonstration of unilateral or bilateral renal agenesis, and a more anterior view can demonstrate the presence of a horseshoe kidney (see below). Color Doppler can also be added to demonstrate the right and left renal arteries arising from the descending aorta (Fig. 13.10). The fetal kidneys can be identified in 86% to 99% of fetuses at 12 weeks of gestation and in 92% to 99% of fetuses at 13 weeks of gestation.[4,6]

## Genitalia

Although genitalia can be well seen either in an axial view of the pelvis or in the midsagittal view during the measurement of the CRL, reliable differentiation of fetal gender is of limited

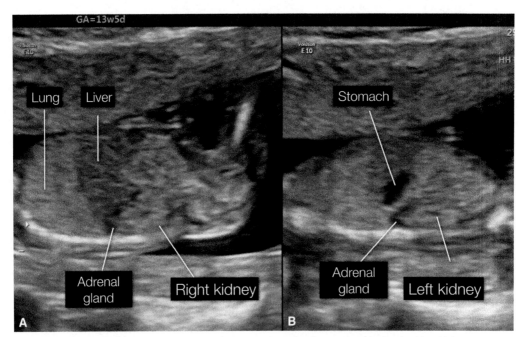

Figure 13.6: Right (A) and left (B) parasagittal planes of a fetus at 13 weeks of gestation obtained with a high-resolution transabdominal transducer showing fetal kidneys. In the right parasagittal plane (A), the right kidney can be seen and appears as echogenic as the lung and is separated from the diaphragm by the hypoechoic adrenal gland. In the left parasagittal plane (B), the left kidney is seen under the left adrenal gland and stomach. The kidneys can also be imaged in the first trimester in a coronal plane of the abdomen and pelvis (see Figs. 13.7 and 13.8).

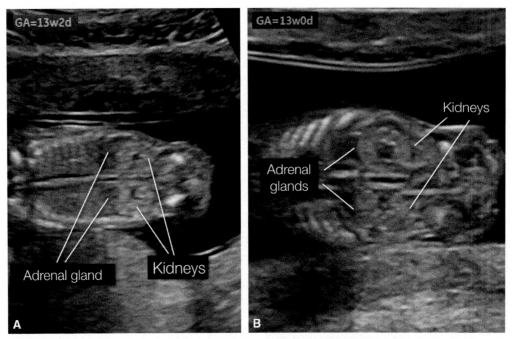

Figure 13.7: Coronal planes of the fetal chest and abdomen, slightly anterior plane to the coronal plane of the spine, in two fetuses (A and B) at 13 weeks of gestation. The coronal plane in A is obtained transabdominally using a convex transducer and the coronal plane in B is obtained transabdominally using a high-resolution linear transducer. Note the clear delineation of both kidneys because of the slight increase in echogenicity of renal tissue. Note that both adrenal glands appear as triangular hypoechoic structures on the cranial poles of the kidneys.

diagnostic accuracy in the first trimester. Embryologically, sex differentiation is not fully completed until about the 11th week of gestation, and thus, sex determination on ultrasound is relatively inaccurate before the 12th week of gestation. The ability to identify fetal gender on ultrasound increases with advancing gestation, and the accuracy is enhanced after the 13th week of gestation or with CRL measurements greater than 70 mm. The midsagittal view of the fetus is most reliable for the identification of gender in the first trimester because it shows a caudally directed clitoris in females (Fig. 13.11A and B)

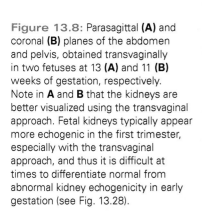

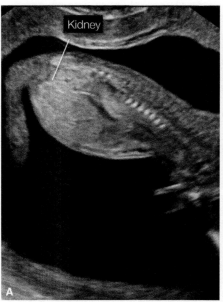

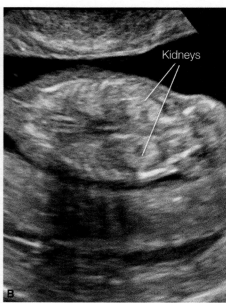

**Figure 13.8:** Parasagittal **(A)** and coronal **(B)** planes of the abdomen and pelvis, obtained transvaginally in two fetuses at 13 **(A)** and 11 **(B)** weeks of gestation, respectively. Note in **A** and **B** that the kidneys are better visualized using the transvaginal approach. Fetal kidneys typically appear more echogenic in the first trimester, especially with the transvaginal approach, and thus it is difficult at times to differentiate normal from abnormal kidney echogenicity in early gestation (see Fig. 13.28).

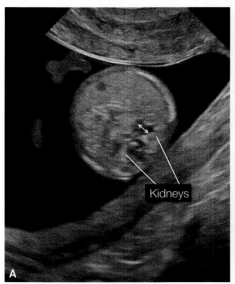

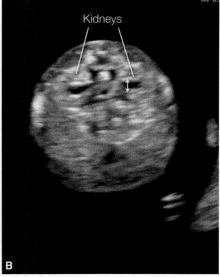

**Figure 13.9:** Axial planes of the fetal abdomen obtained transvaginally in two fetuses at 12 **(A)** and 13 **(B)** weeks of gestation. Note the presence of fetal kidneys in the posterior aspect of the abdomen. The cross-sectional plane is ideally suited for the assessment of the diameter of the renal pelvis, measured as a vertical diameter (*double headed arrow*). It is much easier to see the kidneys in a cross section of the abdomen using the transvaginal approach. The fetus in **A** is in a dorsoposterior position and the fetus in **B** is in a dorsoanterior position.

**Figure 13.10:** Coronal plane of the fetal abdomen and pelvis with color Doppler in two fetuses at 13 **(A)** and 12 **(B)** weeks of gestation. Image in **A** is obtained transabdominally and image in **B** is obtained transvaginally. The use of color Doppler in a coronal plane of the abdomen and pelvis, as shown here in **A** and **B**, demonstrates the two renal arteries arising from the aorta. This approach is helpful in the presence of suspected unilateral or bilateral renal agenesis as the absence of a kidney is associated with an absence of the corresponding renal artery (see Figs. 13.33 and 13.34).

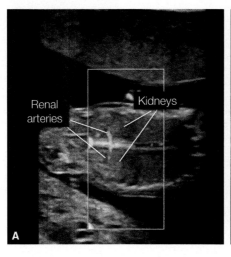

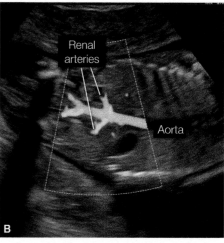

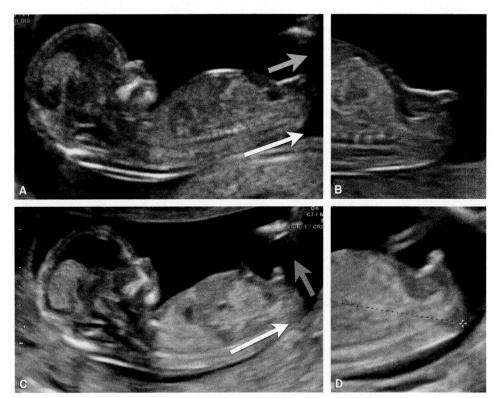

**Figure 13.11:** In some clinical situations, it may be important to determine the fetal gender in the first trimester. The anatomic orientation of the genitalia in relation to the spine (*white arrow*) in the first trimester is helpful in that regard. In female fetuses **(A and B)**, the developing labia and clitoris have an orientation that is parallel (*pink arrow*) to the longitudinal spine. In male fetuses **(C and D)**, the developing penis has an orientation that is almost perpendicular (*blue arrow*) to the spine. Sex determination is more reliable after the 12th weeks of gestation, when the crown-rump length is >65 mm.

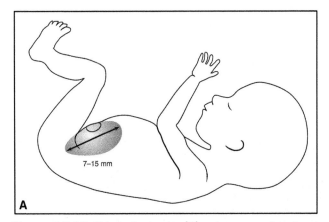
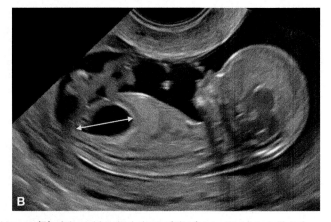

**Figure 13.12:** Schematic drawing **(A)** and corresponding ultrasound image **(B)** of the midsagittal plane of the fetus, showing a dilated bladder with a bladder longitudinal diameter of greater than 7 mm. Dilation of the bladder in the first trimester fetus is defined by a longitudinal diameter of 7 mm or greater and is referred to as megacystis or megavesica (see text for details). The presence of megacystis with bladder longitudinal diameter between 7 and 15 mm is associated with fetal aneuploidy, renal abnormalities, albeit a large number of fetuses with bladder diameter between 7 and 15 mm are normal.

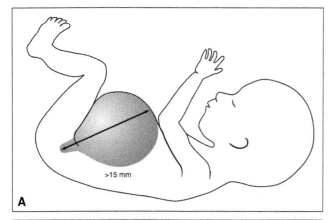

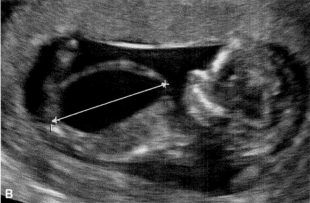

Figure 13.13: Schematic drawing **(A)** and corresponding ultrasound image **(B)** of the midsagittal plane of the fetus, showing a dilated bladder (megacystis) with a bladder longitudinal diameter of greater than 15 mm. The presence of megacystis with bladder longitudinal diameter of greater than 15 mm is associated with fetal aneuploidy and renal abnormalities, along with distension of the anterior abdominal wall. See text for details.

and a cranially directed penis in males (Fig. 13.11C and D). Labia majora and minora appear as parallel lines in females when compared to a nonseptated dome-shaped structure, corresponding to the scrotum in males. Accuracy of fetal gender determination in the first trimester varies from 60% to 100%, being inaccurate before 12 weeks, and reaches >95% after 13 weeks of gestation.[7]

## UROGENITAL SYSTEM ABNORMALITIES

### Megacystis and Lower Urinary Tract Obstruction

#### Definition

The term megacystis is used to describe an unusually dilated bladder (Figs. 13.12 and 13.13). Megacystis is defined in the first trimester by a longitudinal bladder diameter of 7 mm or more obtained on a midline sagittal plane of the fetus.[2,3] Spontaneous resolution of megacystis has been described when the longitudinal bladder length is less than 15 mm and in the absence of associated chromosomal abnormalities.[8] In the first large study on megacystis between 10 and 14 weeks,[3] 145 fetuses with a bladder length ≥7 mm were evaluated: In the group with bladder length between 7 and 15 mm (Fig. 13.12), the incidence of chromosomal defects was 23.6% versus 11.4% for a bladder diameter >15 mm (Figs. 13.13 and 13.14).[3] In the remaining group with bladder diameter between 7 and 15 mm and normal chromosomes, 90% showed spontaneous resolution and 10% developed renal problems. In contrast, in all fetuses with a bladder diameter

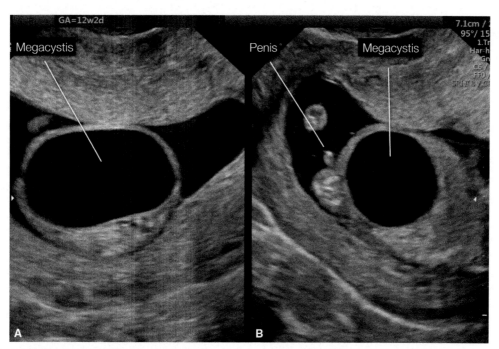

Figure 13.14: Axial **(A)** and sagittal **(B)** planes of the fetal pelvis, obtained transvaginally in a fetus at 12 weeks of gestation with significant megacystis. Megacystis occurs more commonly in male fetuses. See text for details.

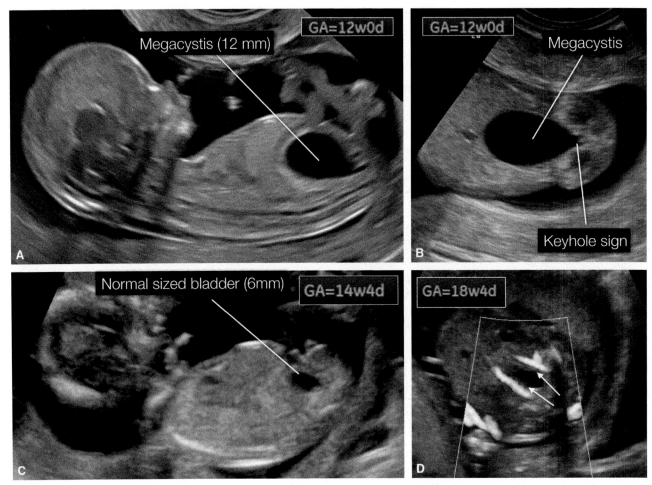

**Figure 13.15: A:** A midline sagittal plane of a fetus at 12 weeks of gestation with megacystis, with a longitudinal bladder diameter of 12 mm. **B:** The corresponding axial plane at the level of the pelvis at 12 weeks of gestation showing the presence of a keyhole sign, suggesting a posterior urethral valves. The fetus had no additional anatomic or chromosomal abnormalities. **C:** The follow-up ultrasound at 14 weeks of gestation showing resolution of the megacystis with a longitudinal bladder diameter of 6 mm. **D:** An axial plane of the pelvis in color Doppler at 18 weeks of gestation showing normal bladder and umbilical arteries with no bladder wall hypertrophy, as evidenced by the proximity of the umbilical arteries to the internal bladder wall (*arrows*). Resolution of first trimester megacystis is a common event. Compare with Figure 13.16.

>15 mm and normal chromosomes, megacystis progressed into obstructive uropathy (Fig. 13.14).[3]

As noted, megacystis in the first trimester can be transient (Figs. 13.15 and 13.16), but can also be a sign of a lower urinary tract obstruction (LUTO). LUTO, previously referred to as bladder outlet obstruction, is an abnormality involving an obstruction of the lower urinary tract at the level of the urethra, resulting from either a membrane-like structure (valves) in the posterior urethra or urethral atresia. LUTO is usually sporadic, and when severe, it is associated with oligohydramnios, pulmonary hypoplasia, and renal damage. Posterior urethral valves (PUV), which represent the most common form of LUTO, affect males almost exclusively with varying degrees of obstruction. Urethral atresia on the other hand occurs in males and females and is extremely rare.

PUV occurs in about 1:8,000 to 1:25,000 of males,[9,10] and its etiology is thought to result from either an exaggerated development of the urethral folds (type 1 and 2) or failure to create a continuous channel within the urethra with the persistence of an obstructive urogenital membrane (type 3).[10] Prenatal therapeutic interventions with placement of a vesicoamniotic shunt or ablation of the obstructive tissue through cystoscopy is reserved to the second trimester of pregnancy. Transient megacystis and PUV will be the primary focus of discussion in this segment.

### Ultrasound Findings

Megacystis is probably the easiest and most commonly diagnosed abnormality of the genitourinary system in the first trimester. It is based on the identification of a large bladder, measuring 7 mm or more in sagittal view (Figs. 13.12 to 13.15). In some cases of resolving megacystis, a thickened bladder wall may still be observed (Fig. 13.16C and D). The presence of progressive obstructive uropathy is common when the longitudinal bladder length measures greater than 15 mm (Figs. 13.13 and 13.17).[3]

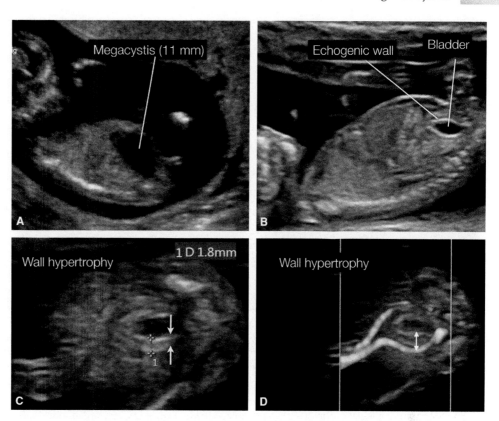

**Figure 13.16: A:** A parasagittal plane of a fetus at 12 weeks of gestation with megacystis, with a longitudinal bladder diameter of 11 mm. **B:** A parasagittal plane of the same fetus at 13 weeks of gestation demonstrating a normal bladder size and echogenic bladder wall. Chorionic villous sampling in this male fetus showed no aneuploidy. **C:** An axial plane of the pelvis at 13 weeks of gestation showing bladder wall hypertrophy, with bladder wall thickness of 1.8 mm. **D:** An axial plane of the pelvis in color Doppler at 13 weeks of gestation confirming the presence of bladder wall hypertrophy as evidenced by the distance between the umbilical arteries and the internal bladder wall (*double headed arrow*).

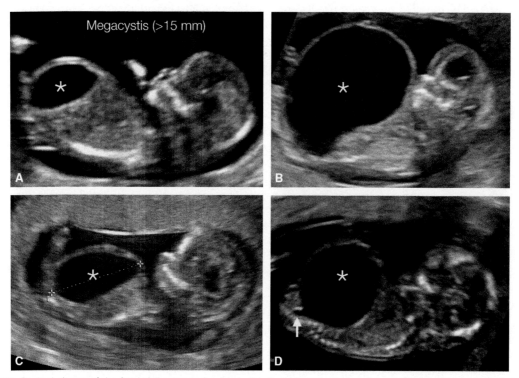

**Figure 13.17:** Sagittal planes of the fetal abdomen and pelvis in the first trimester, in four fetuses **(A–D)** with megacystis (*asterisks*), exceeding 15 mm in longitudinal diameter. This finding is associated with significant risk for aneuploidy and renal abnormalities. Amniotic fluid appears normal in all fetuses, as expected in the first trimester in the presence of significant uropathy, and oligohydramnios is not expected before 16 weeks of gestation. Note the presence of keyhole sign in **D** (*arrow*). Follow-up ultrasound examinations often demonstrate the presence of renal abnormalities and underdeveloped lungs, expected here in fetuses **B**, **C,** and **D** because of significant megacystis with abdominal wall distention.

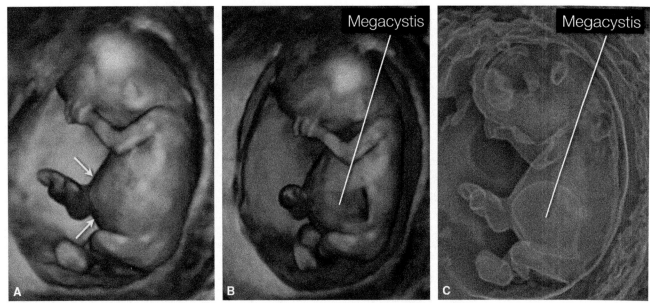

**Figure 13.18:** Three-dimensional ultrasound in surface mode in a fetus with megacystis and trisomy 13 at 13 weeks of gestation. Note the presence of normal amniotic fluid volume surrounding the fetus **(A–C)**. Also note the presence of distended abdominal wall (*arrows*) in **A**. In **B**, the anterior abdominal wall and bladder were opened digitally using postprocessing volume cutting tools to provide an insight into the dilated bladder. **C:** Postprocessing with transparency tool (silhouette ®), thus facilitating the visualization of the megacystis.

The sonographic identification of PUV is possible in the first trimester, especially in severe cases (**Figs. 13.17 and 13.18**). In the first trimester, amniotic fluid is commonly normal in PUV cases, and the diagnosis is typically suspected by the presence of an enlarged bladder (megacystis) (**Figs. 13.17 and 13.18**). PUV in the first trimester is often associated with hydronephrosis and renal dysplasia in severe cases (**Figs. 13.19 and 13.20**).

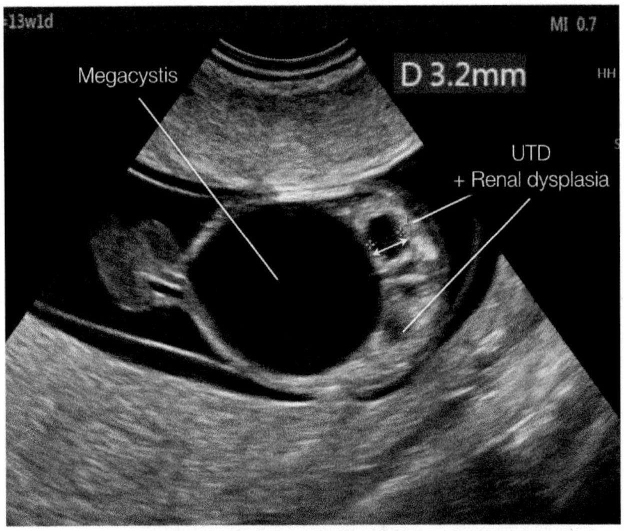

**Figure 13.19:** Axial plane of the fetal pelvis in a fetus at 13 weeks of gestation with megacystis, posterior urethral valves, and trisomy 13. Note the presence of urinary tract dilation (UTD) (*double headed arrows*) and increased renal parenchyma echogenicity, suggesting the presence of renal dysplasia. In this case, it is not feasible to relate the presence of increased renal parenchyma echogenicity to urologic obstruction or trisomy 13.

PUV markers of poor prognosis, such as the presence of renal cortical cysts and increased renal echogenicity, are already present in the first trimester (**Fig. 13.19**), but their absence cannot predict a good prognosis. The keyhole sign, related to a dilated proximal urethra, supports the diagnosis of PUV in the first trimester (**Figs. 13.15B, 13.17D, 13.20B, and 13.21B**).

### Associated Malformations

Megacystis in the first trimester has been associated with chromosomal malformations, primarily trisomy 13 and 18.[3] Outcome of persistent megacystis in the first trimester is poor compared with second and third trimesters.[11,12] Associated malformations are seen in about 40% of PUV fetuses, and chromosomal abnormalities occur in 10% to 24% of cases.[3] In chromosomally abnormal fetuses, thickened nuchal translucency and intracerebral, facial, or cardiac anomalies are common. In a recently published large study on 108,982 first trimester fetuses including 870 fetuses with abnormal karyotypes, megacystis was found in 81 fetuses for a prevalence of 1:1,345.[13] Of all fetuses with megacystis, 63/81 (77.7%) had a bladder length between 7 and 15 mm, with the remainder (18/81; 22.3%) having a bladder larger than 15 mm. The rate of aneuploidy in megacystis was 18% (15/81) and, in this study, was similar in both subgroups.[13] Interestingly, aneuploidies in megacystis were almost equally distributed between trisomy 18 (33%), trisomy 13 (27%), trisomy 21 (27%), and others (20%).[13] Differential diagnosis includes urethral atresia, megacystis microcolon intestinal hypoperistalsis syndrome, which occurs in 75% in female fetuses, cloacal malformation, and other cystic anomalies in the pelvis (**Figs. 13.22 and 13.23**).[14]

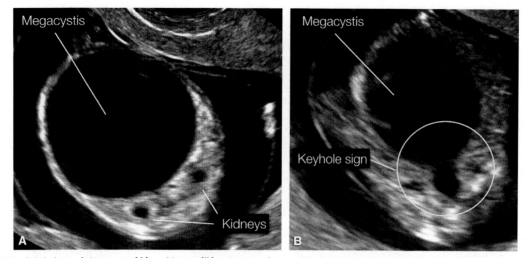

**Figure 13.20:** Axial view of the upper **(A)** and lower **(B)** pelvis in a fetus with megacystis because of posterior urethral valves at 14 weeks of gestation. Note the presence of a massively distended bladder (megacystis) in **A** and **B** and a keyhole sign (*circle* in **B**) typical for the presence of urethral obstruction.

## Urinary Tract Dilation

### Definition

Urinary tract (UT) dilation is a term used to describe the presence of dilation of the renal pelvis and occasionally the ureter. Terms such as pyelectasis, renal pelvis dilation, and hydronephrosis have been used to describe dilation of the UT system. With the apparent confusion associated with all these terms, a multidisciplinary consensus panel recently recommended avoiding the use of nonspecific terms in describing UT dilation, and proposed the consistent use of the term urinary tract dilation, or "UT dilation,"[15,16] which can also be used in the first trimester. The renal pelvis is considered normal when it measures <4 mm at <28 weeks gestation and <7 mm at >28 weeks gestation.[16] Although there are no specific measurements of the renal pelvis in the first trimester, a cutoff

of 1.5 mm was suggested in one study[17] (Fig. 13.24). When UT dilation is noted, additional sonographic features should be evaluated to include the presence of calyceal dilation, renal parenchymal appearance and thickness, ureteral dilation, and bladder abnormalities (see previous section). The evaluation for the presence of many of these additional sonographic features is important in order to further classify the severity of the UT dilation. It is important to note, however, that these features are difficult to assess in the first trimester, and several may not be evident until the second or third trimester of pregnancy. UT dilation is present in 1% to 5% of pregnancies,[15,18,19] with a 2:1 male-to-female prevalence.[19]

The presence of UT dilation in the first trimester is commonly a transient finding, with resolution noted in a significant number of cases upon follow-up into the second and third trimesters of pregnancy.[18] The presence of UT dilation in the first trimester has

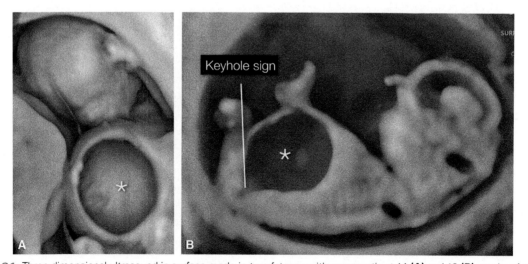

**Figure 13.21:** Three-dimensional ultrasound in surface mode in two fetuses with megacystis at 14 **(A)** and 13 **(B)** weeks of gestation. Postprocessing volume cutting is performed in **A** and **B** to display the dilated bladders (*asterisks*). Note the keyhole sign in fetus **B**, suggesting the presence of posterior urethral valves.

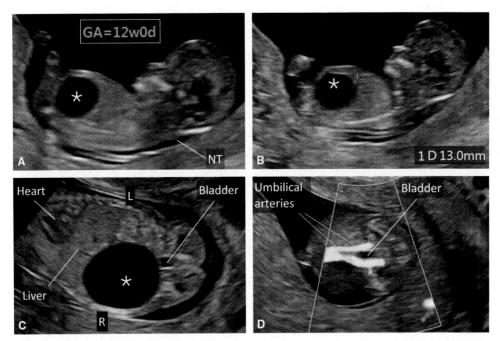

**Figure 13.22:** Sagittal views **(A and B)** of a fetus at 12 weeks of gestation demonstrating the presence of suspected megacystis (*asterisks*) with a longitudinal "bladder" diameter of 13 mm **(B)**. Nuchal translucency (NT) was thickened (3 mm) and tricuspid regurgitation was demonstrated (not shown). Transvaginal ultrasound was performed **(C and D)** to better assess the urogenital organs. Neither a keyhole sign nor abnormal kidneys were found, and the cystic structure was noted to be located in the middle right abdomen under the liver and cranial to a small bladder **(C)**. Color Doppler confirmed the presence of a small filled bladder, normally located between the two umbilical arteries, as shown in **D**. The cystic structure was classified as a "cyst of unknown origin." Chorionic villous sampling revealed trisomy 21. Etiology of abdominal cyst was not revealed because of pregnancy termination. L, Left; R, right. See Figure 13.23.

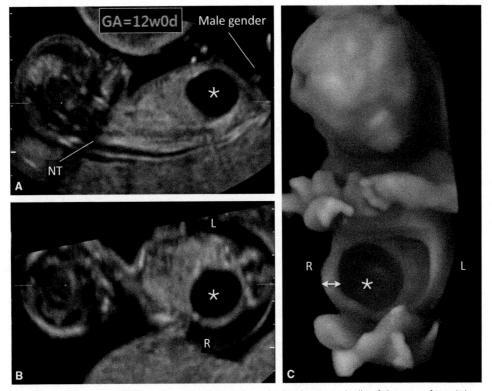

**Figure 13.23:** Three-dimensional ultrasound at 12 weeks of gestation, obtained transvaginally of the same fetus (trisomy 21) as in Figure 13.22. **A and B:** Multiplanar displays and **C** represents display in surface mode. **A:** A midsagittal view with a large cyst (*asterisk*) mimicking megacystis. The corresponding orthogonal coronal view in **B** shows that the cystic structure (*asterisk*) is located laterally in the right abdominal cavity and not midline as expected in megacystis. In **C**, postprocessing volume cutting tools are used to display the cyst (*asterisk*) and visualize its proximity to the right abdominal wall (*double headed arrow*). NT, nuchal translucency; L, Left; R, right.

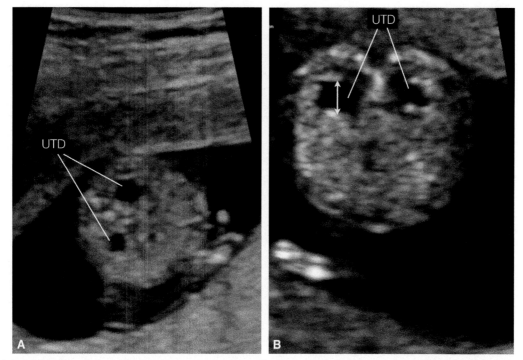

**Figure 13.24:** Axial planes of the fetal abdomen in two fetuses with urinary tract dilation (UTD) at 12 **(A)** and 13 **(B)** weeks of gestation. The assessment for the presence of UTD is obtained in an axial plane of the pelvis **(A and B)** by measuring the renal pelvis in an anterior to posterior diameter as shown in **B** (*double headed arrow*). A clear cutoff for UTD in the first trimester has not been established yet and some suggested a cutoff of greater than 1.5 mm. UTD in the first trimester can resolve spontaneously or be a marker of urinary tract abnormalities or aneuploidy.

been associated with a slight increase in the risk for chromosomal anomalies **(Figs. 13.25 and 13.26)**[17]; it can also be a transient finding or can be associated with the presence of UT dilation later in gestation **(Fig. 13.27)**. A close follow-up in the second trimester is thus recommended to document any progression or resolution. When UT dilation persists into the neonatal period, ureteropelvic junction obstruction is the most common associated abnormality followed by vesicoureteral reflux (VUR).[15,16]

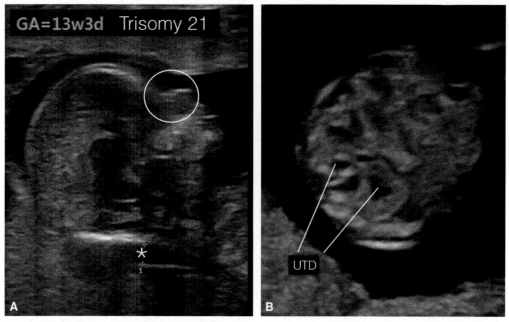

**Figure 13.25:** Midsagittal plane of the fetal head **(A)** and axial plane of the abdomen **(B)** in a fetus at 13 weeks of gestation with trisomy 21. Note in **A** the presence of thickened nuchal translucency (3.3 mm) (*asterisk*) and absent nasal bone (*circle*) and in **B**, urinary tract dilation (UTD) with an anterioposterior diameter of 3.6 mm. (Measurement not shown).

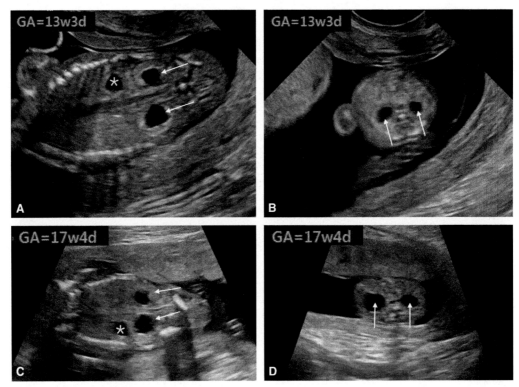

**Figure 13.26:** Coronal **(A)** and axial **(B)** planes, obtained transvaginally, in a fetus at 13 weeks of gestation with urinary tract dilation (UTD) (*arrows*). This patient was referred for diagnostic testing because of maternal balanced translocation. The patient decided to wait for amniocentesis. Follow-up transabdominal ultrasound at 17 weeks of gestation **(C and D)** shows the persistence of UTD (*arrows*). Amniocentesis revealed the presence of an unbalanced translocation in the fetus. *Asterisk* points to the stomach in **A** and **C**.

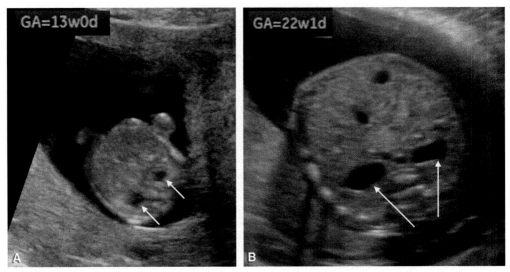

**Figure 13.27:** Axial planes of the fetal abdomen in the same fetus at 13 **(A)** and 22 **(B)** weeks of gestation with fluid accumulation in the renal pelves (*arrows*). The presence of fluid in the renal pelves helps to identify kidneys in the first trimester on transabdominal ultrasound **(A)**. No other associated abnormalities were seen, and isolated urinary tract dilation was confirmed postnatally.

## Ultrasound Findings

Using the transvaginal approach, the renal pelvis can be demonstrated in the first trimester as an anechoic center, surrounded by renal parenchyma. When UT dilation is present in early gestation, it can be recognized on abdominal ultrasound as well (Fig. 13.26). The ideal technique for the measurement of the renal pelvis is based on images of

the kidney obtained from an axial plane of the fetus in an anterior–posterior orientation, with optimal measurements obtained with the fetal spine at the 12 or 6 o'clock positions (Figs. 13.9 and 13.24). In addition, the measurement should be taken in an anterior to posterior orientation of the pelvis at the maximal diameter of the intrarenal pelvis dilation.[16] The calipers should be placed on the inner border of the fluid collection. Evaluating the fetal kidneys in the coronal and parasagittal approach enhances visualization, especially when the fetal spine shadows a posterior kidney (Fig. 13.26). Ureteral dilation is rarely seen in the first trimester, and its presence should suspect LUTO. Grading of the renal pelvis dilation is not applicable in the first trimester because most noted dilations are mild and are not associated with calyceal abnormalities. Amniotic fluid volume is commonly normal in association with renal pelvis dilation in the first trimester.

### Associated Malformations

Associated malformations typically involve chromosomal anomalies and abnormalities of the urogenital system. The presence of renal pelvis dilation in the first trimester of pregnancy has been described as a soft marker for trisomy 21, similar to the second trimester.[17,20] When UT dilation is noted in the first trimester, further assessment of aneuploidy risk with nuchal translucency, biochemical markers, or cell-free DNA along with a comprehensive anatomic survey is an important step in pregnancy management. Follow-up ultrasound examination

in the second trimester is essential to assess fetal anatomy in more detail. Differential diagnosis of UT dilation includes transient finding, ureteral–pelvic or vesicoureteral junction obstruction, vesicoureteral reflux, PUV, or other urogenital malformations.

## Hyperechogenic Kidneys

### Definition

The term "hyperechogenic kidneys" is used in the second trimester to describe increased echogenicity of the renal parenchyma, typically with renal tissue appearing more echogenic than the surrounding liver. As stated in the section on normal anatomy, the kidneys appear slightly more echogenic in the first trimester than later on in pregnancy. There is currently no objective definition on what represents hyperechogenic kidneys in the first trimester, and the diagnosis is based on subjective assessment of experienced operators (Fig. 13.28). Indeed, improvement in ultrasound

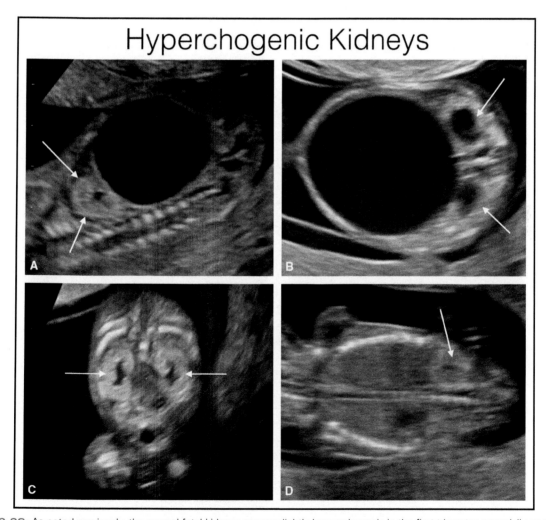

**Figure 13.28:** As noted previously, the normal fetal kidneys appear slightly hyperechogenic in the first trimester, especially on transvaginal ultrasound (see Figs. 13.6 to 13.8). Increased echogenicity of fetal kidneys in the first trimester can be a sign of associated renal dysplasia, aneuploidy, or cystic renal disease. **A and B:** Hyperechogenic kidneys (*arrows*) in the first trimester in association with posterior urethral valves. **C and D:** Hyperechogenic kidneys (*arrows*) in the first trimester in association with trisomy 13. See also Figures 13.29 to 13.32.

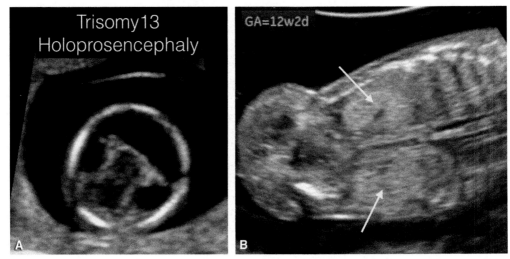

**Figure 13.29:** Axial plane of the head **(A)** and coronal plane of the abdomen in a fetus with trisomy 13 at 12 weeks of gestation. Note the presence of holoprosencephaly in **A**. Facial dysmorphism, cardiac anomaly, and other abnormalities were also seen on ultrasound (not shown). Note in **B**, the presence of hyperechogenic kidneys, a common finding in trisomy 13.

technology has resulted in improved tissue characterization in the first trimester and, in some cases, in increased echogenicity of kidneys. The suspicion of hyperechogenic kidneys is particularly relevant in pregnancies at high risk for renal disease because of the presence of additional ultrasound signs (Figs. 13.28 to 13.30) or to a prior family history (Figs. 13.30 to 13.32). As in the second trimester, hyperechogenic kidneys can be a transient finding, but may also be a marker for renal abnormalities. Detailed sonographic evaluation of the fetus and follow-up examinations are recommended when hyperechogenic kidneys are noted in the first trimester of pregnancy.

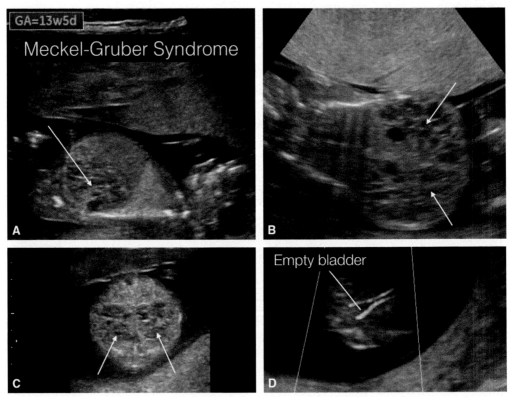

**Figure 13.30:** Meckel–Gruber syndrome in a fetus at 13 weeks of gestation. Note the presence of bilaterally enlarged polycystic kidneys, seen transabdominally in **A** and **C** and transvaginally in **B**. The large kidneys lead to the distension of the abdomen **(A–C)**. **D:** An axial plane of the lower pelvis in color Doppler shows the two umbilical arteries with no bladder seen in between. Amniotic fluid is still normal at this gestation and typically disappears around 16 weeks. This pregnancy was the result of consanguineous couple with recurrence risk of 25%.

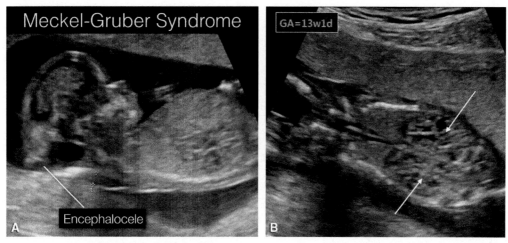

**Figure 13.31:** Midsagittal plane **(A)** and coronal plane **(B)** of a fetus with Meckel–Gruber syndrome at 13 weeks of gestation. Note in **A** the presence of an occipital encephalocele and in **B** the presence of bilateral polycystic kidneys (*arrows*). Similar to the pregnancy in Figure 13.30, amniotic fluid is still present.

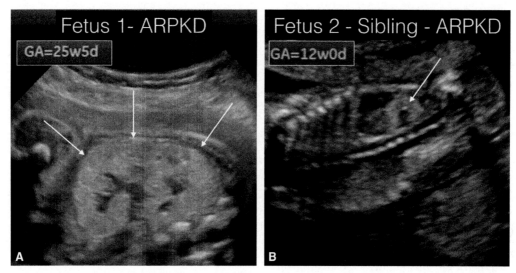

**Figure 13.32: A:** A parasagittal plane of the abdomen at 25 weeks of gestation in a fetus with autosomal recessive polycystic kidney disease (ARPKD), showing one of the two enlarged hyperechogenic kidneys with the typical texture of microcystic dysplasia (*arrows*). The baby died shortly after birth and ARPKD was confirmed genetically with carrier status in both parents. **B:** A coronal plane of the abdomen in the next pregnancy at 12 weeks of gestation, showing normal size kidneys (*one shown—arrow*) with mild hyperechogenicity: within the echogenicity range of normal kidneys in early gestation (compare with Fig. 13.8). Genetic testing confirmed ARPKD and the pregnancy was terminated.

## Ultrasound Findings

Ideally, the kidneys should be visualized in a sagittal or coronal view in order to demonstrate large segments of renal parenchyma and enable a comparison with the surrounding lung, liver, and bowel. Enlarged hyperechogenic kidneys in the first trimester are particularly concerning because of the possibility of polycystic kidney disease or the association with aneuploidies (Fig. 13.29). The association of hyperechogenic kidneys with UT dilation warrants follow-up in the second trimester and can be seen with megacystis or PUV (Figs. 13.28 A and B).

## Associated Malformations

Hyperechogenic kidneys in the first trimester have been described as a marker for the presence of inherited autosomal recessive polycystic kidney disease (ARPKD).[21] We have also seen hyperechogenic, enlarged kidneys at 13 weeks of gestation in an affected fetus of a mother with autosomal dominant polycystic kidney disease (ADPKD). It is important to note, however, that the presence of ARPKD or ADPKD is not commonly associated with hyperechogenic or enlarged kidneys in the first trimester. Figure 13.32 presents a case of ARPKD where the fetal kidneys appeared "normal" at 12 weeks of gestation, but molecular genetics confirmed ARPKD, given a previously affected sibling. Interestingly, other polycystic kidneys, such as in Meckel–Gruber syndrome (Figs. 13.30 and 13.31), can be detected in the first trimester by the presence of enlarged hypoechoic renal parenchyma with cysts. Hyperechogenic kidneys can also be noted in the first trimester in the presence of renal dysplasia in association with PUV, trisomy 13, or trisomy 18 (Figs. 13.28 and 13.29). Hyperechogenic kidneys are an isolated finding in association with *HNF1B* (or *TCF2*) gene mutation, but the earliest suspected case to date was reported at 18 weeks of gestation.[22]

## Autosomal Recessive Polycystic Kidney Disease

### Definition

ARPKD, also referred to as infantile polycystic kidney disease, is an autosomal recessive disease involving cystic dilation of the renal collecting tubules with associated congenital hepatic fibrosis. ARPKD is caused by mutation of the *PKHD1* gene, located on the short arm of chromosome 6, with complete penetrance and variable phenotypic expressivity, given the large size of the gene. The prevalence of ARPKD is around 1:20,000 births.[23] Disease manifestation in childhood or in adulthood is the most common presentation.[24,25] ARPKD is thus generally diagnosed prenatally after 20 weeks of gestation or in the neonatal period in only 30% of cases.[24,25] ARPKD can be isolated, but is also found in association with syndromic diseases of the group of ciliopathies. Out of the ciliopathies group is Meckel–Gruber syndrome, with the triad of polycystic kidneys, encephalocele, and polydactyly (Figs. 13.30 and 13.31).

### Ultrasound Findings

The classic ultrasound findings in ARPKD in late second trimester are symmetrically enlarged hyperechogenic kidneys (Fig. 13.32A) that fill the fetal abdomen and in some conditions in association with oligohydramnios and absent bladder. The prenatal diagnosis of ARPKD has been observed in early gestation around 14 weeks,[21] owing to increased hyperechogenicity, but most cases become apparent only after 25 weeks when kidney enlargement occurs (Fig. 13.32A). The presence of normal appearing kidneys in early gestation, however, does not rule out ARPKD even in previously affected families (Fig. 13.32B). When normal or mildly hyperechogenic kidneys are noted in the first trimester in at-risk families, follow-up ultrasound examinations into the second and third trimester is important because progression of ultrasound findings tend to occur after mid-gestation. An empty bladder on repeated ultrasound examinations in the first trimester was also reported as an important sign for ARPKD, with follow-up examination in the second trimester revealing the diagnosis.[1] In fetuses with Meckel–Gruber syndrome, enlarged cystic kidneys are commonly seen in the first trimester along with the presence of a posterior encephalocele

and polydactyly[21] (Figs. 13.30 and 13.31). Given the lack of morphologic manifestation of ARPKD before the second trimester of pregnancy, along with its variable expressivity, the overall detection of ARPKD in early gestation remains low.[1]

### Associated Findings

Differential diagnosis of enlarged echogenic kidneys in the first trimester includes normal variant, trisomy 13, trisomy 18, adult-onset polycystic kidney disease, Meckel–Gruber syndrome, and/or other ciliopathies.

## Autosomal Dominant Polycystic Kidney Disease

ADPKD is characterized by the presence of enlarged kidneys with multiple cysts of variable size. ADPKD is one of the most common genetic disorders with recurrence risk of 50% and is a common cause of renal dysfunction. The disease manifests itself in adulthood, and the prenatal diagnosis of ADPKD is typically performed when a family history of ADPKD is present. The presence of enlarged hyperechogenic kidneys can occasionally be seen in early gestation, typically in the presence of a family history. The presence of normal appearing kidneys in the first and second trimester of pregnancy, however, is not uncommon in ADPKD.

## Multicystic Dysplastic Kidney

Multicystic dysplastic kidney (MCDK) is a severe nonfunctioning renal malformation in which the kidney contains multiple noncommunicating cysts of varying size, dense central stroma, and an atretic ureter. The pathogenesis of MCDK is unknown. To our knowledge, MCDK has not yet been diagnosed in the first trimester. Bilateral MCDK, which occurs in 25% of cases, is associated with oligohydramnios after about the 16th week of gestation. The presence in the first trimester of an absent bladder on repeated examinations is also possible, given the lack of renal function. The presence of discrepancy in echogenicity of renal parenchyma between the right and left kidney on transvaginal ultrasound is another marker for the possible presence of a unilateral MCKD in early gestation. Unilateral MCDK is associated with contralateral renal anomalies in 30% to 40% of cases and nonrenal anomalies in about 25% of cases.[26] Extrarenal anomalies include central nervous system, cardiac, and gastrointestinal.[26] The risk of aneuploidy is high when MCDK is associated with multiple extrarenal malformations.

## Bilateral Renal Agenesis

### Definition

Bilateral renal agenesis is defined by the congenital absence of both kidneys and ureters, and results from a developmental failure of the ureteric bud and/or the metanephric mesenchyme. Bilateral renal agenesis has a prevalence of 1:4,000 to 1:7,000 pregnancies at the routine obstetric ultrasound examination.[27] The absence of both kidneys results in anhydramnios, which is typically first noted after 16 weeks of gestation. Anhydramnios leads to Potter sequence, which is a constellation of findings including pulmonary hypoplasia, facial abnormalities, and deformities of extremities. Bilateral renal agenesis is more common in males and is a uniformly lethal malformation.

### Ultrasound Findings

The prenatal diagnosis of bilateral renal agenesis is a straightforward diagnosis after 16 weeks, because of associated oligohydramnios, as a leading ultrasound clue. The onset of oligo- or anhydramnios starts between 15 and 16 weeks of gestation when amniotic fluid production is primarily renal in origin. Therefore, the suspicion of bilateral renal agenesis in the first trimester is a challenge and primarily relies on the identification of an absent bladder and kidneys (Figs. 13.33 and 13.34). Absent bladder in the pelvis on repeated ultrasound examinations may alert the examiner to the presence of bilateral renal agenesis in the first trimester.[28] Color Doppler applied on an axial view of the pelvis will identify the two umbilical arteries and help to localize the anatomic site of the bladder (Figs. 13.4, 13.33, and 13.34). On rare occasions, a small "bladder" maybe visible in the pelvis in

early gestation despite the presence of bilateral renal agenesis. Although the exact etiology of this finding is currently unclear, possibilities include retrograde filling of the bladder or the presence of a midline urachal cyst mimicking the bladder.[28] A coronal plane of the abdomen and pelvis in color Doppler will identify the descending aorta and the absence of renal arteries (Figs. 13.33 and 13.34). The "lying down" or "flat" adrenal sign, an important second trimester sign showing the flattened adrenal gland on the psoas muscle, is not easily seen in the first trimester (Fig. 13.35). When bilateral renal agenesis is suspected in the first trimester, follow-up ultrasound in the early second trimester is recommended to confirm the diagnosis by the onset of anhydramnios.

### Associated Malformations

Associated malformations have been frequently reported and include gastrointestinal, vascular, and laterality defects. Several syndromes are associated with bilateral renal aplasia to include VACTERL association, Fraser syndrome, and sirenomelia, to name a few. Chromosomal aneuploidy is present in about 7% of prenatal cases,[27] and several causative gene mutations have been described. The absence of a bladder on ultrasound in the first trimester should also alert the examiner to the presence of other urogenital malformations such as bladder exstrophy or bilateral cystic renal dysplasia.[1]

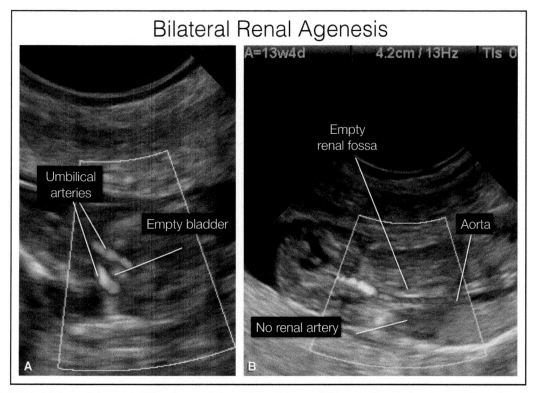

**Figure 13.33:** Axial plane of the pelvis **(A)** and coronal plane of the abdomen **(B)** in color Doppler in a fetus at 13 weeks of gestation with renal agenesis diagnosed on routine first trimester ultrasound. Note in **A** the absence of a bladder between the two umbilical arteries. In **B**, renal arteries could not be imaged with empty renal fossa and absence of renal arteries bilaterally. Amniotic fluid is normal. The presence of a pelvic kidney could not be ruled out, and the patient had a follow-up ultrasound at 16 weeks of gestation (not demonstrated) showing anhydramnios and confirming the diagnosis of bilateral renal agenesis.

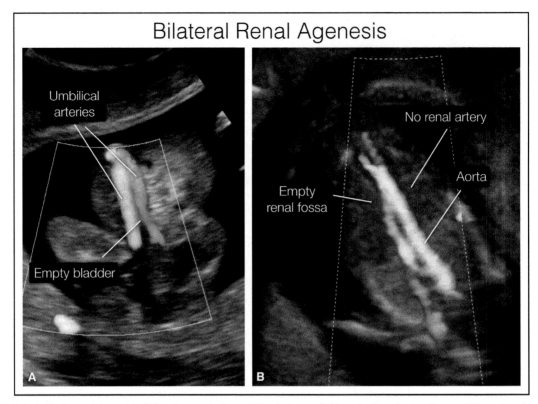

**Figure 13.34:** Axial plane of the pelvis **(A)** and coronal plane of the abdomen **(B)** in color Doppler in a fetus at 13 weeks of gestation with renal agenesis. Similar to Figure 13.33, note the absent bladder in **A** and empty renal fossa with absence of renal arteries in **B**. This fetus also had radial aplasia (not shown).

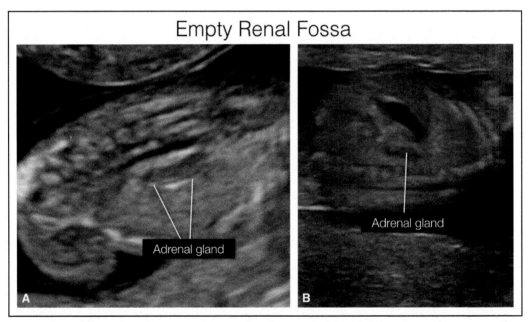

**Figure 13.35:** Parasagittal plane of the fetal abdomen in two fetuses **(A and B)** with empty renal fossa, diagnosed at 12 weeks of gestation in both fetuses. Note the presence of the typical flat adrenal gland (labeled) in **A** and **B** and compare with the normal shape of the adrenal gland in Figure 13.7. Fetus in **A** also had a single umbilical artery, which led us to perform a transvaginal detailed ultrasound. Unilateral renal agenesis was confirmed in fetus **A** at 17 weeks of gestation. Fetus in **B** had a cardiac defect, diagnosed at 12 weeks of gestation and detailed first trimester ultrasound revealed the presence of an empty renal fossa with flat adrenal gland (*asterisk*). The final diagnosis of a pelvic kidney was made and is shown in Figure 13.36.

## Unilateral Renal Agenesis

Unilateral renal agenesis results when one kidney fails to develop and is absent. This is primarily because of failure of development of the ureteric bud or failure of induction of the metanephric mesenchyme. The prenatal diagnosis in the first trimester is initially suspected when one kidney is not seen in the renal fossa (Fig. 13.35). A search for a pelvic kidney or crossed ectopia should be performed before the diagnosis of unilateral renal agenesis is confirmed. Color Doppler of the abdominal aorta, obtained in a coronal plane of the abdomen and pelvis, is helpful to confirm the diagnosis because it shows the absence of a renal artery on the suspected renal agenesis side. In high-resolution ultrasound, visualization of the renal fossa can reveal the presence of the horizontal flat (lying down) adrenal gland instead of the kidney (Fig. 13.35). Follow-up in the second trimester is important in order to confirm the diagnosis. Compensatory hypertrophy of the contralateral kidney is present in the second and third trimester of pregnancy. The diagnosis of a single umbilical artery in the first trimester presents an increased risk for renal malformations.

## Pelvic Kidney, Crossed Renal Ectopia, and Horseshoe Kidney

Abnormal kidney location, also referred to as renal ectopia, encompasses three types of abnormalities: pelvic kidney, crossed renal ectopia, and horseshoe kidney. Abnormal kidney location results from failure of proper migration of the metanephros from the pelvis to the abdomen during embryogenesis. Pelvic kidney refers to a kidney that is located in the pelvis below the aortic bifurcation (Fig. 13.36). Crossed renal ectopia refers to two kidneys on one side of the abdomen, with fusion of the kidneys. Horseshoe kidney, the most common form of renal ectopia, refers to fusion of the lower poles of the kidneys in the midline abdomen, typically below the origin of the inferior mesenteric artery (Fig. 13.37). Other renal abnormalities are common in association with renal ectopia and include UT dilation. In the first trimester, the slightly bright appearance of kidneys helps in the identification of kidney location in the pelvis when the renal fossa appears empty (Fig. 13.36). Bridging of renal tissue over the fetal spine helps in the identification of a horseshoe kidney in the first trimester (Fig. 13.37). In our experience, the presence of trisomy 18, Turner syndrome, and single umbilical artery increases the risk for an association with horseshoe kidneys (Fig. 13.37). Careful evaluation of fetal anatomy in the first trimester is important when renal ectopia is suspected, given a high association with other fetal malformations as VACTERL association, open and closed spina bifida, and chromosomal abnormalities.

## Duplex Kidney

Duplex kidney, also referred to as duplicated collecting system, occurs when a kidney is divided into two separate moieties, an

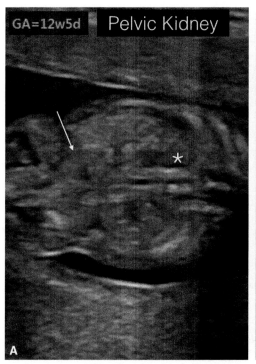
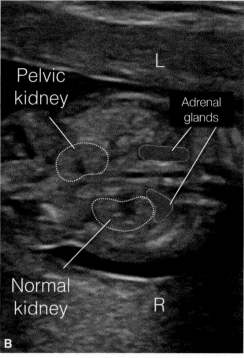

**Figure 13.36:** Coronal plane of the fetal abdomen, obtained with the transabdominal linear probe, in a fetus with a left pelvic kidney diagnosed at 12 weeks of gestation (same fetus as in Fig. 13.35). Note the presence in **A** of a left pelvic kidney (*arrow*) and a flat adrenal gland (*asterisk*). **B:** The same figure as in **A**, with annotations to display both kidneys and adrenals. The kidneys are encircled and the adrenal glands are highlighted in *red*. Note the normal triangular shape of the adrenal on the right (R) side and the flat left (L) adrenal. The left pelvic kidney is shown in the pelvis as opposed to the abdominal location of the right kidney.

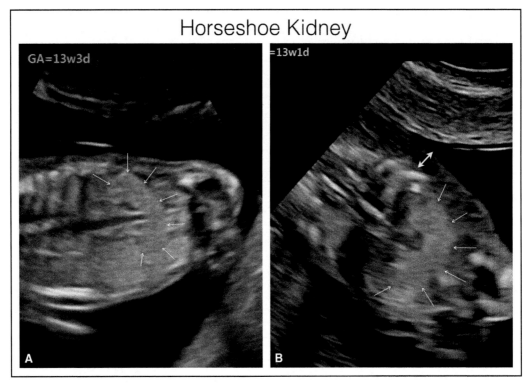

**Figure 13.37:** Coronal planes of the fetal abdomen in two fetuses with horseshoe kidneys (*arrows*) at 13 weeks of gestation. Because of the increased echogenicity in the kidneys in the first trimester, the renal bridge between the right and left kidney across the midline can be well appreciated. The fetus in **A** had other anomalies and trisomy 18 was confirmed. Fetus in **B** also had cystic hygroma and body edema (*double headed arrow*) and the diagnosis of monosomy X was confirmed.

upper moiety and a lower moiety. Duplex kidney is thought to occur during embryogenesis when an additional ureteric bud arises from the mesonephric duct and fuses with the metanephric mesenchyme. The ureter arising from the upper renal moiety is commonly dilated and may form an ureterocele in the bladder, which is a common sign leading to its prenatal diagnosis. The renal pelvis of the upper moiety is also commonly dilated and has a "cyst-like" appearance on prenatal sonography.[29] VUR is commonly seen in the lower moiety. Duplex kidney is more common in females and is present bilaterally in about 15% to 20% of cases. The suspicion of duplex kidney in the first trimester is rare, and the diagnosis is, however, feasible when alerted by family history. The presence of two renal pelves in one kidney on coronal view suggests the diagnosis.

## Bladder Exstrophy and Cloacal Abnormalities

Bladder exstrophy is a defect of the anterior lower abdominal wall, inferior to the insertion of the umbilical cord, and involving the protrusion of the urinary bladder. Typically, the umbilical cord inserts low on the abdominal wall, and the bladder mucosa is eventrated directly below the umbilical

cord. Bladder exstrophy occurs more commonly in males than in females, and is associated with abnormalities in fetal gender with bifid clitoris or penis or with epispadia. In addition, pelvic and pubic bones are widened. Bladder exstrophy can be isolated or can be part of cloacal malformation, as discussed in detail in Chapter 12. The diagnosis of isolated cases of bladder exstrophy can be easily missed on ultrasound. As reported in a literature review of 10 cases, typical clues to the presence of bladder exstrophy include a nonvisible fetal bladder during the first trimester ultrasound examination, along with the presence of normal kidneys and low umbilical cord insertion.[30] In the presence of bladder exstrophy, axial plane of the pelvis in color Doppler will show an absent bladder along with the presence of a "mass of tissue," resulting from bladder exteriorization. The presence of other fluid-filled structures in the pelvis, including urachal remnant, may be misleading in cases of bladder exstrophy.[31] **Figure 13.38A** is a midsagittal plane of a normal fetus, and **Figure 13.38B** is a fetus with bladder exstrophy showing the presence of a low insertion of the umbilical cord along with abnormal tissue inferior to the cord insertion. During the first trimester ultrasound, the diagnosis of bladder exstrophy can be easily missed if imaging of the lower anterior wall of the abdomen and the bladder with the surrounding umbilical arteries is not performed. Bladder

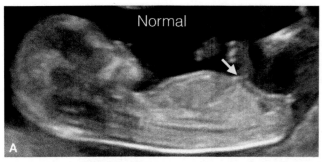 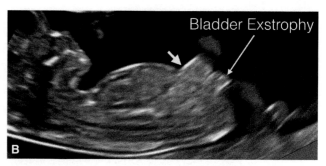

**Figure 13.38:** Midsagittal plane in a normal fetus **(A)** at 12 weeks of gestation and in a fetus with bladder exstrophy **(B)** at 13 weeks of gestation. The bladder could not be visualized in fetus **B** during the detailed ultrasound examination. When compared with the normal fetus **A**, note the presence of a low abdominal cord insertion (*short arrow*) in **B**. Also note the presence of irregular tissue inferior to the cord insertion in **B**, which represents bladder exstrophy. Fetal gender could not be well identified in **B**.

exstrophy is a sporadic anomaly, which could be part of syndromic conditions and other more complex malformations, thus making fetal counseling difficult,[30,31] especially in the first trimester. We recommend a close follow-up ultrasound examination at 16 weeks of gestation if the diagnosis of bladder exstrophy is suspected in the first trimester. This is important to confirm the diagnosis and to exclude additional urogenital, gastrointestinal, and other anomalies.

Cloacal abnormalities refer to a spectrum of anomalies where the gastrointestinal, urinary, and genital tracts share a common cavity for discharge. Embryologically, a cloaca persists beyond the fourth to sixth week of gestation when the partition of the cloaca into the urogenital sinus and the rectum fails to occur. The diagnosis of cloacal abnormalities is possible in the first trimester, especially in its severe forms. The presence of a cystic structure in the mid- or lower abdomen in the first trimester should alert for the possible presence of cloacal abnormalities, because the cystic structure may represent a communication between the bladder and bowel (Figs. 12.44 to 12.46). Association of cloacal abnormalities with enlarged nuchal translucencies has been reported.[32] In its severe form, bladder exstrophy can be part of cloacal exstrophy, and include an omphalocele, bladder exstrophy, imperforate anus, and spinal defects: a constellation of malformations referred to as OEIS (see Chapter 12). The presence of ambiguous genitalia is a common association.

## Abnormal Genitalia

There are currently no comprehensive studies or reports on the diagnosis of abnormal genitalia in the first trimester. As described earlier in this chapter, the reliable assessment of the normal genitalia can be achieved from 12 weeks onward in optimal imaging. It is, however, difficult to achieve a definitive diagnosis on any gender malformation in the first trimester, with the exception of cloacal abnormalities. Once a renal malformation is suspected in the first trimester, however, ultrasound assessment of the genitalia should be performed because this may help in confirming the diagnosis. For instance, PUV is typically found in males, whereas megacystis microcolon peristalsis syndrome is found more commonly in females. The absence of one kidney, in combination with a single umbilical artery and abnormal genitalia, may raise the suspicion for a syndromic condition. Gender discrepancy between chorionic villous sampling and ultrasound in a male fetus could suspect the presence of sexual reversal, as in Smith–Lemli–Opitz syndrome, campomelic dysplasia, chodrodysplasia punctata, and others. **Figure 13.39** shows a case of a thickened nuchal translucency in a male fetus with suspected aortic coarctation, where chorionic villous sampling revealed Turner syndrome mosaic.

## Abnormal Adrenal Gland

The adrenal gland appears as an anechoic structure between the kidney and diaphragm, with an adrenal length about half the length of the kidney.[5,18] In the second and third trimester of pregnancy, the adrenal glands are commonly abnormal in association with neuroblastoma or hemorrhage, conditions that are not existent in the first trimester. On the other hand, a flat adrenal gland can be a marker for the presence of an empty renal fossa (**Figs. 13.35 and 13.36**), in renal agenesis or a pelvic kidney. In addition, we reported on enlarged adrenal glands[5] in a fetus with congenital adrenal hyperplasia and found the adrenals to be larger than the kidneys (**Fig. 13.40**). It is important to note that most cases of congenital adrenal hyperplasia do not have significantly enlarged adrenal glands and remain undetected in utero.

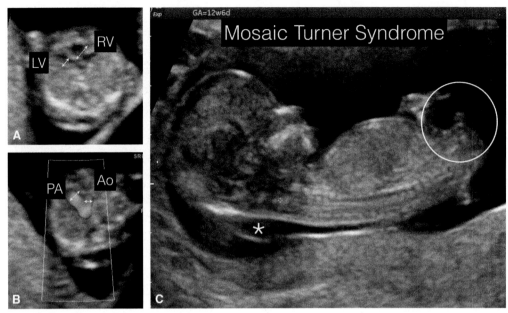

**Figure 13.39:** Axial plane of the chest at the level of the four-chamber view **(A)**, the three-vessel-trachea view **(B)**, and nuchal translucency **(C)** in a fetus at 12 weeks of gestation. Note the presence of ventricular **(A)** and great vessel **(B)** disproportion, suggesting the diagnosis of an aortic coarctation. Also note in **C** the presence of a thickened nuchal translucency of 4 mm (*asterisk*). The combination of a thickened NT with left ventricular outflow obstruction suggests the diagnosis of monosomy X. The fetal gender was male, however, as shown in **C** (*circle*). The diagnosis of mosaic 46 XY and 45 XO was confirmed on invasive testing. PA, pulmonary artery; LV, left ventricle; RV, right ventricle; Ao, aorta.

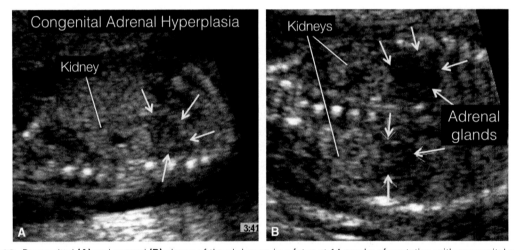

**Figure 13.40:** Parasagittal **(A)** and coronal **(B)** planes of the abdomen in a fetus at 14 weeks of gestation with congenital adrenal hyperplasia (CAH). Note the enlarged size of the adrenal glands bilaterally (*arrows*) and compare with normal first trimester adrenal glands, shown in Figure 13.7. In the previous pregnancy, the diagnosis of CAH was performed, which resulted in a detailed evaluation of the adrenal glands in this pregnancy.

## REFERENCES

1. Syngelaki A, Chelemen T, Dagklis T, et al. Challenges in the diagnosis of fetal non-chromosomal abnormalities at 11-13 weeks. *Prenat Diagn.* 2011;31:90–102.
2. Sebire NJ, Kaisenberg von C, Rubio C, et al. Fetal megacystis at 10–14 weeks of gestation. *Ultrasound Obstet Gynecol.* 1996;8:387–390.
3. Liao AW, Sebire NJ, Geerts L, et al. Megacystis at 10–14 weeks of gestation: chromosomal defects and outcome according to bladder length. *Ultrasound Obstet Gynecol.* 2003;21:338–341.
4. Rosati P, Guariglia L. Transvaginal sonographic assessment of the fetal urinary tract in early pregnancy. *Ultrasound Obstet Gynecol.* 1996;7:95–100.
5. Esser T, Chaoui R. Enlarged adrenal glands as a prenatal marker of congenital adrenal hyperplasia: a report of two cases. *Ultrasound Obstet Gynecol.* 2004;23:293–297.
6. Whitlow BJ, Economides DL. The optimal gestational age to examine fetal anatomy and measure nuchal translucency in the first trimester. *Ultrasound Obstet Gynecol.* 1998;11:258–261.
7. Odeh M, Granin V, Kais M, et al. Sonographic fetal sex determination. *Obstet Gynecol Surv.* 2009;64:50–57.

8. Kagan KO, Staboulidou I, Syngelaki A, et al. The 11-13-week scan: diagnosis and outcome of holoprosencephaly, exomphalos and megacystis. *Ultrasound Obstet Gynecol.* 2010;36:10–14.

9. Casale AJ. Early ureteral surgery for posterior urethral valves. *Urol Clin North Am.* 1990;17:361–372.

10. Dinneen MD, Duffy PG. Posterior urethral valves. *Br J Urol.* 1996;78:275–281.

11. Jouannic J-M, Hyett JA, Pandya PP, et al. Perinatal outcome in fetuses with megacystis in the first half of pregnancy. *Prenat Diagn.* 2003;23:340–344.

12. Bornes M, Spaggiari E, Schmitz T, et al. Outcome and etiologies of fetal megacystis according to the gestational age at diagnosis. *Prenat Diagn.* 2013;33:1162–1166.

13. Syngelaki A, Guerra L, Ceccacci I, et al. Impact of holoprosencephaly, exomphalos, megacystis and high NT in first trimester screening for chromosomal abnormalities. *Ultrasound Obstet Gynecol.* 2016. doi:10.1002/uog.17286.

14. Taipale P, Heinonen K, Kainulainen S, et al. Cloacal anomaly simulating megalocystis in the first trimester. *J Clin Ultrasound.* 2004;32:419–422.

15. Nguyen HT, Herndon CDA, Cooper C, et al. The Society for Fetal Urology consensus statement on the evaluation and management of antenatal hydronephrosis. *J Pediatr Urol.* 2010;6:212–231.

16. Nguyen HT, Benson CB, Bromley B, et al. Multidisciplinary consensus on the classification of prenatal and postnatal urinary tract dilation (UTD classification system). 2014;10:982–998.

17. Dagklis T, Plasencia W, Maiz N, et al. Choroid plexus cyst, intracardiac echogenic focus, hyperechogenic bowel and hydronephrosis in screening for trisomy 21 at 11 + 0 to 13 + 6 weeks. *Ultrasound Obstet Gynecol.* 2007;31:132–135.

18. Bronshtein M, Bar-Hava I, Lightman A. The significance of early second-trimester sonographic detection of minor fetal renal anomalies. *Prenat Diagn.* 1995;15:627–632.

19. Ismaili K, Hall M, Donner C, et al. Results of systematic screening for minor degrees of fetal renal pelvis dilatation in an unselected population. *Am J Obstet Gynecol.* 2003;188:242–246.

20. Benacerraf BR. The role of the second trimester genetic sonogram in screening for fetal Down syndrome. *Semin Perinatol.* 2005;29:386–394.

21. Bronshtein M, Bar-Hava I, Blumenfeld Z. Clues and pitfalls in the early prenatal diagnosis of "late onset" infantile polycystic kidney. *Prenat Diagn.* 1992;12:293–298.

22. Gondra L, Décramer S, Chalouhi GE, et al. Hyperechogenic kidneys and polyhydramnios associated with HNF1B gene mutation. *Pediatr Nephrol.* 2016;31:1705–1708.

23. Zerres K, Mücher G, Becker J, et al. Prenatal diagnosis of autosomal recessive polycystic kidney disease (ARPKD): molecular genetics, clinical experience, and fetal morphology. *Am J Med Genet.* 1998;76:137–144.

24. Gunay-Aygun M, Avner ED, Bacallao RL, et al. Autosomal recessive polycystic kidney disease and congenital hepatic fibrosis: summary statement of a first National Institutes of Health/Office of Rare Diseases conference. *J Pediatr.* 2006;149:159–164.

25. Zerres K, Rudnik-Schöneborn S, Deget F, et al. Autosomal recessive polycystic kidney disease in 115 children: clinical presentation, course and influence of gender. *Acta Paediatr.* 1996;85:437–445.

26. Schreuder MF, Westland R, van Wijk JAE. Unilateral multicystic dysplastic kidney: a meta-analysis of observational studies on the incidence, associated urinary tract malformations and the contralateral kidney. *Nephrol Dial Transplant.* 2009;24:1810–1818.

27. Garne E, Loane M, Dolk H, et al. Prenatal diagnosis of severe structural congenital malformations in Europe. *Ultrasound Obstet Gynecol.* 2005;25:6–11.

28. Bronshtein M, Amit A, Achiron R, et al. The early prenatal sonographic diagnosis of renal agenesis: techniques and possible pitfalls. *Prenat Diagn.* 1994;14:291–297.

29. Abuhamad AZ, Horton CE, Horton SH, et al. Renal duplication anomalies in the fetus: clues for prenatal diagnosis. *Ultrasound Obstet Gynecol.* 1996;7:174–177.

30. Cacciari A, Pilu GL, Mordenti M, et al. Prenatal diagnosis of bladder exstrophy: what counseling? *J Urol.* 1999;161:259–261; discussion 262.

31. Goldstein I, Shalev E, Nisman D. The dilemma of prenatal diagnosis of bladder exstrophy: a case report and a review of the literature. *Ultrasound Obstet Gynecol.* 2001;17:357–359.

32. Keppler-Noreuil K, Gorton S, Foo F, et al. Prenatal ascertainment of OEIS complex/cloacal exstrophy—15 new cases and literature review. *Am J Med Genet A.* 2007;143A:2122–2128.

# CHAPTER 14

# The Fetal Skeletal System

## INTRODUCTION

Ultrasound in the first trimester provides a distinct advantage over ultrasound in the second and third trimester of pregnancy for the evaluation of the fetal skeletal system, especially the upper and lower extremities. With advancing gestation, fetal crowding makes evaluation of the extremities and spine more challenging. Sonographic evaluation of the skeletal system in the first trimester includes imaging of the cranium, the ribs, the spine, and the four extremities. An understanding of the gestational progression of bone ossification is important in order to differentiate normal from abnormal findings. In this chapter, we present a brief description of embryology of the skeletal system, its normal sonographic examination, along with common skeletal system abnormalities that can be diagnosed in the first trimester of pregnancy.

## EMBRYOLOGY

The skeletal system includes the axial and appendicular skeleton. The axial skeleton comprises the skull, spine, and rib cage, and the appendicular skeleton is made of the upper and lower extremities along with the shoulder and pelvic girdles. The skeletal system is primarily derived from the mesoderm, which appears during the third week of embryogenesis. The mesoderm gives rise to mesenchymal cells, which differentiate into fibroblasts, chondroblasts, and osteoblasts to form the tissue of the musculoskeletal system. The embryonic mesoderm is divided into three distinct regions: paraxial mesoderm (medially), intermediate mesoderm (middle part), and lateral plate mesoderm (laterally). The skeletal system is formed from the paraxial and lateral plate mesoderm, along with neural crest cells, derived from ectoderm. The paraxial mesoderm forms the axial skeleton and lateral plate mesoderm forms the appendicular skeleton.

The paraxial mesoderm segments into somites along the neural tube by the third week of embryogenesis. The somites differentiate into the sclerotome (ventromedial part) and the dermomyotome (dermatome and myotome) (dorsolateral part) (Fig. 14.1). During the fifth week of embryogenesis, the upper and lower limb buds are seen as outpocketings from the ventrolateral body wall at the spinal levels of C5–C8 and L3–L5, respectively (Fig. 14.2A). The terminal portions of limb buds flatten out in the fifth week to form hand and foot plates (Fig. 14.2B). Circular constrictions are noted between the proximal portions and the plates, representing the future wrist and ankle creases (Fig. 14.2B). During the fifth week, the upper limbs rotate 90 degrees laterally, whereas the lower limbs rotate 90 degrees medially. Growth of the limb buds continues between the fifth and the eighth week until the extremities take their definitive form (Fig. 14.2C).

Bone ossification occurs in two types: membranous and intracartilaginous. The membranous type is the process of bone formation directly from mesenchyme and is typically seen in flat bone such as the skull, whereas intracartilaginous ossification is the process of ossification from cartilaginous cells and is seen in the spine and long bones. By the end of the fourth week, the cartilaginous centers appear in the long bones, and bone ossification starts by the end of the sixth week. Bone ossification continues postnatally into the second decade of life. The muscles of developing limbs and the axial skeleton are formed from myotomes, derived from the somatic mesoderm. Retinoic acid appears to be important for the initiation of limb bud outgrowth, and appropriate differentiation of the skeletal system has been demonstrated to require sequential *Hox* gene expression.[1,2]

Abnormal development of the skeletal system results in numerous congenital anomalies such as reduction or duplication defects and skeletal dysplasia. Normal anatomy of the skeletal system on ultrasound along with skeletal anomalies that can be seen in the first trimester will be discussed in the following sections.

## NORMAL SONOGRAPHIC ANATOMY

The first evidence of development of extremities includes the limb buds, which are first seen on ultrasound at around

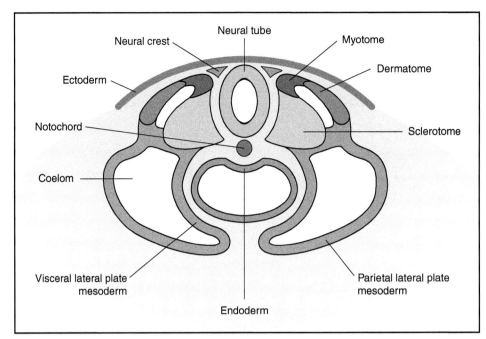

**Figure 14.1:** Embryogenesis of the skeletal system. Note that during the third week of embryogenesis, the paraxial mesoderm segments into somites along the neural tube. The somites differentiate into the sclerotome (ventromedially) and the dermomyotome (dorsolaterally). The dermomyotome includes the dermatome and myotome as shown in this figure. Refer to the embryology section in the chapter for more details on this subject.

## Limb Bud Development

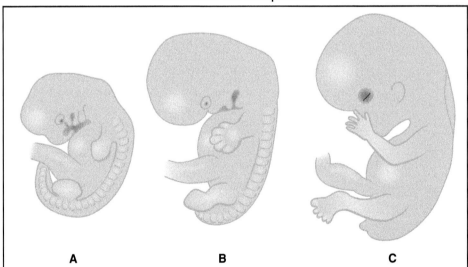

**Figure 14.2:** Development of limb buds in the embryo between the fifth and eighth week of embryogenesis. During the early fifth week of embryogenesis **(A)**, the upper and lower limb buds are seen as outpocketings from the ventrolateral body wall. Circular constrictions are noted at the sixth week **(B)** between the proximal portions and the plates, representing the future wrist and ankle creases. Growth of the limb buds continues between the fifth and the eighth week **(C)** until the extremities take their definitive form. Refer to the embryology section in the chapter for more details on this subject.

the eighth week of gestation, with the upper limb buds seen before the lower limb buds[3] (Figs. 14.3 and 14.4). Three-dimensional (3D) ultrasound in surface mode is very helpful in the identification of limb buds and four extremities in the first trimester (Figs. 14.5 and 14.6). Visualization of

the normal fetal extremities in the first trimester ultrasound includes the demonstration of four limbs, each with three segments along with normal orientations of hands and feet. This is easily accomplished by obtaining a ventral view of the fetus (Fig. 14.6A and C) (see also Chapter 5). Evaluation of a

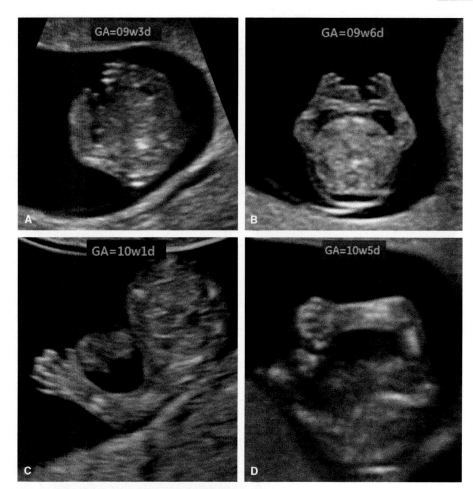

Figure 14.3: Development of arms and hands between 9 and 10 weeks (A–D) of gestation visualized on two-dimensional ultrasound. Note the position of the arms at 9 weeks gestation (A and B) in close proximity to the anterior chest wall. More upper extremity movements are seen by the 10th week of gestation, and the upper arms' segments are then clearly identified (C and D). Note that at 10 weeks of gestation, the hands maintain their proximity to the anterior chest wall and are best imaged in a superior–inferior view.

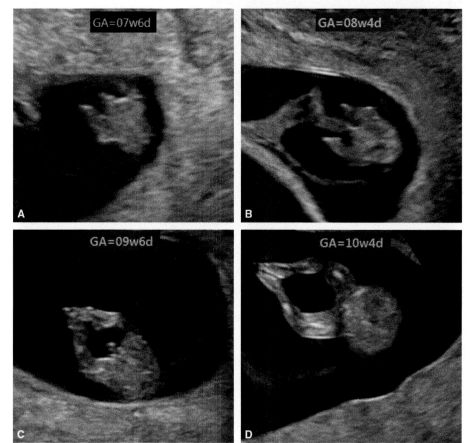

Figure 14.4: Development of legs and feet between 7 and 10 weeks (A–D) of gestation visualized on two-dimensional gray-scale ultrasound. Note that between the 7th and the 8th week (A and B), the legs are straight and short, and by the 9th and 10th week, the feet are in close proximity and touch each other. Before 10 weeks of gestation, the most optimum approach to image the lower extremities is a view inferior to the pelvis (looking from below). Three-dimensional ultrasound is also very helpful in early gestation to assess upper and lower extremities. See Figures 14.5 and 14.6 for more detail.

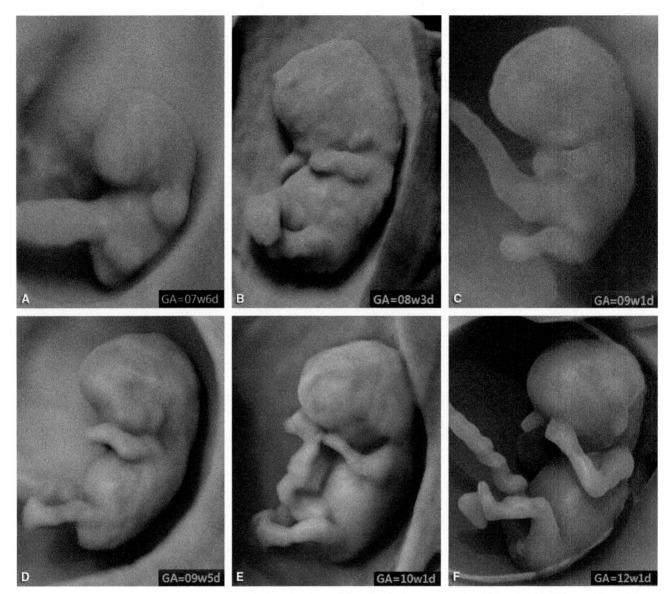

**Figure 14.5:** Three-dimensional ultrasound in surface mode of the embryo/fetus at 7 to 12 weeks of gestation **(A–F)** imaged from the lateral view, demonstrating the development of the arms and legs. See text for details.

single extremity is commonly demonstrated in a longitudinal view (Figs. 14.7 and 14.8). Digits of the hands and feet are reported to be seen from the 11th week of gestation onward[3]; with the new high-resolution transducers however, they can be visualized from 9 weeks onward (Fig. 14.3). Imaging of the fingers may help in the identification of abnormal conditions (polydactyly) and is accomplished by using a high-resolution transducer, either transabdominally or transvaginally (Fig. 14.9). A ventral view of the feet also helps in the demonstration of terminal phalanges (Fig. 14.8D and E). By around the 10th week of gestation, ossification centers within all long bones can be demonstrated. Note that when the lower legs are extended at the knees, the whole lower extremities are seen

on ultrasound obtained from the ventral aspect of the fetus (Fig. 14.10A and B). When the legs are flexed at the knees, only the upper segments (thighs) are seen (Fig. 14.10C). 3D ultrasound at 12 weeks or beyond, obtained from the ventral or lateral approach, can clearly demonstrate upper and lower extremities including both hands and feet (Fig. 14.11).

The fetal spine is difficult to image before the 11th week of gestation because of lack of bone ossification (Fig. 14.12). At 12 weeks of gestation and beyond, the spine is imaged on ultrasound with such details to allow for diagnosis of major spinal deformities (Fig. 14.13). In the first trimester, the fetal spine can be evaluated in the sagittal (Figs. 14.13 and 5.22) and coronal views (Fig. 5.23), but also where possible in

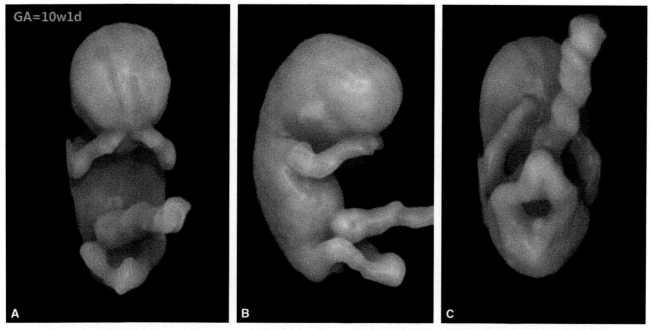

**Figure 14.6:** Three-dimensional ultrasound in surface mode of an embryo at 10 weeks of gestation imaged from the frontal **(A)**, right lateral **(B)**, and inferior **(C)** approach. Note in **A** and **C** the close proximity of the hands and feet at this gestation. See text for details.

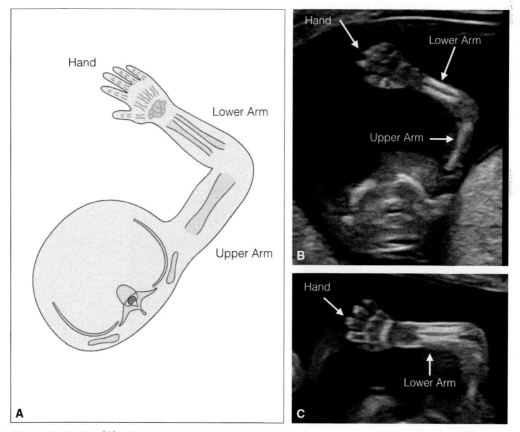

**Figure 14.7:** Schematic drawing **(A)** and corresponding two-dimensional ultrasound images of the upper extremity visualized near a cross-section of the chest in two fetuses at 13 weeks of gestation **(B and C)**. Note the upper arm, lower arm, and hand (all labeled).

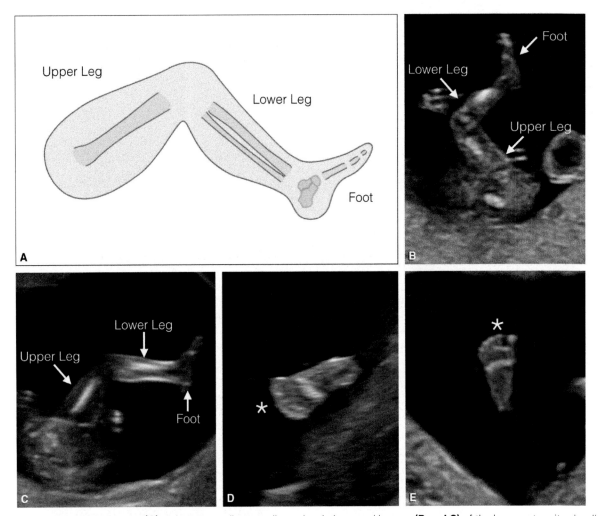

**Figure 14.8:** Schematic drawing **(A)** and corresponding two-dimensional ultrasound images **(B and C)** of the lower extremity visualized in a parasagittal plane in two fetuses at 13 weeks of gestation. Note the upper leg, lower leg, and foot (all labeled). Planes **D** and **E** show a ventral view of the foot. Note that the toes can be visualized at this early gestation (*asterisk*).

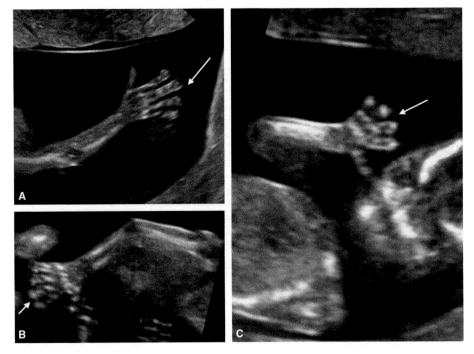

**Figure 14.9:** Two-dimensional ultrasound of the upper extremity at 13 weeks of gestation imaged from different angles (A–C). Note the visualization of arms and hands. Note that at this early gestation all five fingers can be well seen (*arrows*) because the hand is always open.

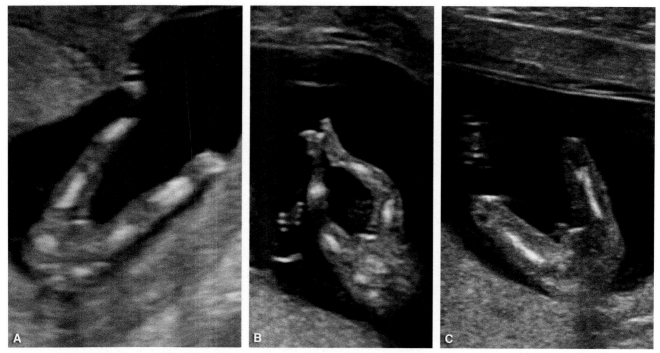

**Figure 14.10:** Axial views **(A–C)** of the fetal pelvis demonstrating the lower extremities. Note that when the lower legs are extended at the knees **(A and B)**, the whole lower extremities are seen. When the legs are flexed at the knee **(C)**, only the upper segments (thighs) are seen.

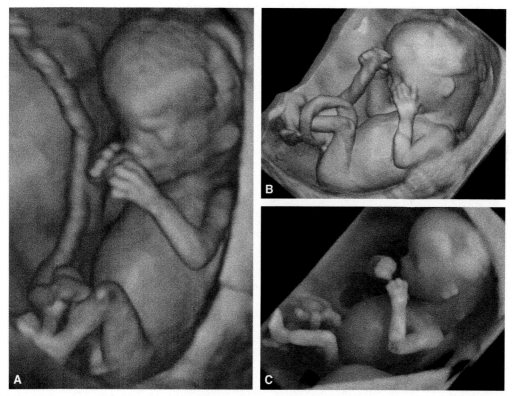

**Figure 14.11:** Three-dimensional ultrasound in surface mode of the entire fetus in three fetuses **(A–C)** at 12 weeks of gestation. Note that the upper and lower extremities can be clearly seen. With high-resolution transducers, the fingers and toes can also be seen. Note the common position of the hands and feet in front of the fetus at this early gestation, which makes visualization easier than later on in pregnancy.

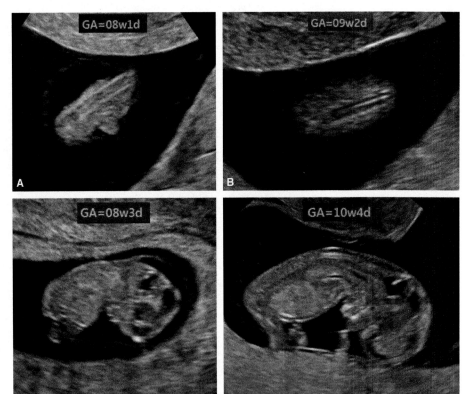

**Figure 14.12:** Visualization of the fetal spine between 8 and 10 weeks of gestation **(A–D)** on two-dimensional transvaginal ultrasound with high resolution. Note that the spine is not yet ossified before 11 weeks of gestation, which makes its assessment somewhat difficult in a midline sagittal plane. The combination of a coronal plane **(A and B)** along with a midline sagittal plane **(C and D)** is occasionally needed to evaluate the spine in early gestation. When technically feasible, three-dimensional ultrasound in surface mode allows for an excellent evaluation of the fetal back and spine.

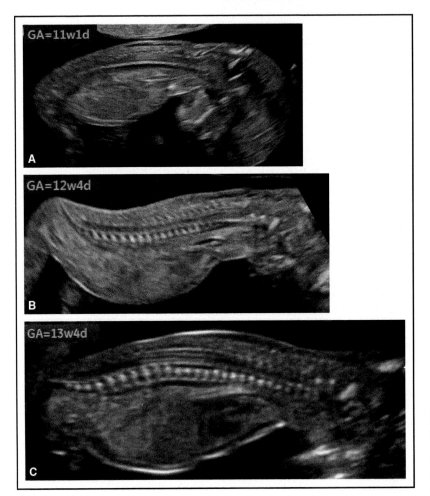

**Figure 14.13:** Midline sagittal planes of the fetal spine in two-dimensional ultrasound in three fetuses at 11 **(A)**, 12 **(B)**, and 13 **(C)** weeks of gestation. Note the progressive ossification of the spine between 11 **(A)** and 13 **(C)** weeks of gestation. Compare the spine ossification with Figure 14.12.

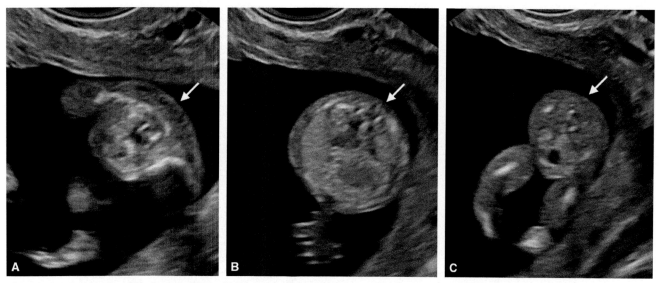

**Figure 14.14:** Cervical **(A)**, thoracic **(B)**, and lumbosacral **(C)** axial planes of the spine in a fetus at 12 weeks of gestation. Note the normal spine and the overlying skin (*arrow*). Along with a sagittal and coronal view of the spine, these planes allow for a comprehensive evaluation of the fetal spine in the first trimester.

axial views at the cervical, thoracic, and lumbosacral regions (Fig. 14.14). This approach is important when spinal abnormalities are suspected such as spina bifida. When technically feasible, 3D ultrasound in surface mode allows for an excellent evaluation of the integrity of the fetal back and spine for open spina bifida in the first trimester (Figs. 14.15, 8.45, and 8.47). Furthermore, 3D ultrasound in skeletal mode of a coronal view of the fetus allows for the evaluation of the spine and thoracic cavity (Fig. 14.16A). 3D ultrasound in skeletal mode also allows for an evaluation of facial and cranial bones

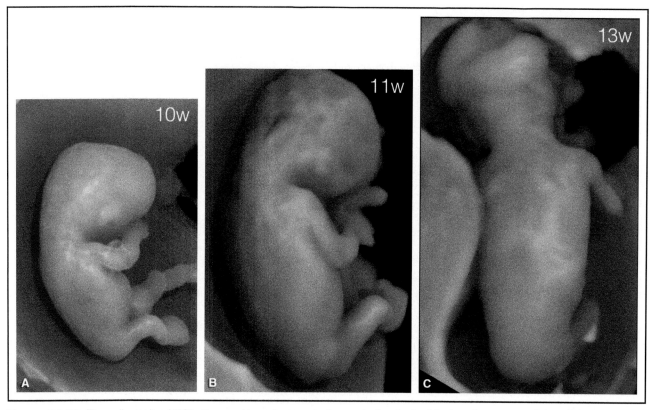

**Figure 14.15:** Three-dimensional (3D) ultrasound in surface mode demonstrating the back in three fetuses at 10 **(A)**, 11 **(B)**, and 13 **(C)** weeks of gestation. Note the absence of a defect in the back, confirming the lack of an open spina bifida. When technically feasible, 3D ultrasound in surface mode allows for an excellent evaluation of the fetal back and spine for open spina bifida.

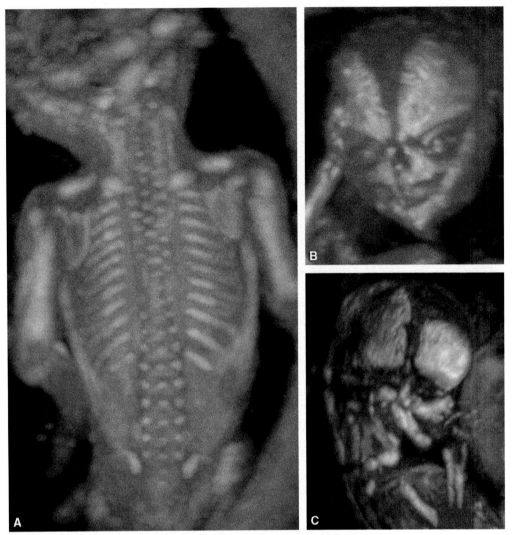

**Figure 14.16:** Three-dimensional (3D) ultrasound in maximum mode in a fetus at 13 weeks of gestation demonstrating the ossified spine, ribs, and scapulae **(A)**, the facial **(B)** and skull **(C)** bones.

in the first trimester (Fig. 14.16B and C). Imaging of the fetal cranium has been discussed in Chapter 8.

# SKELETAL SYSTEM ABNORMALITIES

When compared to the second and third trimester of pregnancy, fewer abnormalities of the skeletal system can be diagnosed in the first trimester primarily because of delayed ossification of bone. In general, the more severe the skeletal abnormality, the more evident it is on ultrasound in the first trimester. Furthermore, confirming the exact type of skeletal abnormality can be challenging in the first trimester. There are two major types of skeletal abnormalities: generalized and localized. Generalized skeletal abnormalities refer to skeletal dysplasia(s), and localized abnormalities refer to more focal malformations of spine and limbs.

## Skeletal Dysplasias

### Definition

Skeletal dysplasias are a large mixed group of bone and cartilage abnormalities resulting in abnormal growth, shape, and/or density of the skeleton. The birth prevalence of skeletal dysplasias ranges from 2 to 7 per 10,000 births.[4] The first trimester diagnosis of a case of skeletal dysplasia (thanatophoric dwarfism) was originally performed in 1988,[5] and since then, several cases have been diagnosed by ultrasound in the first trimester[6–14] (Table 14.1). When technically feasible, the first trimester diagnosis of skeletal dysplasia is helpful because it allows for fetal karyotyping and for molecular genetic testing. Molecular genetic testing takes time, and thus, its performance in the first trimester allows for the results to be available in the second trimester for appropriate patient counseling. Mutation in the *FGFR3* gene is responsible for a spectrum of skeletal dysplasias to include thanatophoric dysplasia on one end and

**Table 14.1 • Skeletal Dysplasias That Can Be Diagnosed by 14 Weeks of Gestation**

Achondrogenesis I and II
Ellis–van Creveld syndrome
Osteogenesis imperfecta II
Thanatophoric dysplasia
Campomelic dysplasia
Diastrophic dysplasia
Congenital hypophosphatasia
Jeune asphyxing thorax dysplasia
Short-rib polydactyly syndromes
Roberts syndrome
Cleidocranial dysplasia

Adapted from Khalil A, Pajkrt E, Chitty LS. Early prenatal diagnosis of skeletal anomalies. *Prenat Diagn.* 2011;31:115–124; copyright John Wiley & Sons, Ltd., with permission.

about the 14th week of gestation, and thus, suspecting its presence is possible in most cases. Suspicion for and/or detection of skeletal dysplasia in the first trimester has been reported in up to 80% in some series,[16] with lethal abnormalities having the highest detection rates. Accurate diagnosis of the specific subtype of skeletal dysplasia is often difficult in the absence of a relevant family history.[14] Enlarged nuchal translucency (NT) and/or hydrops is commonly seen in fetuses with skeletal dysplasias in the first trimester.[14,16,17] There is considerable phenotypic overlap between various types of skeletal dysplasia, and the specific diagnosis may be difficult to make in the first trimester.

### Ultrasound Findings

Common ultrasound features of skeletal dysplasia in the first trimester include short femur, abnormal skull shape and mineralization, and abnormal fetal profile or chest.[14] In our experience, the presence on the first trimester ultrasound of shortened, misshapen, or fractured long bones is typically the first clue for the presence of skeletal dysplasia in the fetus (Fig. 14.17). A small thorax with shortened ribs, when seen at 14 weeks of gestation, should also raise the suspicion for skeletal dysplasia (Fig. 14.18). Fetal biometric measurements, especially when performed at 14 to 15 weeks, may give a clue to the presence of skeletal dysplasia. For instance, the combination of long bone measurements at less than the 5th percentile along with a head circumference greater than the 75th percentile is highly suspicious for the presence of

achondroplasia and hypochondroplasia on the other end.[15] When a lethal skeletal dysplasia is suspected in the first trimester, a follow-up ultrasound examination is recommended at around 15 to 17 weeks of gestation, because detailed sonographic features of the malformation are commonly present by then. It is important to note, however, that the typical sonographic features of many significant skeletal dysplasias are present by

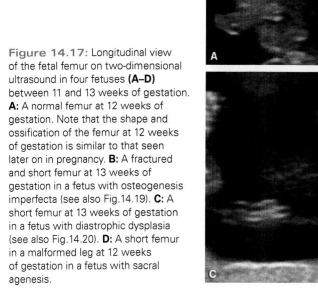
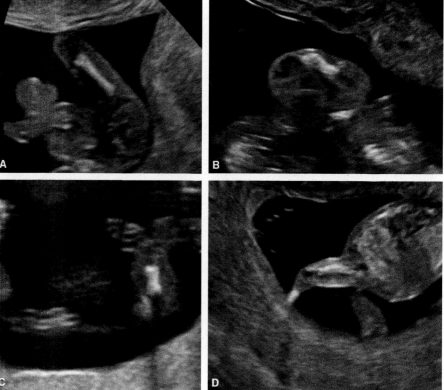

**Figure 14.17:** Longitudinal view of the fetal femur on two-dimensional ultrasound in four fetuses **(A–D)** between 11 and 13 weeks of gestation. **A:** A normal femur at 12 weeks of gestation. Note that the shape and ossification of the femur at 12 weeks of gestation is similar to that seen later on in pregnancy. **B:** A fractured and short femur at 13 weeks of gestation in a fetus with osteogenesis imperfecta (see also Fig. 14.19). **C:** A short femur at 13 weeks of gestation in a fetus with diastrophic dysplasia (see also Fig. 14.20). **D:** A short femur in a malformed leg at 12 weeks of gestation in a fetus with sacral agenesis.

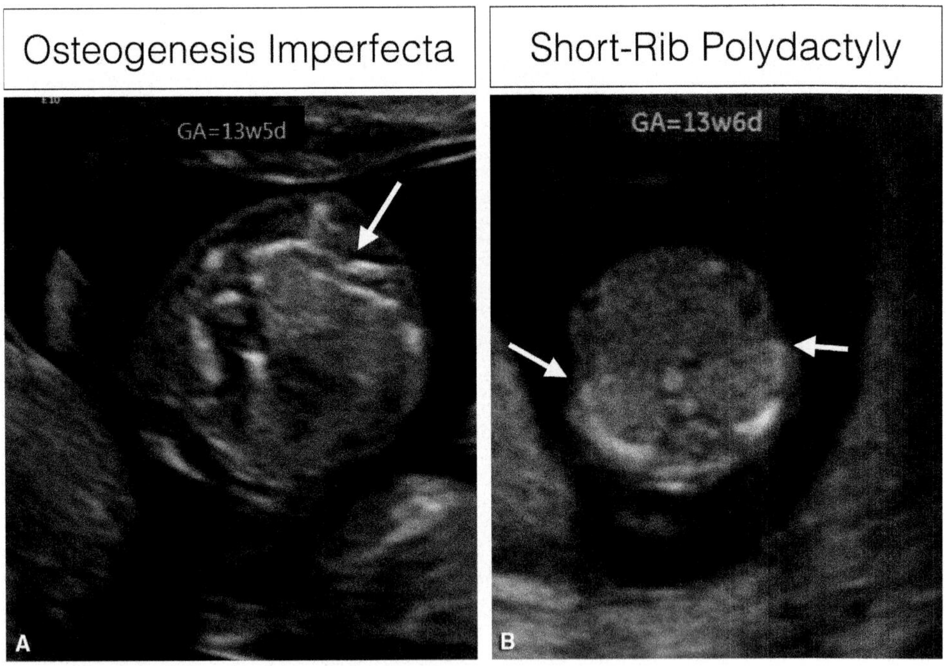

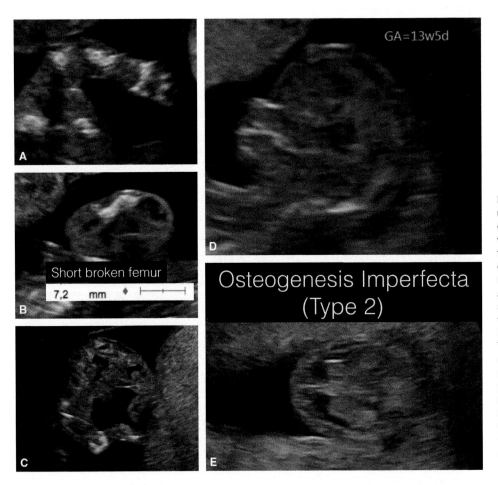

**Figure 14.18:** Axial plane of the fetal chest in two-dimensional ultrasound at 13 weeks of gestation in two fetuses **(A)** and **(B)** with skeletal dysplasia and abnormal ribs. Note in **A**, the presence of broken ribs (*arrow*) in a fetus with osteogenesis imperfecta and in **B**, short ribs (*arrows*) in a fetus with short-rib polydactyly syndrome. Compare with Figure 14.22 and note that short ribs may not appear at less than 14 weeks of gestation.

**Figure 14.19:** Two-dimensional ultrasound images of the extremities and head in a fetus with osteogenesis imperfecta type 2, diagnosed at 13 weeks of gestation and confirmed by molecular genetic testing. Note in **A–C** the presence of abnormally shortened and bowed long bones with discrepant length and shape between the left and right side. The fetal ribs also appeared abnormal and broken and are shown in Figure 14.18A. Note the presence of a hypomineralized skull in **D** and **E**, which also suggested the diagnosis. Compare with the fetus in Figure 14.21 with thanatophoric dysplasia, with shortened long bones but with increased mineralization of skull.

skeletal dysplasia.[18] When bone abnormalities are suspected in the first trimester, detailed evaluation by high-resolution ultrasound transducers (transvaginal when feasible) is helpful in order to assess the fetal skeletal system in its entirety. Evaluation of the cranium, spine, ribs, long bones, and digits should be performed. Along with genetic and molecular testing, a follow-up ultrasound at 15 to 16 weeks of gestation is recommended in order to assess the severity of the skeletal abnormality and to ascertain the specific subtype of skeletal dysplasia. Figures 14.19 to 14.23 show typical sonographic

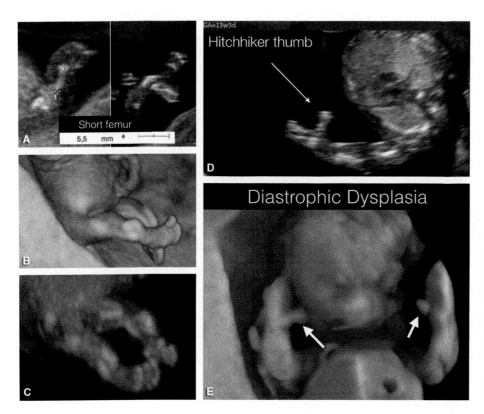

Figure 14.20: Two-dimensional and three-dimensional ultrasound images of the upper and lower extremities in a fetus with diastrophic dysplasia, diagnosed at 13 weeks of gestation and confirmed by molecular genetic testing. Note the presence of short long bones **(A)** along with abnormal long bone shape and overall short extremities **(B and C)**. The presence of an abducted thumb, known as "hitchhiker" thumb, in **D** and **E**, suggested the diagnosis of diastrophic dysplasia.

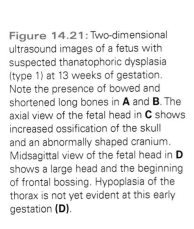

Figure 14.21: Two-dimensional ultrasound images of a fetus with suspected thanatophoric dysplasia (type 1) at 13 weeks of gestation. Note the presence of bowed and shortened long bones in **A** and **B**. The axial view of the fetal head in **C** shows increased ossification of the skull and an abnormally shaped cranium. Midsagittal view of the fetal head in **D** shows a large head and the beginning of frontal bossing. Hypoplasia of the thorax is not yet evident at this early gestation **(D)**.

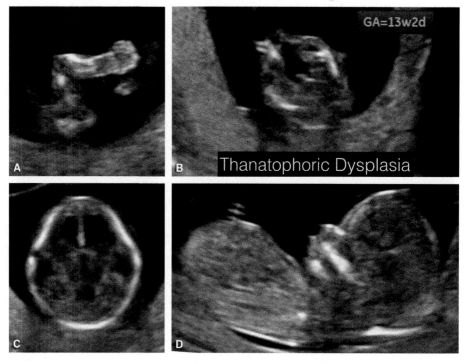

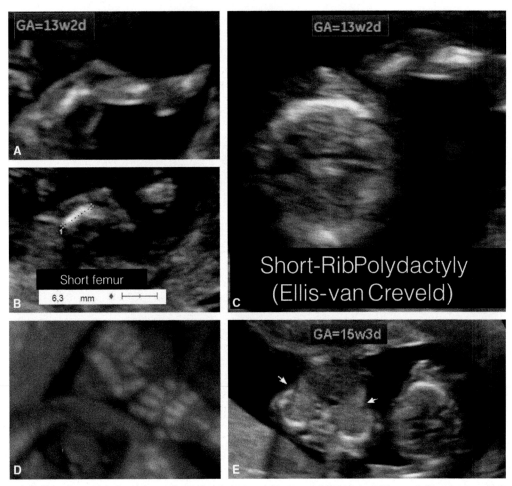

**Figure 14.22: A–D:** Two-dimensional and three-dimensional ultrasound images of fetal extremities and chest in a monochorionic twin pregnancy at 13 weeks of gestation. Note the presence of short femurs in **A** and **B**, normal-appearing ribs in **C**, and polydactyly in **D**. Follow-up ultrasound examination at 15 weeks **(E)** shows a new finding of short ribs, thus suspecting the diagnosis of short-rib polydactyly syndrome. Molecular genetic diagnosis confirmed the presence of Ellis–van Creveld syndrome, belonging to the group of short-rib polydactyly syndromes.

features of some major skeletal dysplasias in the first trimester. Table 14.2 lists ultrasound findings that are helpful in the evaluation of suspected skeletal dysplasia in early gestation.

Making a diagnosis in the first trimester of a specific type of skeletal dysplasia is challenging. The presence of typical features of some skeletal dysplasias, however, can be helpful in that regard (Tables 14.1 and 14.2). In general, the main leading sign for the presence of a skeletal abnormality in the first trimester is short limbs or short femur(s) (Fig. 14.17). Absent, or significantly reduced, cranial ossification is typical for osteogenesis imperfecta type 2 (Fig. 14.19), whereas an increased cranial ossification is an important finding in thanatophoric dysplasia (Fig. 14.21). Careful examination of the hands is crucial, because the presence of hitchhiker thumbs, in addition to short and bowed femurs, suggests the diagnosis of diastrophic dysplasia (Fig. 14.20). The presence of polydactyly with short femurs not only can be suggestive for chromosomal aneuploidy but also is a very important early clue for the presence of short rib polydactyly or Ellis–van Creveld syndrome

(Fig. 14.22). The latter is typically associated with cardiac defects, but their absence does not exclude this diagnosis. In our experience, short ribs are first evident around 14 weeks of gestation (Fig. 14.18), as shown in the case presented in Figure 14.22 with normal-appearing fetal ribs at 13 weeks and short ribs noted on follow-up ultrasound at 15 weeks. A short and bowed femur with a clubfoot with a normal-appearing humerus suggests the diagnosis of campomelic dysplasia (Fig. 14.23). When campomelic dysplasia is suspected, look for the presence of sex reversal in males, where female genitalia are found, and hypoplastic scapulae (Fig. 14.23). In a fetus with a significantly thickened NT with short femur and micrognathia, the diagnosis of achondrogenesis should be suspected, especially when the spine shows near-absent ossification. Despite all these anatomic markers, a detailed ultrasound examination in the early second trimester along with fetal echocardiogram is indicated when a skeletal dysplasia is suspected in the first trimester, because additional anatomic findings can become more apparent with the growth of the fetus.

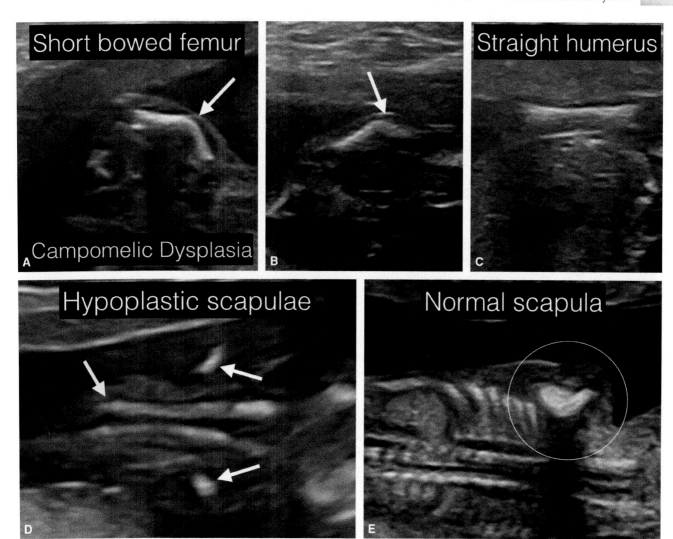

**Figure 14.23:** Two-dimensional ultrasound images of a fetus with campomelic dysplasia at 14 weeks of gestation. The diagnosis was suspected because of the presence of a thickened nuchal translucency with short bowed femurs (*arrow*) **(A and B)** and clubfeet. The upper limbs appear normal **(C)** with a straight humerus. Visualization of hypoplastic scapulae (*arrows*) as shown in **D** in addition to hemivertebra (*yellow arrow*) confirmed the diagnosis of campomelic dysplasia. This male fetus had male genitalia. Chorionic villous sampling confirmed the diagnosis with the *SOX*-9 gene mutation. **E:** A scapula in a normal fetus at 13 weeks of gestation for comparison sake.

| **Table 14.2 •** First Trimester Ultrasound Findings in Skeletal Dysplasias |
| --- |

Thickened nuchal translucency

Abnormality of ductus venosus flow

Femur: short, bowed, broken, absent

Arms and legs: short, abnormal shape, asymmetric

Thorax: small, narrow, short ribs, broken ribs

Skull ossification: decreased or increased

Abnormal hands: polydactyly, oligodactyly, hitchhiker thumb, radius aplasia, club hands, cleft hand, absent hand

Abnormal feet: clubfeet, polydactyly, oligodactyly, absent foot, cleft foot

Spine: reduced ossification, abnormal shape, convex angle

## Associated Malformations

Enlarged NT and abnormal ductus venosus Doppler are common associated findings.[14,16,17] Associated fetal malformations are common and are typically related to the specific type of skeletal dysplasia.

## Abnormalities of Fetal Limbs

### Definition

Congenital abnormalities of fetal limbs include limb reduction defects such as complete absence of an extremity, absence of a hand or foot or radial ray abnormalities, limb deformities such as clubfoot, abnormalities of digits such as polydactyly and syndactyly, and fusion of lower extremities as in sirenomelia, among others. Limb abnormalities can be isolated or more commonly seen in association with structural and chromosomal

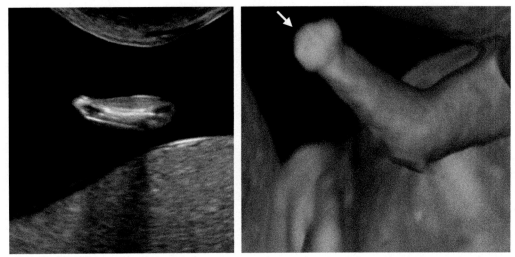

**Figure 14.24:** Two- (*left image*) and three-dimensional (*right image*) ultrasound in surface mode of a fetus with distal transverse limb reduction with an absent hand (*arrow*) at 13 weeks of gestation. This fetus also had a thickened nuchal translucency (not shown), and genetic testing revealed trisomy 21.

malformations and syndromic conditions. The overall incidence of fetal limb abnormalities was reported as 0.38% in a large retrospective cohort of pregnancies undergoing fetal NT and detailed fetal anatomic survey in the first trimester.[19] In this study, a total of 36 fetal limb abnormalities were identified in the cohort, with 23 (63.9%) diagnosed in the first trimester by transabdominal ultrasound.[19] Limb abnormalities are more commonly detected in the first trimester when associated with other fetal abnormalities.[19,20] An enlarged NT is an uncommon finding when fetal limb anomalies are isolated.[19] A detailed

classification of limb abnormalities is beyond the scope of this chapter. Detailed discussion on forearm anomalies are presented in the overview of Pajkrt et al.[21]

## Ultrasound Findings

A combined transabdominal and transvaginal ultrasound examination increases detection of limb abnormalities in the first trimester.[22–24] The authors recommend the use of high-frequency transducers and magnification of ultrasound images in order

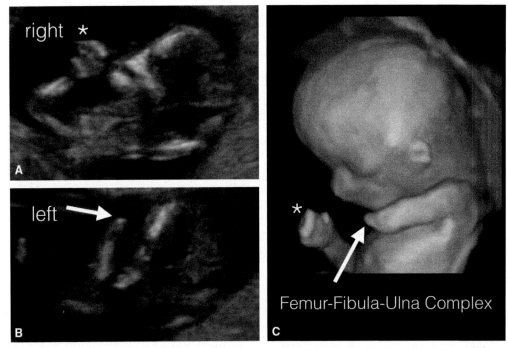

**Figure 14.25:** Two-dimensional (2D) ultrasound **(A and B)** and three-dimensional (3D) ultrasound in surface mode **(C)** in a fetus at 13 weeks of gestation with femur-fibula-ulna complex and unilateral **(left)** forearm abnormality shown in **B** on 2D and in **C** on 3D ultrasound (*arrows*). The right upper extremity appears normal as shown in **A** and **C** (*asterisk*). It is important to image both upper and lower extremities in order to detect such anomalies.

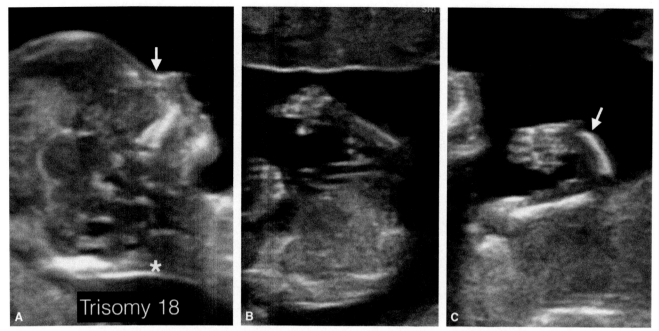

**Figure 14.26:** Fetus with trisomy 18 at 13 weeks of gestation. Note the presence in **A** of a normal nuchal translucency (*asterisk*) and hypoplastic nasal bone (*arrow*). **B:** A normal left upper extremity, and **C** shows an abnormal right upper extremity with radial aplasia (*arrow*). In addition to these findings, early growth restriction and a cardiac defect were also present.

to allow detailed evaluation of fetal extremities in early gestation. Limb reduction defects appear to be the most common abnormalities detected in the first trimester[19,20] and include absence of a hand (Fig. 14.24) or foot (transverse limb reduction), unilateral ray abnormalities (Figs. 14.25 and 14.26), bilateral radial ray abnormalities (Figs. 14.27 to 14.29), among others. Transverse limb reduction defect can be an isolated finding, a sign of vascular disruption, or seen in combination with amniotic bands.

There is inconsistency in the literature with regard to the ability to make the diagnosis of clubfoot in the first trimester,

and this may be related to the nonossification of the ankle in early gestation. In some studies,[20,22,23] clubfoot was diagnosed in each case in the first trimester, whereas in others, most if not all cases were missed.[25] In our experience, careful attention to the position of the foot is required in order to make the diagnosis of clubfoot in the first trimester (Fig. 14.30). The addition of 3D ultrasound in surface mode is helpful to confirm the diagnosis when suspected on the two-dimensional ultrasound examination (Fig. 14.30). It is important to note, however, that a normal anatomic position of the foot in the first trimester does not preclude the presence of clubfoot later on in

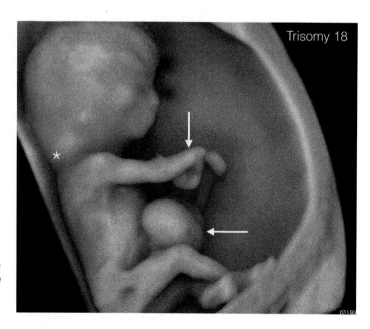

**Figure 14.27:** Three-dimensional ultrasound in surface mode of a fetus with trisomy 18 at 13 weeks of gestation. Note the presence of bilateral radius ray abnormalities (*vertical arrow*) in the upper extremities and an omphalocele (*horizontal arrow*). Also note the abnormal facial profile and the thickened region of the neck (*asterisk*).

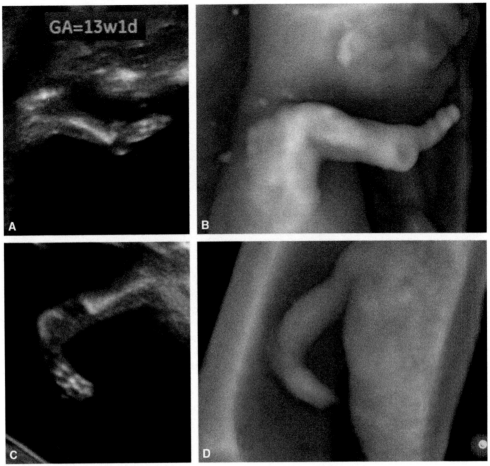

**Figure 14.28:** Two-dimensional (2D) **(A and C)** and three-dimensional (3D) ultrasound **(B and D)** in a fetus at 13 weeks of gestation with bilateral radial ray abnormalities. Note the correlation between the 2D images in **A** and **B** and 3D images in **C** and **D**.

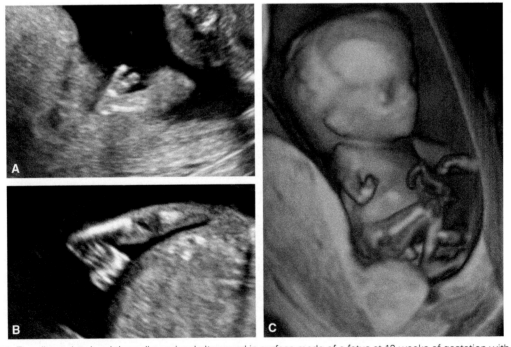

**Figure 14.29:** Two-dimensional and three-dimensional ultrasound in surface mode of a fetus at 12 weeks of gestation with multiple malformations. Bilateral radial ray abnormalities are noted with radial aplasia in one upper extremity shown in **A** and **C** and radius dysplasia in the other upper extremity shown in **B**. The fetus also had short stature because of spinal abnormalities (see Fig. 14-41). The authors suspected Roberts syndrome, which could not be confirmed on molecular genetics testing.

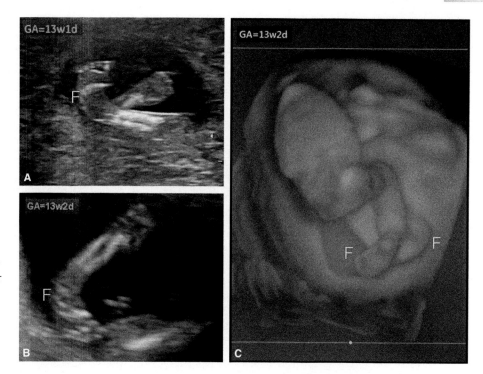

**Figure 14.30:** Two-dimensional ultrasound of the lower extremity in two fetuses **(A and B)** at 13 weeks of gestation with clubfoot (F). Close examination of the lower extremities in the first trimester is needed in order to diagnose clubfoot. Second trimester ultrasound follow-up examination is required to confirm this finding. Three-dimensional ultrasound in surface mode of the back and lower extremities of a fetus **(C)** at 13 weeks of gestation with bilateral clubfeet (F).

pregnancy.[22] Other major abnormalities of the lower extremities, such as sirenomelia (Fig. 14.31) and femur-fibula-ulna complex (Fig. 14.32), can also be diagnosed in the first trimester. In the presence of a prior family history of a genetic abnormality that involves limb deformities, careful evaluation of the extremities in the first trimester can help in the early gestation diagnosis of a recurrence (Fig. 14.33).

Abnormalities of the fingers and toes that have been diagnosed in the first trimester include polydactyly (Fig. 14.34), syndactyly, overlapping digits, split hand as in ectrodactyly

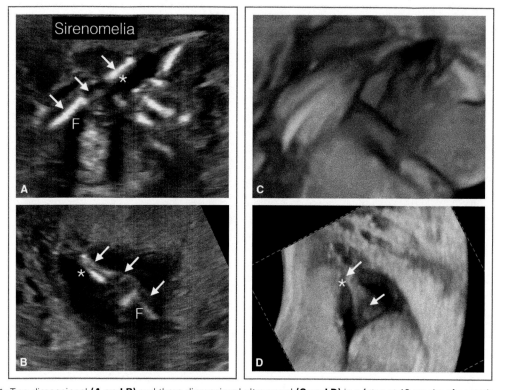

**Figure 14.31:** Two-dimensional **(A and B)** and three-dimensional ultrasound **(C and D)** in a fetus at 13 weeks of gestation with sirenomelia. Both legs are fused into one lower limb (*arrows*), with no feet. One femur (F) bone is seen along with fused bones in the lower segment (*asterisk*). Some fetuses with sirenomelia have only one femur, whereas others may have two femurs. Renal agenesis is part of the disease.

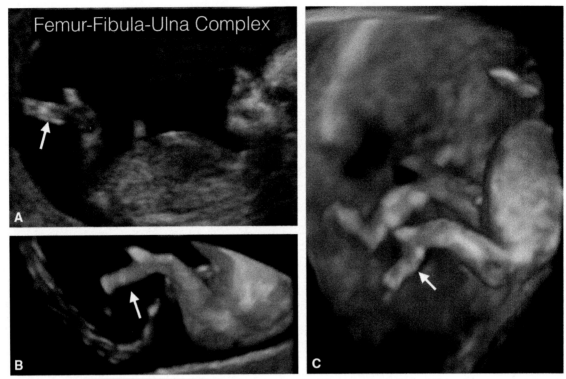

**Figure 14.32:** Two-dimensional (2D) **(A)** and three-dimensional ultrasound in surface mode **(B and C)** in a fetus at 12 weeks of gestation with femur-fibula-ulna complex. Note that the left leg and foot is malformed as shown on 2D **(A)** and 3D ultrasound **(B and C)** (*arrows*).

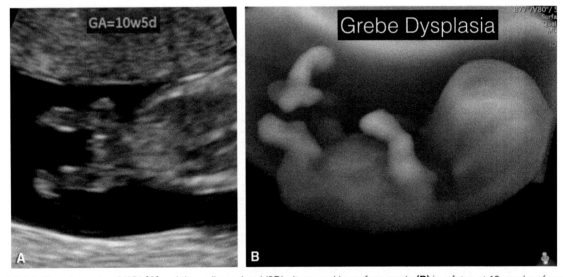

**Figure 14.33:** Two-dimensional (2D) **(A)** and three-dimensional (3D) ultrasound in surface mode **(B)** in a fetus at 10 weeks of gestation with Grebe dysplasia. Grebe dysplasia has an autosomal recessive inheritance resulting from mutation of the *GDF*-5 gene. This pregnancy was a recurrent case of Grebe dysplasia with a previous child with severely malformed legs and feet. The patient presented at 10 weeks of gestation for chorionic villous sampling and on 2D and 3D ultrasound, the images were clearly similar to the limbs of the previous child. Note that after 10 weeks of gestation, the normal feet should be touching each other as shown in Figure 14.4.

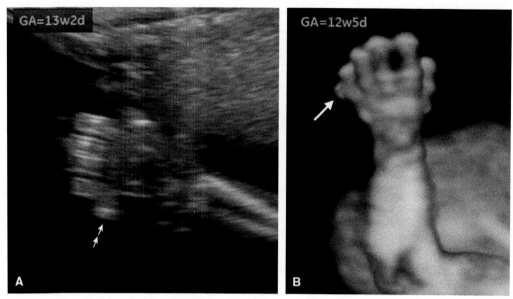

**Figure 14.34:** Two-dimensional ultrasound at 13 weeks **(A)** and three-dimensional ultrasound in surface mode at 12 weeks **(B)** of the upper extremity in two fetuses with postaxial polydactyly (*arrows*). Note that with high-resolution ultrasound, polydactyly can be seen as early as 12 weeks of gestation.

(Fig. 14.35), adactyly, and thumb abnormalities (Fig. 14.20).[22] Polydactyly is one of the most common skeletal findings in the first trimester.[25] Polydactyly can be present in both hands and feet or only in hands or feet (Fig. 14.36), bilateral and unilateral. The presence of a family history is a common clue for the diagnosis of polydactyly in the first trimester.

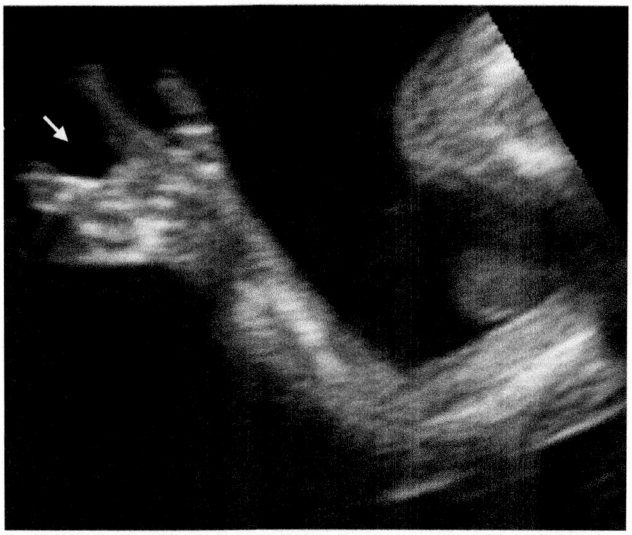

The combination of polydactyly with multiple anomalies mainly of the heart, face, and kidneys can be typical for aneuploidy such as trisomy 13 or 18 (Fig. 14.37).[21] On the other hand, if polydactyly is found together with other signs of skeletal dysplasia such as a short femur, short-rib poly-dactyly syndrome should be considered (Fig. 14.22), even if the ribs appear normal in the first trimester. Polydactyly is commonly seen in the first trimester in association with other malformations.[22] Forearm anomalies are more common than anomalies of lower extremities, and their differential diagnosis includes chromosomal anomalies and genetic syndromes, especially if present bilaterally or in association with other anomalies.[21]

### Associated Malformations

It is important to note that most limb anomalies reported in the literature in the first trimester were described in association with other fetal malformations. Common associated abnormalities include hydrops, single umbilical artery, cardiac abnormalities, and megacystis.[19,20] As stated, the presence of an enlarged NT is a common finding in limb anomalies, especially when associated with other findings. Bilateral oc-currence of limb anomalies is concerning for the presence of a genetic or chromosomal etiology, and a detailed first trimester ultrasound along with follow-up in the second trimester is recommended.[21] A search for the presence of fetal limb abnor-malities should be performed when other fetal malformations are diagnosed in the first trimester. Table 14.3 lists typical conditions associated with forearm anomalies.

**Figure 14.35:** Ectrodactyly (split hand) in a fetus at 11 weeks of gestation (*arrow*). Ectrodactyly can be diagnosed in the first trimester with high-resolution ultrasound transducers and with the transvaginal approach when feasible.

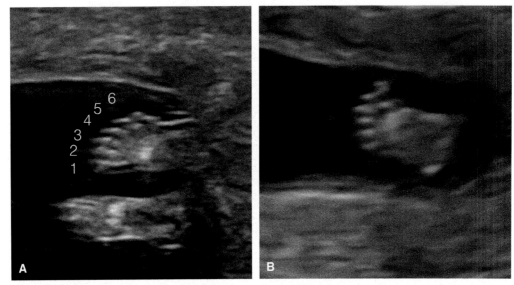

**Figure 14.36:** Two-dimensional (2D) ultrasound of fetal feet in two fetuses **(A,B)** at 13 weeks of gestation with polydactyly. Note that high-resolution transducers and magnification of the foot is required to image the toes in early gestation.

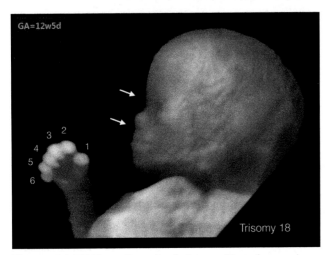

**Figure 14.37:** Three-dimensional ultrasound in surface mode of a fetus with trisomy 18 at 12 weeks of gestation. Note the presence of a flat facial profile (*arrows*) and postaxial polydactyly (6 digits).

## Abnormalities of Spine

### Definition

The most common spinal abnormality in the fetus is spina bifida, with a reported incidence of 1/1,000 live births. Body stalk anomaly is also a malformation that is associated with significant spinal deformity and is commonly diagnosed in the first trimester. Spina bifida along with body stalk anomaly has been discussed in detail in Chapters 8 and 12, respectively. Other spinal abnormalities include isolated or multiple hemivertebrae, iniencephaly, an interrupted lower spine in segmental spinal dysplasia, caudal regression, and severe sacral agenesis. Although sacrococcygeal teratoma is not a spinal defect, we will include it in this section for completeness sake.

**Table 14.3 •** Selected Etiologies of Fetal Forearm Anomalies Listed Alphabetically

Amniotic band
Cornelia de Lange syndrome
Femur-fibula-ulna (FFU) complex
Gallop syndrome
Holt–Oram
Isolated bilateral
Isolated unilateral
Roberts syndrome
Thrombocytopenia absent radius (TAR)
Trisomy 13
Trisomy 18
VACTERL (vertebral, anal, cardiac, tracheo-esophageal, renal, limbs)
Vascular incident

Adapted from Pajkrt E, Cicero S, Griffin DR. Fetal forearm anomalies: prenatal diagnosis, associations and management strategy. *Prenat Diagn.* 2012;32:1084–1093; Copyright John Wiley & Sons, Ltd., with permission.

### Ultrasound Findings

Evaluation of fetal spine biometry on ultrasound has been reported between 11 and 14 weeks of gestation.[26] With the exception of large spina bifida, body stalk anomaly, or severe spinal deformity, the prenatal diagnosis of other spinal abnormalities is rather uncommon in the first trimester because of the lack of spinal ossification.[27] In general, spinal abnormalities detected in the first trimester are likely to represent severe spinal deformities associated with other fetal anatomic

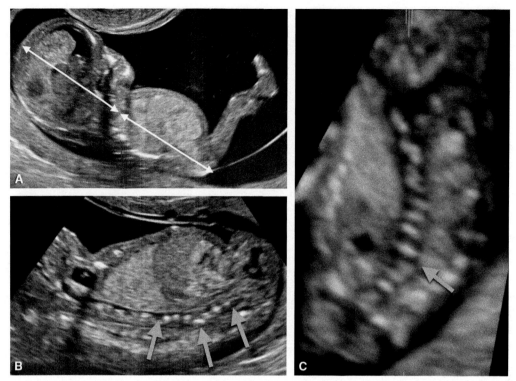

**Figure 14.38:** Two-dimensional (2D) ultrasound in **A** and **B** and three-dimensional (3D) ultrasound in maximum mode in **C** of a fetus with multiple abnormalities at 12 weeks of gestation (same fetus as in Fig. 14.29). Note the presence of abnormal proportions (*double-headed arrows*) of head to chest and abdomen in the midsagittal view in **A**. Note also the presence of a severely malformed spine with multiple hemivertebrae and scoliosis, shown in **B** and **C** (*arrows*). This fetus also had significant abnormalities in the upper and lower extremities as shown in Figure 14.29.

(Figs. 14.38 and 14.39) and chromosomal abnormalities. Suboptimal visualization of the fetal spine in the first trimester has been reported in about 15% of cases because of unfavorable fetal position, decreased ossification, and maternal body habitus.[28] Small and isolated spinal defects typically escape first trimester detection unless there is a high index of suspicion and optimal imaging conditions. In a review of the sonographic

features of spinal anomalies in first trimester fetuses presenting for screening for chromosomal abnormalities, a total of 21 fetuses were diagnosed including 8 with body stalk anomaly, 7 with spina bifida, 2 with vertebral, anal, cardiac, tracheal, esophageal, renal, and limb (VACTERL) association, and 1 case each of isolated kyphoscoliosis, tethered cord, iniencephaly, and sacrococcygeal teratoma.[29] Sacral agenesis in the first

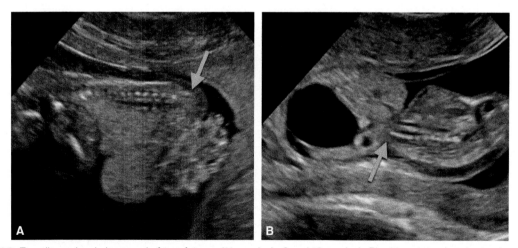

**Figure 14.39:** Two-dimensional ultrasound of two fetuses (11 weeks in **A** and 12 weeks in **B**) with an interrupted spine (*arrow*), abdominal wall defect, and absent bladder and kidneys representing an OEIS complex. OEIS complex include an omphalocele, exstrophy of the bladder, imperforate anus, and spinal defects.

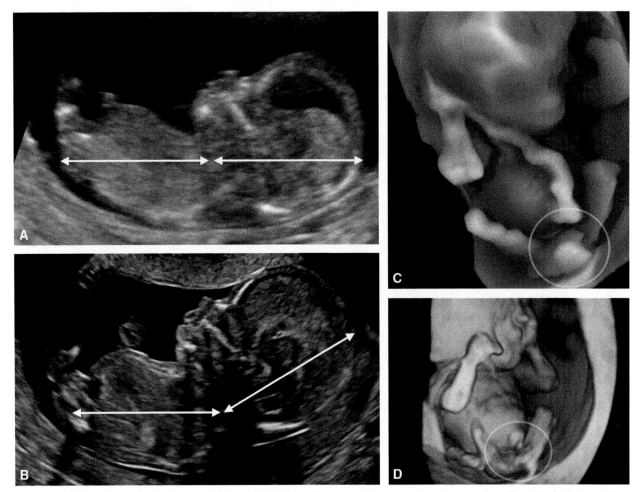

**Figure 14.40:** Two-dimensional ultrasound in **A** and **B** and three-dimensional ultrasound in surface mode in **C** and **D** of a fetus at 12 weeks of gestation with sacral agenesis. Note the abnormal proportions (*double-headed arrows*) of head to chest and abdomen in the midsagittal views in **A** and **B**. This disproportion along with a shortened crown-rump length should alert for the presence of sacral agenesis. In sacral agenesis, the lower extremities are in a typical position with the knees wide apart and the feet touching **(C and D)** (*open circle*), a position referred to as the "Buddha position."

trimester is associated with abnormal proportions of the head to body, short crown-rump length, interruption of spine in the lumbar region, and multiple lower extremity abnormalities[30] (Figs. 14.40 to 14.42). The presence of hemivertebrae is first suspected by the presence of spinal deformities, such as kyphoscoliosis[31] (Fig. 14.43). 3D ultrasound in maximum or skeleton mode is helpful in the evaluation of the spine when hemivertebrae are suspected (Fig. 14.43C and D). Iniencephaly is a very rare fetal anomaly that typically belongs to the neural tube defects category. Typically, it is associated with an extreme retroflexion of the head, in association with an occipital encephalocele (Fig. 14.44) or rachischisis of the cervical or thoracic spine. Sacrococcygeal teratoma is diagnosed in the first trimester when a mass is seen protruding below the spine on a sagittal view (Fig. 14.45). Color Doppler can help assess the vascularity of the sacrococcygeal teratoma and identify feeding vessel(s) (Fig. 14.45).

## Associated Malformations

Congenital vertebral defects can be a prominent feature of several syndromes including the VACTERL and others such as an OEIS complex in association with an omphalocele, exstrophy of the bladder, imperforate anus, and spine abnormalities (Fig. 14.39) (Chapters 12 and 13). Increased NT was found in about a third of spinal abnormalities diagnosed in the first trimester.[29]

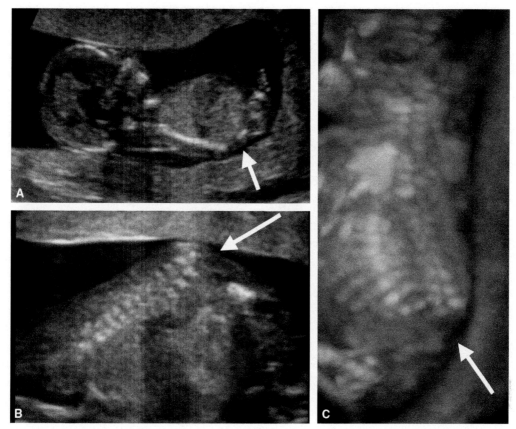

**Figure 14.41:** Two-dimensional ultrasound in **A** and three-dimensional (3D) ultrasound in maximum mode in **B** and **C** in a fetus at 14 weeks of gestation with sacral agenesis. This pregnancy was complicated by maternal diabetes. Note that the spine is interrupted at the level of the lumbar region as shown in **A–C** (*arrows*). A short crown-rump length for gestational age along with body disproportion as shown in **A** suspected the presence of spinal abnormality. 3D ultrasound in **B** and **C** clearly shows the level of spine interruption (*arrows*).

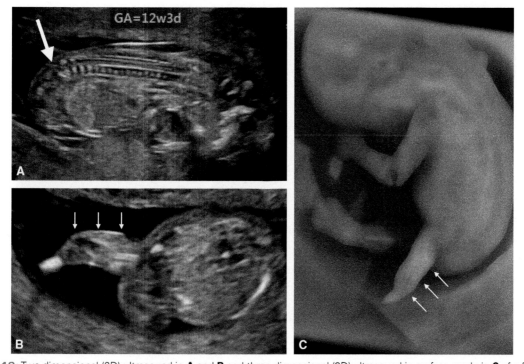

**Figure 14.42:** Two-dimensional (2D) ultrasound in **A** and **B** and three-dimensional (3D) ultrasound in surface mode in **C** of a fetus at 12 weeks of gestation with sacral agenesis. Note in **A** that the spine is interrupted at the lumbar region (*arrow*). In **B** and **C**, abnormal pelvic bones are noted along with a severely malformed lower extremity (*small arrows*), which also appears to arise from the lateral lower abdomen. Fetal death occurred 1 week later following this ultrasound examination.

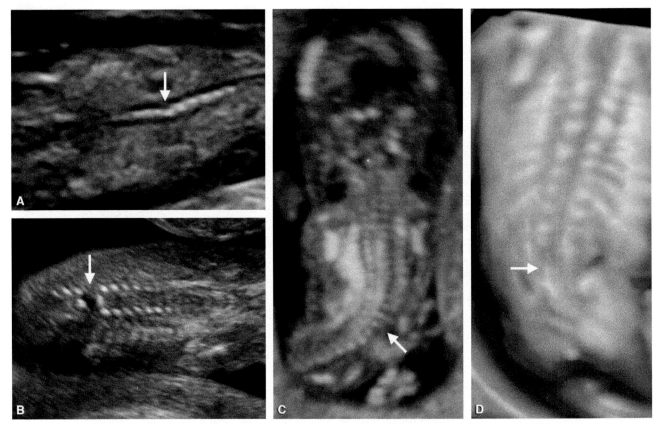

**Figure 14.43:** Two-dimensional (2D) ultrasound in **A** and **B** and three-dimensional (3D) ultrasound in maximum mode in **C**, and **D** of four fetuses at 12 to 14 weeks of gestation with spinal deformities because of hemivertebrae (*arrows*). Note the presence of scoliosis in **C**, and **D**. 3D ultrasound in maximum or skeleton mode is helpful in the evaluation of the spine in early gestation when spinal abnormalities are suspected on 2D ultrasound.

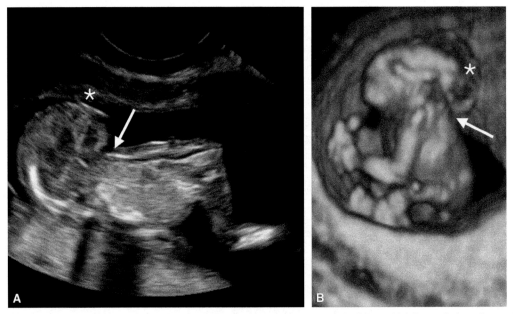

**Figure 14.44:** Two-dimensional (**A**) and corresponding three-dimensional ultrasound of a fetus with iniencephaly and encephalocele at 13 weeks of gestation. Note the presence of significant dorsal flexion of the head and spine (*arrow*) and the presence of a large encephalocele (*asterisks*).

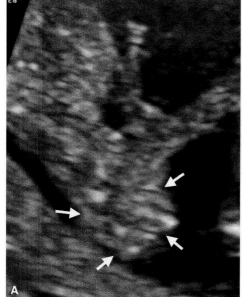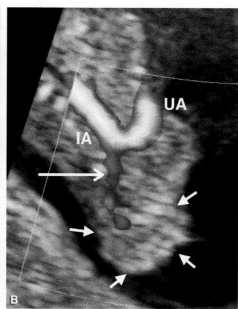

**Figure 14.45:** Two-dimensional (2D) ultrasound in gray scale **(A)** and color Doppler **(B)** of a sagittal view of a fetus at 13 weeks of gestation with sacrococcygeal teratoma (*small arrows*). Note in **A** and **B** that the sacrococcygeal teratoma is a mass that is posterior and inferior to the pelvis. **B:** Color Doppler of the feeding artery (*long arrow*) arising from the iliac artery (IA). UA, umbilical artery.

# REFERENCES

1. Stratford T, Horton C, Maden M. Retinoic acid is required for the initiation of outgrowth in the chick limb bud. *Curr Biol*. 1996;6:1124–1133.
2. Pineault KM, Wellik DM. Hox genes and limb musculoskeletal development. *Curr Osteoporos Rep*. 2014;12:420–427.
3. van Zalen-Sprock RM, Brons JT, Van Vugt JM, et al. Ultrasonographic and radiologic visualization of the developing embryonic skeleton. *Ultrasound Obstet Gynecol*. 1997;9:392–397.
4. Gabrielli S, Falco P, Pilu G, et al. Can transvaginal fetal biometry be considered a useful tool for early detection of skeletal dysplasias in high-risk patients? *Ultrasound Obstet Gynecol*. 1999;13:107–111.
5. Benacerraf BR, Lister JE, DuPonte BL. First-trimester diagnosis of fetal abnormalities. A report of three cases. *J Reprod Med*. 1988;33:777–780.
6. Fisk NM, Vaughan J, Smidt M, et al. Transvaginal ultrasound recognition of nuchal edema in the first-trimester diagnosis of achondrogenesis. *J Clin Ultrasound*. 1991;19:586–590.
7. Soothill PW, Vuthiwong C, Rees H. Achondrogenesis type 2 diagnosed by transvaginal ultrasound at 12 weeks' gestation. *Prenat Diagn*. 1993;13:523–528.
8. DiMaio MS, Barth R, Koprivnikar KE, et al. First-trimester prenatal diagnosis of osteogenesis imperfecta type II by DNA analysis and sonography. *Prenat Diagn*. 1993;13:589–596.
9. Ben-Ami M, Perlitz Y, Haddad S, et al. Increased nuchal translucency is associated with asphyxiating thoracic dysplasia. *Ultrasound Obstet Gynecol*. 1997;10:297–298.
10. Petrikovsky BM, Gross B, Bialer M, et al. Prenatal diagnosis of pseudothalidomide syndrome in consecutive pregnancies of a consanguineous couple. *Ultrasound Obstet Gynecol*. 1997;10:425–428.
11. Hill LM, Leary J. Transvaginal sonographic diagnosis of short-rib polydactyly dysplasia at 13 weeks' gestation. *Prenat Diagn*. 1998;18:1198–1201.
12. Stewart PA, Wallerstein R, Moran E, et al. Early prenatal ultrasound diagnosis of cleidocranial dysplasia. *Ultrasound Obstet Gynecol*. 2000;15:154–156.
13. Catavorello A, Vitale SG, Rossetti D, et al. Case report of prenatal diagnosis of Stüve-Wiedemann Syndrome in a woman with another child affected too. *J Prenat Med*. 2013;7:35–38.
14. Khalil A, Pajkrt E, Chitty LS. Early prenatal diagnosis of skeletal anomalies. *Prenat Diagn*. 2011;31:115–124.
15. Foldynova-Trantirkova S, Wilcox WR, Krejci P. Sixteen years and counting: the current understanding of fibroblast growth factor receptor 3 (FGFR3) signaling in skeletal dysplasias. *Hum Mutat*. 2012;33:29–41.
16. Grande M, Arigita M, Borobio V, et al. First-trimester detection of structural abnormalities and the role of aneuploidy markers. *Ultrasound Obstet Gynecol*. 2012;39:157–163.
17. Souka AP, Kaisenberg von CS, Hyett JA, et al. Increased nuchal translucency with normal karyotype. *Am J Obstet Gynecol*. 2005;192:1005–1021.
18. Krakow D, Lachman RS, Rimoin DL. Guidelines for the prenatal diagnosis of fetal skeletal dysplasias. *Genet Med*. 2009;11:127–133.
19. Liao Y-M, Li S-L, Luo G-Y, et al. Routine screening for fetal limb abnormalities in the first trimester. *Prenat Diagn*. 2016;36:117–126.
20. Rice KJ, Ballas J, Lai E, et al. Diagnosis of fetal limb abnormalities before 15 weeks: cause for concern? *J Ultrasound Med*. 2011;30:1009–1019.
21. Pajkrt E, Cicero S, Griffin DR, et al. Fetal forearm anomalies: prenatal diagnosis, associations and management strategy. *Prenat Diagn*. 2012;32:1084–1093.
22. Bronshtein M, Keret D, Deutsch M, et al. Transvaginal sonographic detection of skeletal anomalies in the first and early second trimesters. *Prenat Diagn*. 1993;13:597–601.
23. Ebrashy A, Kateb El A, Momtaz M, et al. 13-14-week fetal anatomy scan: a 5-year prospective study. *Ultrasound Obstet Gynecol*. 2010;35:292–296.
24. Souka AP, Pilalis A, Kavalakis Y, et al. Assessment of fetal anatomy at the 11-14-week ultrasound examination. *Ultrasound Obstet Gynecol*. 2004;24:730–734.
25. Syngelaki A, Chelemen T, Dagklis T, et al. Challenges in the diagnosis of fetal non-chromosomal abnormalities at 11-13 weeks. *Prenat Diagn*. 2011;31:90–102.
26. Cheng P-J, Huang S-Y, Shaw S-W, et al. Evaluation of fetal spine biometry between 11 and 14 weeks of gestation. *Ultrasound Med Biol*. 2010;36:1060–1065.
27. Vignolo M, Ginocchio G, Parodi A, et al. Fetal spine ossification: the gender and individual differences illustrated by ultrasonography. *Ultrasound Med Biol*. 2005;31:733–738.
28. De Biasio P, Ginocchio G, Vignolo M, et al. Spine length measurement in the first trimester of pregnancy. *Prenat Diagn*. 2002;22:818–822.
29. Sepulveda W, Wong AE, Fauchon DE. Fetal spinal anomalies in a first-trimester sonographic screening program for aneuploidy. *Prenat Diagn*. 2011;31:107–114.
30. González-Quintero VH, Tolaymat L, Martin D, et al. Sonographic diagnosis of caudal regression in the first trimester of pregnancy. *J Ultrasound Med*. 2002;21:1175–1178.
31. Chen M, Chan B, Lam TPW, et al. Sonographic features of hemivertebra at 13 weeks' gestation. *J Obstet Gynaecol Res*. 2007;33:74–77.

# CHAPTER 15

# Placenta and Umbilical Cord

## INTRODUCTION

The placenta is a highly specialized organ that supports growth and development of the fetus and serves as the interface between the maternal and fetal circulations. The placenta functions as the pregnancy organ that delivers nutrients, exchanges respiratory gas, and eliminates toxic waste. The placenta is also an important endocrine organ producing hormones to support and sustain pregnancy and plays a critical role in prevention of pregnancy rejection. Impairment in placental development and/or function has a profound impact on pregnancy outcome. Accumulating data suggest that the placenta plays a critical role in the future health of the fetus such as the risk for adult-onset cardiovascular disease among other diseases.[1–4] This chapter presents the embryologic development and normal sonographic appearance of the placenta and umbilical cord and discusses common placental and cord abnormalities that can be detected in the first trimester of pregnancy.

## EMBRYOLOGY

The blastocyst reaches the endometrial cavity at 4 to 5 days postfertilization. The outer surface of the blastocyst differentiates into trophoblastic cells and produces an overlying syncytial layer that adheres to the endometrium. Implantation of the blastocyst then commences as the syncytiotrophoblast cells penetrate the decidualized endometrium. Endometrial gland secretions provide nourishment to the embryo at this early stage. Spaces are then developed within the syncytiotrophoblast and form anastomosis with maternal vascular sinusoids, thus establishing the first (lacunar) uteroplacental circulation (Fig. 15.1). The placental circulation then develops with finger-like projections into the maternal blood spaces. These projections extend from the chorion and form the primary villi with an inner layer of cytotrophoblast and an outer layer of syncytiotrophoblast. The primary villi become secondary villi with the invasion of the extraembryonic mesoderm and finally become tertiary villi as embryonic blood vessels develop within them. In the early stages of placental development, cytotrophoblasts invade the endothelium and smooth muscle of endometrial spiral arteries, releasing them from maternal influences. The fully formed human placenta is termed hemochorial because the maternal blood is separated from the fetal blood only by elements of the chorion. Growth in size and thickness of the placenta continues rapidly in the first trimester and into the second trimester of pregnancy. The term placenta has a fetal portion, the chorion frondosum, and a maternal portion, the decidua basalis, and covers 15% to 30% of the decidua of the endometrial cavity.[5] The placenta at term is about 20 cm in diameter, has a volume of 400 to

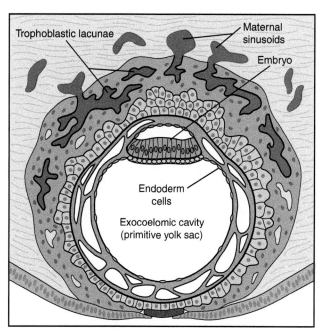

**Figure 15.1:** Schematic drawing of early stages of establishment of the first (lacunar) uteroplacental circulation, shortly after implantation of the blastocyst. Note the presence of spaces developed within the syncytiotrophoblast and forming anastomosis with maternal vascular sinusoids. See text for details.

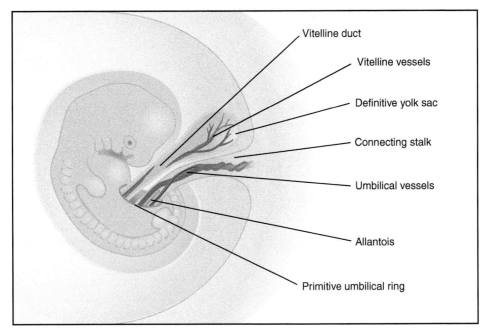

**Figure 15.2:** Schematic drawing of the embryogenesis of the umbilical cord. The umbilical cord is formed by fusion of the connecting stalk (allantois and umbilical vessels) and the vitelline duct and vessels with cephalocaudal flexion of the embryo. See text for details.

600 mL, and weighs approximately one-sixth as much as the fetus.[5,6]

In early embryogenesis, two stalks are seen: the yolk sac, ventrally located and containing the vitelline duct and vessels, and the connecting stalk, caudally located and containing the allantois and the umbilical vessels (Fig. 15.2). With cephalocaudal flexion of the embryo, the connecting stalk fuses with the yolk sac stalk to form the umbilical cord. The

umbilical cord in its early development is inserted in the lower ventral portions of the embryo, is short and thick, and contains the allantois, the vitelline duct and vessels, and the umbilical vessels. The amnion covers the umbilical cord and becomes continuous with the outer epithelial layer of the embryo. The umbilical cord elongates and thins out with the development of the anterior abdominal wall. The umbilical cord initially attaches centrally to the developing

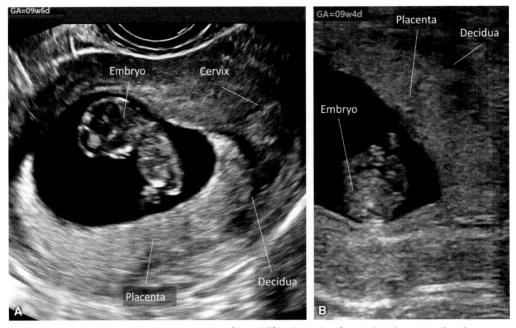

**Figure 15.3:** Two-dimensional ultrasound in two pregnancies **(A and B)** at 9 weeks of gestation demonstrating the appearance of the placenta. Note that the placenta is slightly more echogenic than the surrounding endometrium. The decidua (endometrium behind the placenta) is hypoechogenic in appearance.

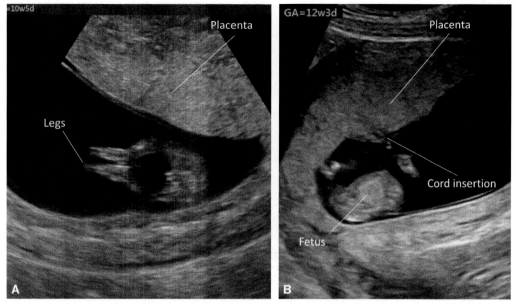

**Figure 15.4:** Two-dimensional ultrasound in two pregnancies at 10 **(A)** and 12 **(B)** weeks of gestation, respectively, demonstrating the appearance of the placenta. Note that the placenta in **A** and **B** has a uniform homogeneous echotexture and is slightly more echogenic than the surrounding endometrium and uterine wall. Placental cord insertion is shown in **B**.

placenta. As the placenta grows, it tends to expand preferentially in regions with sufficient myometrial perfusion and atrophy in areas with suboptimal blood supply. As a result, the cord insertion may become somewhat eccentric. This process is known as trophotropism. The umbilical cord consists of two umbilical arteries and one vein, which are surrounded by mucoid connective tissue—Wharton jelly. The cord at term is usually 1 to 2 cm in diameter and 30 to 90 cm in length.

## NORMAL SONOGRAPHIC ANATOMY

The placenta is first recognized sonographically as a thickened echogenic region on the endometrium by about 9 to 10 weeks of gestation (**Figs. 15.3 and 15.4A**). By 12 to 13 weeks of gestation, the placenta is easily seen on ultrasound and appears slightly echogenic with uniformed homogeneous echotexture (**Figs. 15.4B and 15.5**).

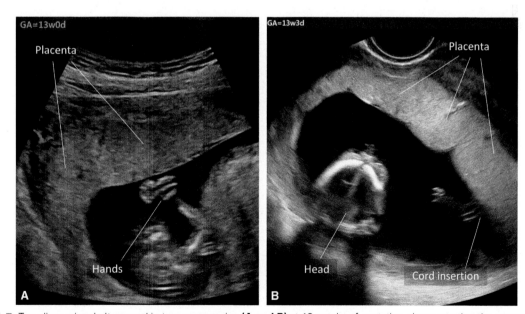

**Figure 15.5:** Two-dimensional ultrasound in two pregnancies **(A and B)** at 13 weeks of gestation, demonstrating the appearance of the placenta. **A:** Image obtained by the transabdominal approach. **B:** Image obtained by the transvaginal approach. Note that the transvaginal approach clearly outlines placental borders because of increased resolution of the transducer. Placental cord insertion is shown in **B**.

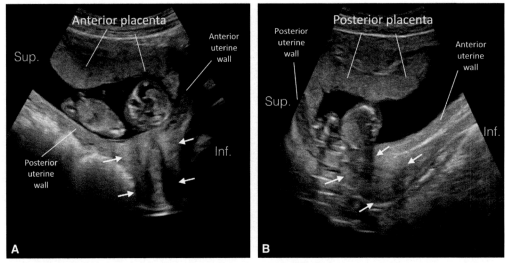

**Figure 15.6:** Placental location in the first trimester is best described after localizing the cervix (*arrows*) and anterior/posterior uterine walls. Transabdominal ultrasound in two pregnancies **(A and B)**, where the placentas appear to be on the anterior uterine walls. In **A**, the placenta is anterior; however, in **B**, because of the presence of uterine anteflexion, the posterior uterine wall is seen as closest to the transducer, and thus the placenta is posterior. Inf, Inferior; Sup, superior.

During the first trimester ultrasound examination (see Chapter 5), the location of the placenta in the uterus should be reported. Identifying the location of the placenta on the first trimester ultrasound is not as easy as in the second trimester given the presence of uterine flexion and extension. Indeed, inaccuracies can be introduced especially when the placenta appears to be in the lower uterine segment. In order to improve accuracy of placental localization on the first trimester ultrasound, we recommend identifying the cervix and the anterior and posterior uterine walls before describing the placental location (**Figs. 15.6 and 15.7**).

The placental size, thickness, location within the endometrial cavity, and echogenicity can also be evaluated by ultrasound in the late first trimester of pregnancy.[7] The normal thickness of the placenta is correlated to gestational age of the embryo/fetus and is approximately 1 mm per week of gestation.[8] With advanced three-dimensional (3D) ultrasound techniques, placental volume can now be measured in the first trimester

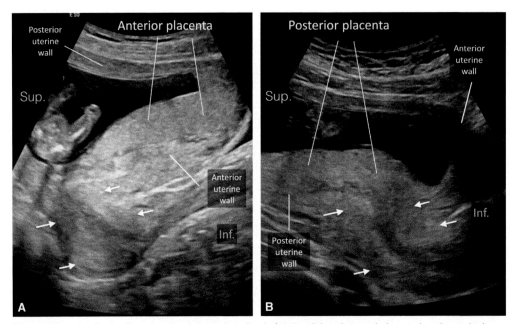

**Figure 15.7:** Placental location in the first trimester is best described after localizing the cervix (*arrows*) and anterior/posterior uterine walls. Transabdominal ultrasound in two pregnancies **(A and B)**, where the placentas appear to be on the posterior uterine walls. In **A**, the placenta is anterior, and the presence of uterine anteflexion gives an erroneous impression of a posterior location of the placenta. In **B**, the placenta is clearly posterior in location. Inf, Inferior; Sup, superior.

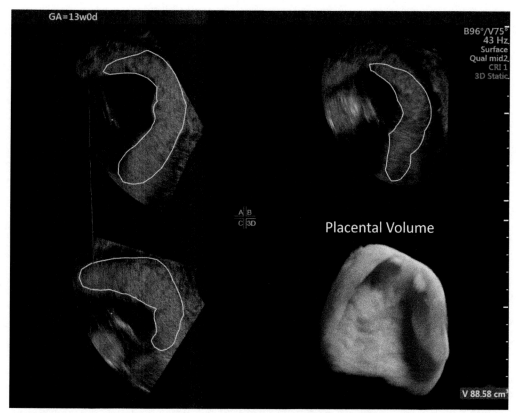

**Figure 15.8:** Three-dimensional (3D) ultrasound volume of a placenta at 13 weeks of gestation shown in multiplayer display with placental volume obtained from the analysis of the 3D volume set. The placental volume is 88.58 cm³.

(Fig. 15.8), and along with placental biometry has been shown to correlate with pregnancy complications.[9,10] Indeed, we believe that first trimester measurement of placental length, width, and volume is more accurate than later on in pregnancy given that the whole placenta is seen in one ultrasound image in early gestation. The assessment of biometric dimensions of the placenta is infrequently performed on prenatal sonography today, unless in rare pathologic conditions or for research purposes. Abnormal placental findings on first trimester ultrasound, such as masses, multiple cystic spaces, or large subchorionic fluid collection, should be noted and followed up.

Maternal blood flow is established within the placenta by 12 weeks of gestation.[11] Blood flow in the maternal and fetal placental vasculature can be demonstrated in the first trimester on color and pulsed Doppler ultrasound (Fig. 15.9).

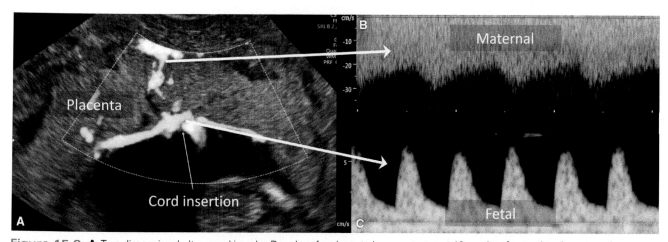

**Figure 15.9: A:** Two-dimensional ultrasound in color Doppler of a placenta in a pregnancy at 12 weeks of gestation demonstrating the maternal and fetal circulation at the level of the cord insertion. **B and C:** The corresponding pulsed Doppler of the maternal and fetal vasculature. Note the differences in blood flow velocities between the maternal and fetal circulation, with the maternal circulation showing a low impedance pattern. Also note the difference in heart rates between the two circulations.

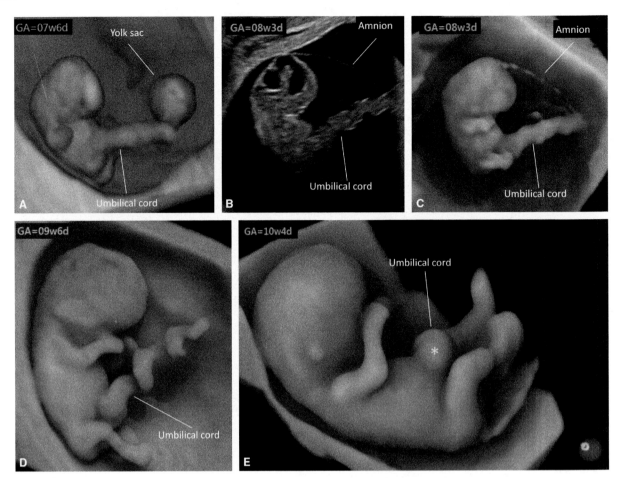

**Figure 15.10:** Three-dimensional ultrasound in surface mode **(A, C–E)** and two-dimensional ultrasound **(B)** of the embryo and umbilical cord at 7 to 10 weeks of gestational age. Note that the umbilical cord in this gestational age window is short and thick and connects the embryo to the placenta. Note in **E**, at 10 weeks of gestation, thickening of the umbilical cord at the abdominal cord insertion (*asterisk*), corresponding to the physiologic hernia.

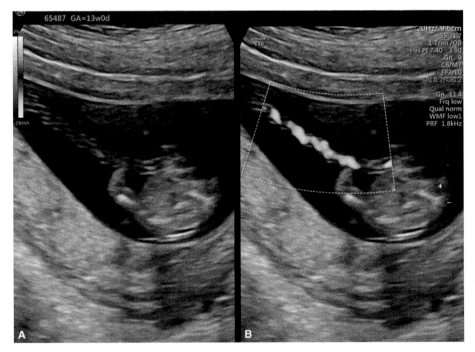

**Figure 15.11:** Two-dimensional ultrasound in gray scale **(A)** and color Doppler **(B)** of the umbilical cord in a pregnancy at 13 weeks of gestation. Note in **A** and **B** that the umbilical cord is elongated and thinned from its appearance between 7 and 10 weeks of gestation (Fig. 15.10). The umbilical cord at 13 weeks of gestation has the same appearance as that in the second trimester of pregnancy.

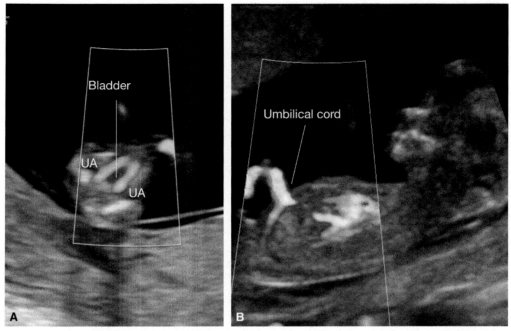

**Figure 15.12: A:** An axial plane (cross-section) of the pelvis in color Doppler in a fetus at 13 weeks of gestation demonstrating the two umbilical arteries (UA) surrounding the fetal bladder. **B:** A midline sagittal plane in color Doppler in a fetus at 12 weeks of gestation demonstrating the umbilical cord insertion into the fetal abdomen.

Quantitative assessment of placental vascularization may be useful for predicting pregnancy complications and adverse events.[12–14]

The umbilical cord can be recognized by ultrasound as early as the seventh week of gestation and appears as a straight thick structure connecting the embryo to the developing placenta (Fig. 15.10). In the first trimester, the length of the umbilical cord is approximately the same as the crown-rump length.[15] The umbilical cord elongates and thins with advancing gestation, and by the 13th week, the cord has the same sonographic appearance as in the second trimester of pregnancy (Fig. 15.11). Umbilical arteries can be seen in the first trimester as branches of the internal iliac arteries, running alongside the fetal bladder in a cross-section view of the fetal pelvis using color or power Doppler (Fig. 15.12A), and the number of umbilical arteries can thus be reliably determined.[16] Midline sagittal plane of the fetus demonstrates the insertion of the umbilical cord into the abdomen, and this plane is also important in the evaluation of the integrity of the abdominal wall in the first trimester (Fig. 15.12B) (see Chapters 5 and 12). 3D ultrasound in surface mode can also clearly demonstrate the umbilical cord (Fig. 15.13).

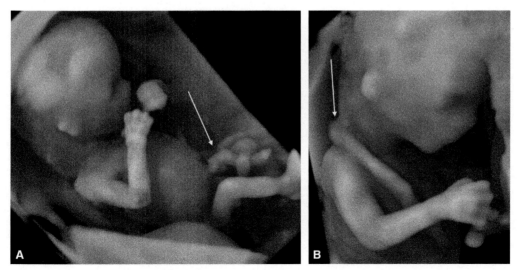

**Figure 15.13:** Three-dimensional ultrasound in surface mode in two fetuses at 12 **(A)** and 13 **(B)** weeks of gestation demonstrating external fetal anatomy along with the umbilical cord (*arrow*).

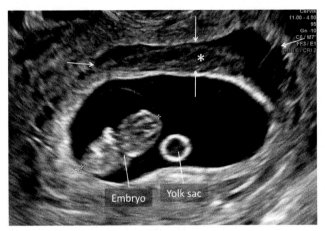

**Figure 15.14:** Two-dimensional ultrasound in a pregnancy at 9 weeks of gestation demonstrating a subchorionic hematoma (*asterisk* and *arrows*) located between the chorion and the uterine wall.

## PLACENTAL ABNORMALITIES

### Intrauterine Hematoma

Intrauterine hematoma is a common finding on routine ultrasound in the first trimester, especially among pregnant women presenting with vaginal bleeding. Intrauterine hematoma usually appears as a crescent-shaped, sonolucent fluid collection behind the fetal membranes or the placenta, but may vary significantly in shape and size. The position of the hematoma relative to the placental site can be described as subchorionic or retroplacental. The subchorionic hematoma is located between the chorion and the uterine wall (Fig. 15.14), whereas the retroplacental hematoma is located behind the placenta (Fig. 15.15). The reported incidence of first trimester hematomas diagnosed by ultrasound varies widely, from as low as 0.5% to as high as 22%, depending on the patient population studied and the ultrasound evaluation.[17,18] In low-risk

general obstetric population, intrauterine hematomas occur in 3.1% of cases in the first trimester.[19] Although approximately 70% of subchorionic hematomas resolve spontaneously by the end of the second trimester without clinical sequelae, some may persist until the end of pregnancy and be associated with increased risk of pregnancy complications.[17]

The clinical significance of an intrauterine hematoma noted on the first trimester ultrasound is currently controversial.[20–24] Systematic review and meta-analysis performed by Tuuli et al.[25] demonstrated that presence of a first trimester intrauterine hematoma is associated with adverse pregnancy outcome, including an increased risk for spontaneous abortion, stillbirth, placental abruption, preterm premature rupture of membranes, and preterm delivery. There is no consistency in study results, however, and the association of an intrauterine hematoma with pregnancy complications such as preeclampsia and fetal growth restriction has not been confirmed.[25] Retroplacental position of the hematoma (Fig. 15.15) appears to carry a higher risk for poor pregnancy outcome.[19] An intrauterine hematoma can be classified based upon its relative size. In a study on this subject, the size of the hematoma was graded according to the percentage of chorionic sac circumference elevated by the hematoma, with small indicating less than one-third of the chorionic sac circumference, moderate indicating one-third to one-half of the chorionic sac circumference, and large indicating two-thirds or greater of chorionic sac circumference.[22] Large intrauterine hematomas (Fig. 15.16) were found to be associated with an almost threefold increase in risk of spontaneous abortion.[22] There is currently sufficient evidence in the literature to suggest that the presence of a first trimester large intrauterine hematoma may increase the pregnancy risk, and follow-up ultrasound examinations in the second and possibly third trimester of pregnancy is thus warranted.

Although a subchorionic hematoma is relatively easy to identify in the first trimester, the diagnosis of a subplacental hematoma is challenging especially in the absence of clinical symptoms. The presence of a transient uterine contraction (see

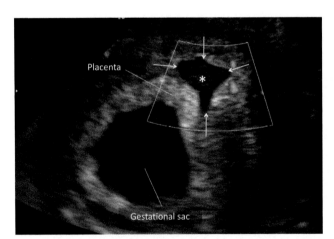

**Figure 15.15:** Two-dimensional ultrasound with color Doppler in a pregnancy at 10 weeks of gestation demonstrating a retroplacental hematoma (*asterisk* and *arrows*) located behind the placenta.

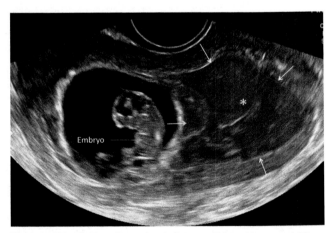

**Figure 15.16:** Two-dimensional ultrasound in a pregnancy at 10 weeks of gestation demonstrating a large intrauterine hematoma (*asterisk* and *arrows*). Note that the size of this hematoma (color overlay) is almost larger than the circumference of the gestational sac.

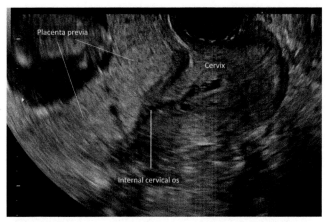

**Figure 15.17:** Two-dimensional transvaginal ultrasound in a pregnancy at 12 weeks of gestation demonstrating a placenta previa. Note that the placenta is covering the internal cervical os.

Fig. 5.1) or thickened uterine wall can mimic the diagnosis of subplacental bleed. The application of color Doppler can help differentiate a subplacental bleed from a uterine contraction or thickening.

## Placenta Previa

The term placenta previa describes a placenta that covers the internal cervical os. In normal pregnancy, the placenta implants in the upper uterine segment. In the case of placenta previa, the placenta is partially or totally implanted in the lower uterine segment and placental tissue covers the internal cervical os (Figs. 15.17 and 15.18). In the second trimester of pregnancy, if the placenta is attached in the lower uterine segment and placental tissue does not cover the internal os, but is within 2 cm from the internal os, the placenta is called low lying.

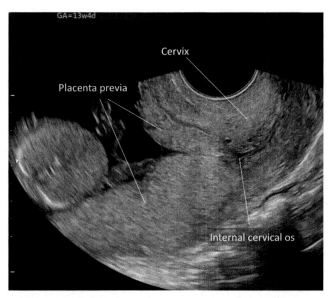

**Figure 15.18:** Two-dimensional transvaginal ultrasound in a pregnancy at 13 weeks of gestation demonstrating a placenta previa. Note that the placenta is covering the internal cervical os.

The incidence of placenta previa varies greatly with gestational age. Placenta previa is more commonly seen in early gestation and presents in approximately 4.5% to 6.2% of pregnancies between 12 and 16 weeks of gestation.[26,27] The proportion of patients with the placenta extending to or covering the internal cervical os significantly decreases with advancing gestation from 5.5% at 12+0 to 12+6 weeks, to 2.4% at 15+0 to 15+6 weeks of gestation and to 0.16% at term.[26] Several studies have shown that if the placenta extends at least 15 mm over the internal cervical os at 12 to 16 weeks of gestation, a placenta previa is present at term with a sensitivity of 80% and a positive predictive value of 5.1%.[26–28] The mechanism resulting in the resolution of a first trimester placenta previa with advancing gestation is poorly understood, but may be related to a preferential growth of the placenta toward a better vascularized upper endometrium (trophotropism). According to current guidelines for performance of first trimester fetal ultrasound, it is not recommended to report the presence of placenta previa or low-lying placenta between 11+0 and 13+6 weeks of gestation because the position of the placenta in relation to the cervix at this stage of pregnancy is of less clinical importance as a result of the "migration" phenomenon.[7]

## Morbidly Adherent Placenta

The term "morbidly adherent placenta" implies abnormal implantation of the placenta into the uterine wall, and this term has been used to describe placenta accreta, increta, and percreta. Placenta accreta occurs when the placental villi adhere directly to the myometrium, a placenta increta involves placental villi invading into the myometrium, and a placenta percreta is defined as placental villi invading through myometrium and into serosa and, sometimes, adjacent organs. About 75% of morbidly adherent placentas are placenta accretas, 18% are placenta incretas, and 7% are placenta percretas,[29] but this differentiation is not always possible on prenatal ultrasound. We will use the term placenta accreta to describe morbidly adherent placenta.

The sonographic markers of placenta accreta in the first trimester primarily include a gestational sac that is implanted in the lower uterine segment (Fig. 15.19), a gestational sac that is embedded in a cesarean section scar (Figs. 15.20 and 15.21) (cesarean scar pregnancy), and the presence of multiple vascular spaces (lacunae) within the placental bed, primarily in the setting of a placenta previa (Figs. 15.22 and 15.23).

Ballas et al.[30] defined lower uterine segment implantation as a gestational sac that is implanted in the lower third of the uterus between 8 and 10 weeks or primarily occupying the lower uterine segment from 10 weeks (Fig. 15.19). In the authors' experience, identifying that a gestational sac is in the lower uterine segment is more difficult at 10 weeks of gestation and beyond as the gestational sac typically expands into the upper uterine segment. One must also differentiate lower uterine segment implantation from an ongoing pregnancy loss (miscarriage). With the application of color Doppler, a failing pregnancy can be clearly distinguished as a sac that lacks

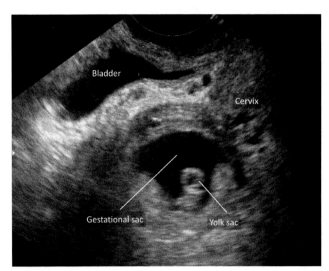

**Figure 15.19:** Two-dimensional transvaginal ultrasound in a pregnancy at 7 weeks of gestation demonstrating a low implantation of the gestational sac. Note that the gestational sac is in the lower uterine segment, posterior to the bladder and next to the cervix. This patient had three prior cesarean deliveries and the placenta was diagnosed as placenta previa and accreta in the second and third trimester of pregnancy.

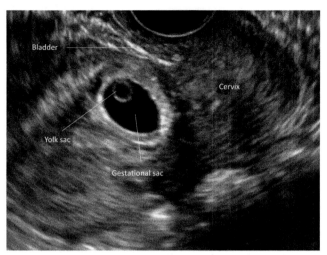

**Figure 15.20:** Transvaginal ultrasound of the midline sagittal plane of the uterus in a pregnancy at 7 weeks of gestation demonstrating a cesarean section scar implantation. Note that the gestational sac is imbedded into the cesarean section scar. Also note the proximity of the empty bladder to the gestational sac.

circumferential blood flow, in addition to a sac that moves when pressure is applied to the anterior surface of the uterus.[31] Not all gestational sacs that implant in the lower uterine segment lead to placenta accretas, because subsequent normal pregnancies in this setting have been reported.[32] In these instances, a normal thick anterior myometrium superior to the gestational sac and a continuous white line representing the bladder–uterine wall interface is seen on ultrasound. The gestational sac should be contiguous with the endometrial cavity.[31]

In patients with a prior cesarean section, pregnancies implanted in or near the cesarean section scar (**Figs. 15.20 and 15.21**)

carry significant risk for placenta accreta and pregnancy complications. In these cases, the gestational sac appears embedded into the cesarean section scar, the anterior myometrium appears thin, and the placental–myometrial and bladder–uterine wall interfaces often appear irregular.[31] In the authors' experience, the gestational sac of a cesarean scar implantation is typically fusiform in shape at 6 to 8 weeks of gestation (**Fig. 15.21**). Color Doppler reveals increased vascularity surrounding the gestational sac (**Fig. 15.21B**).

Many studies combine cesarean scar pregnancies with pregnancies that implant in the lower uterine segment, near the cesarean section scar.[31,33–35] A true cesarean scar pregnancy is defined by the presence of a gestational sac that is

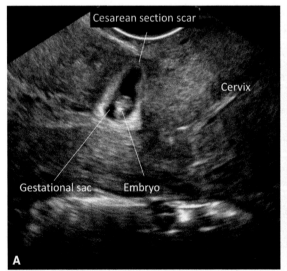

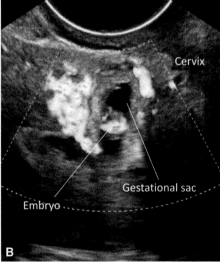

**Figure 15.21:** Transvaginal ultrasound of the midline sagittal plane of the uterus in gray scale (**A**) and color Doppler (**B**) in a pregnancy at 7 weeks of gestation demonstrating a cesarean section scar implantation. Note that the gestational sac is imbedded into the cesarean section scar. Also note the fusiform shape of the gestational sac in **A** and **B**. Color Doppler shows increased vascularity surrounding the gestational sac.

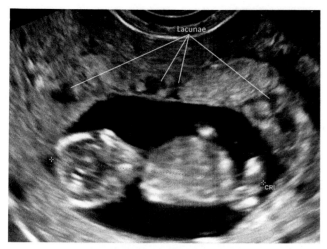

**Figure 15.22:** Transvaginal ultrasound in a pregnancy at 11 weeks of gestation demonstrating the presence of multiple placental lacunae in a patient with two prior cesarean sections. The presence of placental lacunae in the first trimester increases the risk for placenta accreta.

implanted within the myometrium, surrounded on all sides by myometrium, and be separate from the endometrium (Figs. 15.20 and 15.21).

The third marker of placenta accreta in the first trimester is the presence of anechoic areas within the placenta with or without documented blood flow on color Doppler (Figs. 15.22 and 15.23). These anechoic areas have been described as vascular spaces, lacunae, or lakes. Multiple case reports describe the presence of hypoechoic placental vascular spaces on ultrasound at less than 12 weeks of gestation and have linked their presence to the early diagnosis of placenta accreta.[30,36–39] Three examples of irregularly shaped placental lacunae diagnosed at 8, 9, and 12 weeks, respectively, were reported in women presenting with vaginal bleeding and suspicion for abnormal placentation.[36,38,39] Two resulted in hysterectomy secondary to hemorrhage as early as 15 weeks, and placenta accreta was confirmed on pathology.

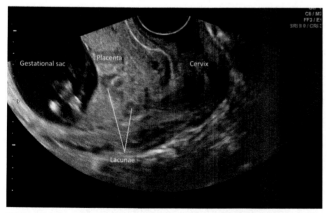

**Figure 15.23:** Transvaginal ultrasound in a pregnancy at 13 weeks of gestation demonstrating the presence of multiple placental lacunae and placenta previa in a patient with one prior cesarean section. The presence of placenta previa with multiple lacunae in the first trimester increases the risk for placenta accreta.

In the third case, the patient elected termination, and the uterus was preserved. A retrospective study by Ballas et al.[30] further confirmed lacunae as a first trimester marker for placenta accreta. They reported on 10 cases of placenta accreta with first trimester ultrasound examinations and noted that anechoic placental areas were present in 8 of 10 (80%).[30] If the pregnancy progresses, these lacunae become more prominent in the second and third trimester of pregnancy and may demonstrate blood flow on low-velocity color Doppler.

## Amniotic Band Syndrome

It is commonly accepted that amniotic band syndrome (ABS) occurs when the inner membrane (amnion) ruptures without injury to the outer membrane (chorion), thus exposing the embryo/fetus to fibrous sticky tissue from the ruptured amnion (bands), which can float in the amniotic fluid. These bands can entangle the fetus, reducing blood supply and causing a variety of fetal congenital abnormalities. The incidence of ABS is approximately 1 in 1,200 live births.[40] Defects caused by ABS range from minor defects of the digits to major complex multiorgan anomalies. The most common findings are constriction rings with lymphedema around the fingers, toes, arms, or legs. ABS should be suspected in case of limbs amputations and in the presence of unusual asymmetric craniofacial (Fig. 15.24) or visceral defects. The direct ultrasound visualization of amniotic bands is challenging and requires high-resolution transducers, preferably by the transvaginal approach (Fig. 15.24). Use of transvaginal 3D/four-dimensional imaging can be particularly helpful in the first trimester for the differential diagnosis of amniotic bands and related fetal abnormalities.[41,42] There are several case reports on the diagnosis of ABS in the first trimester.[41–44]

## CORD ABNORMALITIES

Abnormalities of the umbilical cord are common and may affect the length, size, number, insertion, and course of the umbilical vessels. The use of color Doppler is very helpful in the diagnosis of cord insertion and presence of structural abnormalities of the umbilical cord, between 11 and 14 weeks of gestation.[45] Abnormally short umbilical cord can occur as a result of embryonic infolding failure, which is associated with limb-body-stalk anomalies (see Chapter 13 for details). Abnormally long cord may predispose to cord prolapse, nuchal cord, or true cord knots. True cord knots occur in about 1% of single pregnancies and very rarely can be observed on the first trimester ultrasound (Fig. 15.25). Color Doppler and 3D ultrasound can help confirm the presence of a true knot, when suspected, on gray scale ultrasound in the first trimester (Fig. 15.25).

Cord entanglement is a common complication of the monochorionic–monoamniotic gestation and can be noted as early as 12 to 13 weeks of gestation. The application of color and pulsed Doppler can confirm the diagnosis of cord

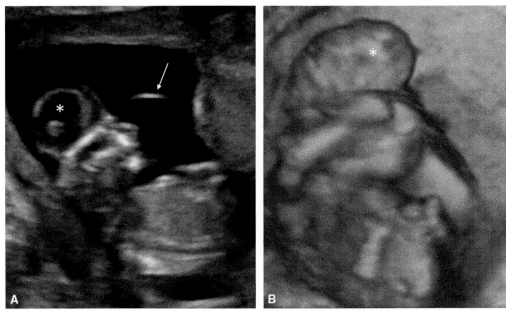

**Figure 15.24:** Transvaginal two-dimensional **(A)** and three-dimensional ultrasound **(B)** of a fetus at 13 weeks of gestation with severe brain malformation (anencephaly—*asterisk*) resulting from amniotic band syndrome. Note the presence in **A** of a reflective membrane within the amniotic cavity (*arrow*) that is attached to the fetal head. This reflective membrane represents an amniotic band.

entanglement in the first trimester of pregnancy (Fig. 15.26A) (see Chapter 7). 3D ultrasound can also confirm the diagnosis and display the entangled cords (Fig. 15.26B).

Excessive or absent coiling of the umbilical cord can be occasionally detected in the first trimester ultrasound. Abnormal insertion of the umbilical cord may result in velamentous cord insertion or vasa previa. Abnormally thickened umbilical cord can be observed in association with fetal hydrops or cord cysts. In the following sections, common umbilical cord abnormalities are discussed in more detail.

## Single Umbilical Artery

The absence of one of the arteries in the umbilical cord is called single umbilical artery (SUA) or two-vessel umbilical cord. The pathogenesis of SUA is uncertain. Aplasia or atrophy of the missing vessel has been suggested as an etiology of SUA.[46] SUA is one of the most common sonographic findings during pregnancy and is more commonly seen in multiple gestations, in the presence of velamentous cord insertion, in advanced maternal age, in maternal diabetes, in hypertensive and seizure disorders, and in smoking.[47,48] The incidence of SUA reported in the first trimester of pregnancy is 1.1% and 3.3% in single and twin gestations, respectively.[45] Detection of SUA in the first trimester ultrasound is possible, with reported sensitivity between 57.1% and 84.2% and specificity 98.9% and 99.8%.[45,49] This is best performed by obtaining an axial plane of the fetal pelvis in color Doppler and identifying a SUA next to the bladder (Fig. 15.27), rather than the two umbilical arteries normally seen (Fig. 15.12A).

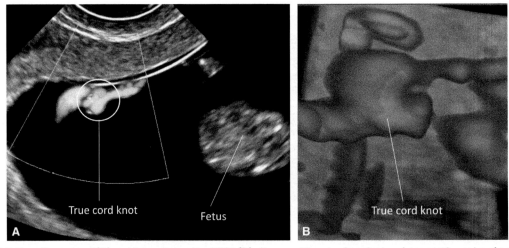

**Figure 15.25:** Two-dimensional **(A)** and three-dimensional (3D) **(B)** ultrasound in color Doppler in a fetus at 12 weeks of gestation with a true cord knot. Note in **A** the presence of a thickening of the cord on color Doppler. The presence of cord thickening (*circle*) suggests the presence of a true knot. **B:** A 3D volume display of the cord in glass body mode demonstrating the cord knot.

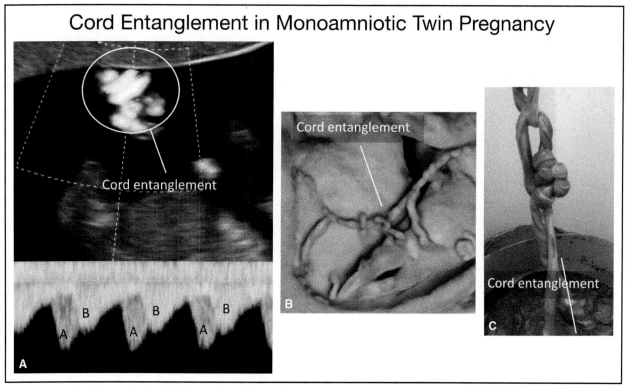

# Cord Entanglement in Monoamniotic Twin Pregnancy

**Figure 15.26: A:** Color and pulsed Doppler of cord entanglement in a monoamniotic twin pregnancy at 13 weeks of gestation. Note the presence of "a mass of cord" on color Doppler suggesting the diagnosis. Pulsed Doppler applied to the mass of cord and displayed in lower panel **A** shows two interposed fetal umbilical Doppler spectrums (A and B in Doppler spectrum), confirming cord entanglement. **B:** A three-dimensional ultrasound in surface mode of another monoamniotic twin pregnancy at 12 weeks of gestation with cord entanglement. **C:** The entangled cords of pregnancy in **B** after delivery at 33 weeks of gestation.

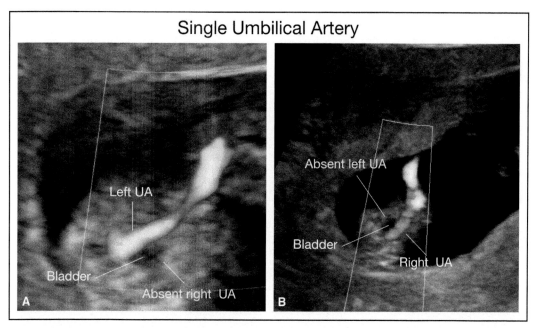

# Single Umbilical Artery

**Figure 15.27:** Axial plane of the pelvis in color Doppler in two fetuses **(A and B)** at 13 weeks of gestation with single umbilical artery. Note in **A** that the right umbilical artery (UA) is absent and in **B**, the left UA is absent. Although earlier studies suggested a significance to the laterality of single umbilical artery, this has not been proven in subsequent studies.

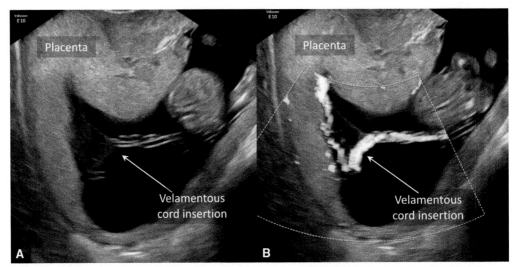

**Figure 15.28:** Gray scale **(A)** and color Doppler **(B)** of a pregnancy at 11 weeks of gestation with velamentous insertion of the umbilical cord. Note that the umbilical cord inserts in the membranes, rather than directly into the placenta.

The association of SUA with fetal anomalies, mainly genitourinary and cardiac, as well as with a wide range of genetic syndromes and chromosomal aberrations has been reported[50–52] and described in various chapters of this book. SUA can also be associated with intrauterine growth restriction, preterm delivery, and poor pregnancy outcomes.[53] The presence of a SUA as an isolated sonographic finding, however, is often associated with a normal pregnancy outcome.[53–55] A study performed by Martínez-Payo et al.[45] demonstrated that about 17.6% of SUA cases diagnosed between 11+0 and 13+6 weeks of gestation had concomitant malformations detected at the first trimester ultrasound, and in an additional 7.7% of SUA cases, anomalies were found in the second trimester of pregnancy. The authors concluded that the assessment of

the number of umbilical cord vessels during the first trimester ultrasound examination is useful given the association of SUA with fetal malformations that can be diagnosed in early gestation.[45] We recommend a detailed first trimester ultrasound examination when SUA is detected in early gestation (see Chapter 5 for more detail).

## Velamentous and Marginal Cord Insertion

The term velamentous umbilical cord describes an insertion of the umbilical cord into the membranes at the placental margin rather than into the placental surface (Figs. 15.28 and 15.29). Velamentous umbilical cord has been reported in about 1% of

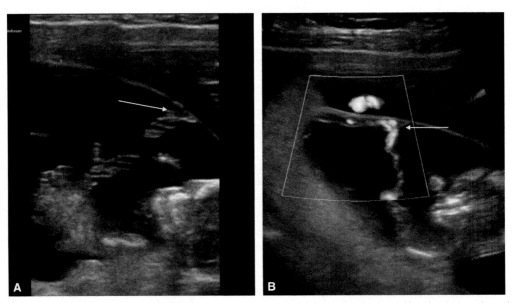

**Figure 15.29:** Gray scale **(A)** and color Doppler **(B)** of a twin pregnancy at 12 weeks of gestation with velamentous insertion of the umbilical cord into the dividing membrane (*arrow*). Velamentous cord insertion is more common in multiple pregnancies. See text for details.

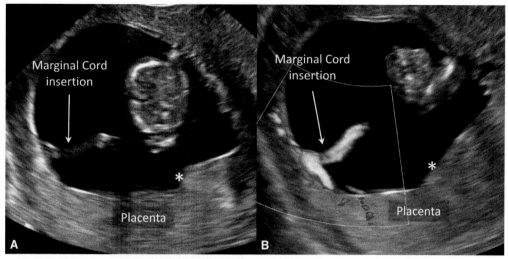

**Figure 15.30:** Gray scale **(A)** and color Doppler **(B)** of a pregnancy at 11 weeks of gestation with marginal insertion of the umbilical cord. Note that the umbilical cord inserts on the lateral margins of the placenta rather than centrally (*asterisk*).

pregnancies.[56–58] High prevalence of velamentous umbilical cord insertion was found in spontaneous abortions occurring in 33% of specimens examined between 9 and 12 weeks and in 27% of specimens examined between 13 and 16 weeks of gestation.[59] Marginal umbilical cord insertion refers to attachment of the umbilical cord to the periphery of the placenta (Fig. 15.30) and is noted in 2% to 10% of pregnancies.[56–58] Common perinatal complications associated with velamentous and marginal umbilical cord insertions include miscarriage, prematurity, fetal growth restriction, fetal malformation, perinatal death, low Apgar scores, and retained placenta.[60–63] Several studies have reported a higher incidence of velamentous cord insertion in pregnancies of assisted reproduction.[64–66] Velamentous cord insertion has a higher prevalence in multiple gestations. Monochorionic pregnancies with velamentous cord insertion should be monitored for signs of twin–twin transfusion or selective fetal growth restriction.

Visualization of the umbilical cord insertion site is feasible in the first trimester and can be successfully achieved in 93.5% of cases between 9 and 11 weeks of gestation and in up to 100% of cases at 11 to 14 weeks of gestation, and can be completed within a 30-second time period.[67,68] Assessment of the placental umbilical cord insertion site should be performed using the appropriate magnification and settings of ultrasound equipment (Fig. 15.31). It is recommended to identify the free loop of the cord and then follow it until it reaches the placental surface. Color or power Doppler imaging can improve visualization of the insertion site (Figs. 15.28 to 15.31) by confirming the presence of branching vessels. This helps to distinguish true insertion site from an adjacent free loop of the umbilical cord.

There is limited information on the detection of abnormal placental umbilical cord insertion by ultrasound in the first trimester. The first case of velamentous cord insertion

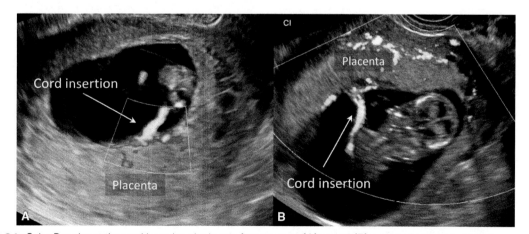

**Figure 15.31:** Color Doppler at the cord insertion site in two fetuses at 13 **(A)** and 12 **(B)** weeks of gestation. Note the normal central insertion of the umbilical cord in the placenta. **A:** Posterior placenta. **B:** Anterior placenta.

diagnosed by transvaginal sonography in the first trimester was published by Monteagudo et al. in 2000.[69] Sepulveda[68] reported five cases of velamentous cord insertions diagnosed in the first trimester and confirmed at term from a group of 533 consecutive singleton pregnancies examined over a 1-year period. Of note, one of the five pregnancies with velamentous cord insertion was complicated by fetal chromosomal abnormality (Turner syndrome) and two other women had a history of infertility, and in one of them, the pregnancy was conceived by intracytoplasmic sperm injection.[68] A study by Hasegawa et al.[67] demonstrated that visualization of cord insertion in the lower third of the uterus between 9 and 13 weeks of gestation was associated with developmental abnormalities of the placenta and the umbilical cord, including velamentous and marginal cord insertions, vasa previa, and placenta previa. Velamentous insertion can be a prerequisite for vasa previa; early prenatal detection of an abnormal umbilical cord insertion requires follow-up ultrasound at 32 weeks of gestation looking for the presence of vasa previa.

## Vasa Previa

Vasa previa refers to the presence of fetal blood vessels between the presenting fetal parts and the cervix. The fetal blood vessels can run in the fetal membranes unprotected or the umbilical cord can be tethered to the membranes at the level of the cervical os. These vessels are prone to compression and bleeding preferentially at the time of delivery and may cause unexpected fetal death because of hypoxia or exsanguination. The incidence of vasa previa is approximately 1 in 2,500 deliveries.[70] When undiagnosed, vasa previa has an associated perinatal mortality of 60%, whereas 97 % of fetuses survive when the diagnosis is made prenatally.[71]

Ultrasound markers for vasa previa described in the second and third trimester include resolving low-lying placenta or placenta previa, presence of an accessory placental lobe (succenturiate lobe), velamentous cord insertion, multiple gestations, or a suspicion of aberrant vessels crossing over the internal os.[72] Pregnancies conceived by assisted reproduction are also at higher risk for vasa previa.

Information regarding the diagnosis of vasa previa in the first trimester ultrasound is currently lacking in the literature. Hasegawa et al.[73] demonstrated that cases of vasa previa detected in the second or third trimester of pregnancy occurred only in pregnancies with cord insertions in the lower third of the uterus between 9 and 13 weeks of gestation. The detection of an abnormal umbilical cord insertion in the first trimester ultrasound examination should prompt further evaluation for possible vasa previa in later pregnancy.

## Cord Cyst

The diagnosis of a cord cyst in the first trimester is based on the visualization of a rounded thin-walled anechoic structure within or adjacent to the umbilical cord, which can be seen from about 8 weeks of gestation (Figs. 15.32 to 15.36). Umbilical cysts

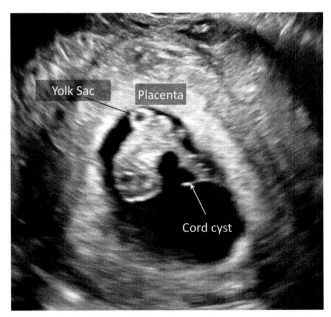

**Figure 15.32:** Gray scale ultrasound of a pregnancy at 9 weeks of gestation with an umbilical cord cyst. Note the location of the umbilical cord cyst close to the placental insertion of the cord. See the corresponding three-dimensional ultrasound image in Figure 15.33.

can be single or multiple (Fig. 15.34) and vary significantly in size (Fig. 15.35). The prevalence of an umbilical cord cyst in the first trimester of pregnancy has been reported between 0.4% and 3.4%.[74,75] Multiple cysts are much less common and

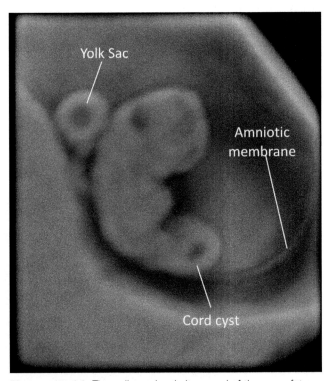

**Figure 15.33:** Three-dimensional ultrasound of the same fetus in Figure 15.32 with a cord cyst at 9 weeks of gestation. The umbilical cord cyst is seen within the amniotic cavity in contrast to the yolk sac seen outside of the amniotic cavity.

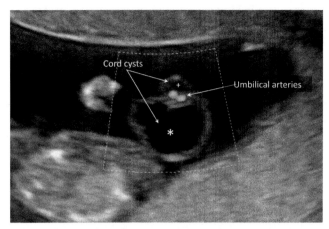

**Figure 15.34:** Color Doppler ultrasound of a pregnancy at 13 weeks of gestation with two umbilical cord cysts. Note the varying size of the umbilical cord cysts with a large (*asterisk*) and a small (*plus sign*) cyst. Color Doppler shows the two umbilical arteries within the cord.

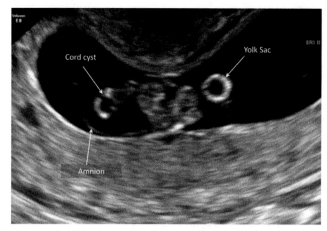

**Figure 15.36:** Gray scale ultrasound of a fetus at 8 weeks of gestation with an umbilical cord cyst (cord cyst). Note that the umbilical cord cyst is seen within the amniotic cavity in contrast to the yolk sac seen outside of the amniotic cavity. Compare with Figures 15.32 and 15.33.

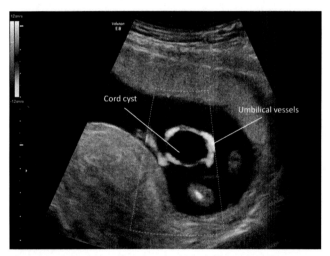

**Figure 15.35:** Color Doppler ultrasound of a pregnancy at 13 weeks of gestation with an umbilical cord cyst. Note that the umbilical vessels surround the cyst on color Doppler.

affect about 0.52% of pregnancies in the first trimester.[76] Most of the umbilical cord cysts appear to be transient, with no effect on pregnancy outcome. The majority of them are incidentally discovered during transvaginal ultrasound between 8 and 9 weeks of gestation and resolve on follow-up ultrasound at 12 to 14 weeks of gestation or later in pregnancy. Attention should be paid to differentiate a single umbilical cord cyst from the yolk sac, which has more echogenic borders and is extraamniotic in location (**Figs. 15.32, 15.33, and 15.36**).[58] Cysts can be found at any location along the length of the umbilical cord; however, most of them are situated at the middle part of the umbilical cord.[76–78]

Initial studies established an association between umbilical cord cysts found in the first trimester and a higher incidence of aneuploidy, congenital abnormalities, and overall poor pregnancy outcomes.[74] More recent large series of first trimester

umbilical cord cysts did not corroborate the same associations with poor pregnancy outcome.[77] Based on the evidence provided by recent literature, the first trimester umbilical cord cyst should not be considered an independent marker of poor pregnancy outcome regardless of its location, size, and number, especially when the cord cysts resolve on follow-up ultrasound examinations in the second trimester of pregnancy.

### REFERENCES

1. Longtine MS, Nelson DM. Placental dysfunction and fetal programming: the importance of placental size, shape, histopathology, and molecular composition. *Semin Reprod Med.* 2011;29:187–196.
2. Barker DJ, Gelow J, Thornburg K, et al. The early origins of chronic heart failure: impaired placental growth and initiation of insulin resistance in childhood. *Eur J Heart Fail.* 2010;12:819–825.
3. Barker DJ, Thornburg KL, Osmond C, et al. The surface area of the placenta and hypertension in the offspring in later life. *Int J Dev Biol.* 2010;54:525–530.
4. Eriksson JG, Kajantie E, Thornburg KL, et al. Mother's body size and placental size predict coronary heart disease in men. *Eur Heart J.* 2011;32:2297–2303.
5. Moore KL, Persaud TVN, Torchia MG. *The Developing Human: Clinically Oriented Embryology.* 10th ed. New York, NY: Elsevier; 2016:109.
6. Fox H. The development and structure of the placenta. In Fox H, ed. *Pathology of the Placenta.* 2nd ed. London: WB Saunders; 1997:1–41.
7. Salomon LJ, Alfirevic Z, Bilardo CM, et al. ISUOG Practice Guidelines: performance of first-trimester fetal ultrasound scan. *Ultrasound Obstet Gynecol.* 2013;41:102–113.
8. Tonsong T, Boonyanurak P. Placental thickness in the first half of pregnancy. *J Clin Ultrasound.* 2004;32:231.
9. Cabezas Lopez E, Martinez-Payo C, Engels Calvo V, et al. Reproducibility of first trimester three-dimensional placental measurements. *Eur J Obstet Gynecol Reprod Biol.* 2016;201:156–160.
10. Farina A. Systematic review on first trimester three-dimensional placental volumetry predicting small for gestational age infants. *Prenat Diagn.* 2016;36(2):135–141.
11. Jaffe R, Jauniaux E, Hustin J. Maternal circulation in the first trimester human placenta—myth or reality? *Am J Obstet Gynecol.* 1997;176:695.
12. Rizzo G, Capponi A, Cavicchioni O, et al. Placental vascularization measured by three-dimensional power Doppler ultrasonography at 11

to 13 + 6 weeks'gestation in normal and aneuploid fetuses. *Ultrasound Obstet Gynecol.* 2007;30:259–262.

13. De Paula CSF, Ruano R, Campos JADB, et al. Quantitative analysis of placental vasculature by three-dimensional power Doppler ultrasonography in normal pregnancies from 12 to 40 weeks of gestation. *Placenta.* 2009;30:142–148.

14. Hafner E, Metzenbauer M, Stümpflen I, et al. First trimester placental and myometrial blood perfusion measured by 3D power Doppler in normal and unfavourable outcome pregnancies. *Placenta.* 2010;31:756–763.

15. Hill LM, DiNofrio DM, Guzick D. Sonographic determination of first trimester umbilical cord length. *J Clin Ultrasound.* 1994;22:435–438.

16. Rembouskos G, Cicero S, Longo D, et al. Single umbilical artery at 11–14 weeks' gestation: relation to chromosomal defects. *Ultrasound Obstet Gynecol.* 2003;22:567–570.

17. Seki H, Kuromaki K, Takeda S, et al. Persistent subchorionic hematoma with clinical symptoms until delivery. *Int J Gynaecol Obstet.* 1998;63:123–128.

18. Borlum KG, Thomsen A, Clausen I, et al. Long-term prognosis of pregnancies in women with intrauterine hematomas. *Obstet Gynecol.* 1989;74:231–233.

19. Nagy S, Bush M, Stone J, et al. Clinical significance of subchorionic and retroplacental hematomas detected in the first trimester of pregnancy. *Obstet Gynecol.* 2003;102:94–100.

20. Sauerbrei EE, Pham DH. Placental abruption and subchorionic hemorrhage in the first half of pregnancy: US appearance and clinical outcome. *Radiology.* 1986;160:109–112.

21. Mandruzzato GP, D'Ottavio G, Rustico MA, et al. The intrauterine hematoma: diagnostic and clinical aspects. *J Clin Ultrasound.* 1989;17:503–510.

22. Bennett GL, Bromley B, Lieberman E, et al. Subchorionic hemorrhage in first-trimester pregnancies: prediction of pregnancy outcome with sonography. *Radiology.* 1996;200:803–806.

23. Tower CL, Regan L. Intrauterine haematomas in a recurrent miscarriage population. *Hum Reprod.* 2001;16:2005–2007.

24. Johns J, Hyett J, Jauniaux E. Obstetric outcome after threatened miscarriage with and without a hematoma on ultrasound. *Obstet Gynecol.* 2003;102:483–487.

25. Tuuli MG, Norman S, Odibo AO, et al. Perinatal outcomes in women with subchorionic hematoma: a systematic review and meta-analysis. *Obstet Gynecol.* 2011;117(5):1205–1212.

26. Taipale P, Hiilesmaa V, Ylöstalo P. Diagnosis of placenta previa by transvaginal sonographic screening at 12-16 weeks in a non-selected population. *Obstet Gynecol.* 1997;89(3):364–367.

27. Hill LM, DiNofrio DM, Chenevey P. Transvaginal sonographic evaluation of first trimester placenta previa. *Ultrasound Obstet Gynecol.* 1995;5(5):301–303.

28. Mustafá SA, Brizot ML, Carvalho MH, et al. Transvaginal ultrasonography in predicting placenta previa at delivery: a longitudinal study. *Ultrasound Obstet Gynecol.* 2002;20(4):356–359.

29. Miller DA, Chollet JA, Goodwin TM. Clinical risk factors for placenta previa-placenta accreta. *Am J Obstet Gynecol.* 1997;177(1):210–214.

30. Ballas J, Pretorius D, Hull AD, et al. Identifying sonographic markers for placenta accreta in the first trimester. *Am J Obstet Gynecol.* 2012;31:1835–1841.

31. Comstock CH, Bronsteen RA. The antenatal diagnosis of placenta accreta. *Br J Obstet Gynecol.* 2014;121:171–182.

32. Comstock CH, Wesley L, Vettraino IM, et al. The early sonographic appearance of placenta accreta. *J Ultrasound Med.* 2003;22(1):19–23.

33. Jurkovic D, Hillaby K, Woelfer B, et al. First-trimester diagnosis and management of pregnancies implanted into the lower uterine segment Cesarean section scar. *Ultrasound Obstet Gynecol.* 2003;21:220–227.

34. Timor-Trisch IE, Monteagudo A, Santos R, et al. The diagnosis, treatment and follow-up of cesarean scar pregnancy. *Am J Obstet Gynecol.* 2012;207:44.e1–44.e13.

35. Sadeghi H, Rutherford T, Rackow BW, et al. Cesarean scar ectopic pregnancy: case series and review of the literature. *Am J Perinatol* 2010;27:111–120.

36. Chen YJ, Wang PH, Liu WM, et al. Placenta accreta diagnosed at 9 weeks' gestation. *Ultrasound Obstet Gynecol.* 2002;19:620–622.

37. Wong HS, Zuccollo J, Tait J, et al. Placenta accreta in the first trimester of pregnancy: sonographic findings. *J Clin Ultrasound.* 2007;37:100–102.

38. Yang JI, Kim HY, Kim HS, et al. Diagnosis in the first trimester of placenta accreta with previous cesarean section. *Ultrasound Obstet Gynecol.* 2009;34:116–118.

39. Shih JC, Cheng WF, Shyu MK, et al. Power Doppler evidence of placenta accreta appearing in the first trimester. *Ultrasound Obstet Gynecol.* 2002;19:623–625.

40. Garza A, Cordero JF, Mulinare J. Epidemiology of the early amnion rupture spectrum of defects. *Am J Dis Child.* 1988;142(5):541–544.

41. Hata T, Tanaka H, Noguchi J. 3D/4D sonographic evaluation of amniotic band syndrome in early pregnancy: a supplement to 2D ultrasound. *J Obstet Gynaecol Res.* 2011;37(6):656–660.

42. Inubashiri E, Hanaoka U, Kanenishi K, et al. 3D and 4D sonographic imaging of amniotic band syndrome in early pregnancy. *J Clin Ultrasound.* 2008;36(9):573–575.

43. Higuchi T, Tanaka M, Kuroda K, et al. Abnormal first-trimester fetal nuchal translucency and amniotic band syndrome. *J Med Ultrason (2001).* 2012;39(3):177–180.

44. Nishi T, Nakano R. Amniotic band syndrome: serial ultrasonographic observations in the first trimester. *J Clin Ultrasound.* 1994;22(4):275–288.

45. Martínez-Payo C, Cabezasc E, Nieto Y, et al. Detection of single umbilical artery in the first trimester ultrasound: its value as a marker of fetal malformation. *Biomed Res Int.* 2014;2014:548729.

46. Monie IW. Genesis of single umbilical artery. *Am J Obstet Gynecol.* 1970;108(3):400–405.

47. Naeye RL. Disorders of the umbilical cord. In: *Disorders of the Placenta, Fetus and Neonate: Diagnosis and Clinical Significance,* St Louis, MO: Mosby-Year Book; 1992:92.

48. Leung AKC, Robson WLM. Single umbilical artery: a report of 159 cases. *Am J Dis Child.* 1989;143(1):108–111.

49. Lamberty CO, Burlacchini de Carvalho MH, Miguelez J, et al. Ultrasound detection rate of single umbilical artery in the first trimester of pregnancy. *Prenat Diagn.* 2011;31:865–868.

50. Hua M, Odibo AO, MacOnes GA, et al. Singleumbilical artery and its associated findings. *Obstet Gynecol.* 2010;115(5):930–934.

51. Gornall AS, Kurinczuk JJ, Konje JC. Antenatal detection of a single umbilical artery: does it matter? *Prenat Diagn.* 2003;23(2):117–123.

52. Prefumo F, Gueven MA, Carvalho JS. Single umbilical artery and congenital heart disease in selected and unselected populations. *Ultrasound Obstet Gynecol.* 2010;35(5):552–555.

53. Murphy-Kaulbeck L, Dodds L, Joseph KS, et al. Single umbilical artery risk factors and pregnancy outcomes. *Obstet Gynecol.* 2010;116(4):843–850.

54. Defigueiredo D, Dagklis T, Zidere V, et al. Isolated single umbilical artery: need for specialist fetal echocardiography? *Ultrasound Obstet Gynecol.* 2010;36(5):553–555.

55. Bombrys AE, Neiger R, Hawkins S, et al. Pregnancy outcome in isolated single umbilical artery. *Am J Perinatol.* 2008;25(4):239–242.

56. Benirschke K, Kaufmann P. *Pathology of the Human Placenta.* New York, NY: Springer-Verlag; 2000:353–359

57. Sepulveda W, Rojas I, Robert JA, et al. Prenatal detection of velamentous insertion of the umbilical cord: a prospective color Doppler ultrasound study. *Ultrasound Obstet Gynecol.* 2003;21:564–569.

58. Sepulveda W, Sebire NJ, Harris R, et al. The placenta, umbilical cord, and membranes. In: Nyberg DA, McGahan JP, Pretorius DH, et al, eds. *Diagnostic Imaging of Fetal Anomalies.* Philadelphia, PA: Lippincott Williams & Wilkins; 2003:85–132.

59. Monie IW. Velamentous insertion of the cord in early pregnancy. *Am J Obstet Gynecol.* 1965;93:276–281.

60. Uyanwah-Akpom P, Fox H. The clinical significance of marginal and velamentous insertion of the cord. *Br J Obstet Gynecol.* 1977;84:941–943.

61. Kouyoumdjian A. Velamentous insertion of the umbilical cord. *Obstet Gynecol.* 1980;56:737–742.

62. Eddleman KA, Lockwood CJ, Berkowitz GS, et al. Clinical significance and sonographic diagnosis of velamentous umbilical cord insertion. *Am J Perinatol.* 1992;9:123–126.

63. Heinonen S, Ryynanen M, Kirkinen P, et al. Perinatal diagnostic evaluation of velamentous umbilical cord insertion: clinical, Doppler, and ultrasonic findings. *Obstet Gynecol.* 1996;87:112–117.

64. Gavriil P, Jauniaux E, Leroy F. Pathologic examination of placentas from singleton and twin pregnancies obtained after in vitro fertilization and embryo transfer. *Pediatr Pathol.* 1993;13:453–462.

65. Hasegawa J, Iwasaki S, Matsuoka R, et al. Velamentous cord insertion caused by oblique implantation after in vitro fertilization and embryo transfer. *J Obstet Gynaecol Res.* 2011;37:1698–1701.

66. Delbaere I, Goetgeluk S, Derom C, et al. Umbilical cord anomalies are more frequent in twins after assisted reproduction. *Hum Reprod.* 2007;22:2763–2767.

67. Hasegawa J, Matsuoka R, Ichizuka K, et al. Cord insertion into the lower third of the uterus in the first trimester is associated with placental and umbilical cord abnormalities. *Ultrasound Obstet Gynecol.* 2006;28:183–186.

68. Sepulveda W. Velamentous insertion of the umbilical cord: a first-trimester sonographic screening study. *Ultrasound Med.* 2006;25:963–968.

69. Monteagudo A, Sfakianaki AK, Timor-Tritsch IE. Velamentous insertion of the cord in the first trimester. *Ultrasound Obstet Gynecol.* 2000;16:498–499.

70. Oyelese KO, Turner M, Lees C, et al. Vasa previa: an avoidable obstetric tragedy. *Obstet Gynecol Surv.* 1999;54:138–145.

71. Francois K, Mayer S, Harris C, et al. Association of vasa previa at delivery with a history of second-trimester placenta previa. *J Reprod Med.* 2003;48:771–774.

72. Lee W, Lee VL, Kirk JS, et al. Vasa previa: prenatal diagnosis, natural evolution, and clinical outcome. *Obstet Gynecol.* 2000;95:572–576.

73. Hasegawa J, Nakamura M, Sekizawa A, et al. Prediction of risk for vasa previa at 9–13 weeks' gestation. *J Obstet Gynecol Res.* 2011;37(10):1346–135.

74. Ross JA, Jurkovic D, Zosmer N, et al. Umbilical cord cysts in early pregnancy. *Obstet Gynecol.* 1997;89:442–445.

75. Skibo LK, Lyons EA, Levi CS. First-trimester umbilical cord cysts. *Radiology.* 1992;82:719–722.

76. Ghezzi F, Raio L, Di Naro E, et al. Single and multiple umbilical cord cysts in early gestation: two different entities. *Ultrasound Obstet Gynecol.* 2003;21:215–219.

77. Hannaford K, Reeves S, Wegner E. Umbilical cord cysts in the first trimester: are they associated with pregnancy complications? *J Ultrasound Med.* 2013;32:801–806.

78. Sepulveda W, Leible S, Ulloa A, et al. Clinical significance of first trimester umbilical cord cysts. *J Ultrasound Med.* 1990;18:95–99.

# Index

Page numbers followed by "f" denote figures; "t," tables